Claus-Peter Adler and Kazimierz Kozlowski

Primary Bone Tumors and Tumorous Conditions in Children

Pathologic and Radiologic Diagnosis

Foreword by Hubert Sissons and Ronald Murray

With 381 Figures

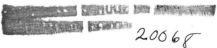
Springer-Verlag
London Berlin Heidelberg New York
Paris Tokyo Hong Kong
Barcelona Budapest

Prof. Dr. med. Claus-Peter Adler
Head, Reference Center of Bone Disease, Institute of Pathology, University of
Freiburg, Ludwig-Aschoff-Haus, Albertstrasse 19, D-7800 Freiburg i. Br., Germany

Kazimierz Kozlowski, FRACR
Senior Staff Specialist, Department of Radiology, The Children's Hospital, Pyrmont
Bridge Road, Camperdown, Sydney 2050, NSW, Australia

Front Cover: The background X-ray shows a large sessile osteochondroma of the right proximal
tibial metaphysis of a 13-year-old girl. The inset illustration is an histological section through an
osteochondroma at low magnification (not from the same patient) – see Figs 2.5 and 2.10.

ISBN 3–540–19731–1 Springer-Verlag Berlin Heidelberg New York
ISBN 0–387–19731–1 Springer-Verlag New York Berlin Heidelberg

British Library Cataloguing in Publication Data
Adler, C.P.
  Primary Bone Tumours and Tumorous
  Condition in Children
  I. Title   II. Kozlowski, Kazimierz
  616.99
  ISBN 3–540–19731–1
Library of Congress Cataloging-in-Publication Data
Adler, C.P.
    Primary bone tumours and tumorous condition in children/Claus Peter Adler and Kazimierz Kozlowski.
      p.   cm.
    Includes index.
    ISBN 3–540–19731–1. — ISBN 0–387–19731–1
    1. Bones—Tumors—Diagnosis.   2. Tumors in children—Diagnosis.
  I. Kozlowski, Kazimierz, 1928–   . II. Title.
    [DNLM: 1. Bone Neoplasms—diagnosis.   2. Bone Neoplasms—in infancy & childhood. WE 258
A237p] RC280.B6A35   1992
618.92'99271—dc20
DNLM/DLC
for Library of Congress   91-5242

Typeset by Best-set Typesetter Ltd., Hong Kong
28/3830-543210 Printed on acid-free paper

To our families
Dr Maria Adler, Elisabeth and Nikola,
Dr Daniela Kozlowski, Ala and Kasia

Foreword

We welcome the publication of this volume, which discusses the diagnosis of bone tumours with particular reference to children and adolescents.

As founder members of the International Skeletal Society we are delighted to learn that the book had its inception at one of the Society's meetings. It reflects, moreover, the combined presentation of radiological and pathological diagnostic information which has been such a feature of the meetings of the International Skeletal Society.

We commend it to all readers with an interest in tumours of the skeleton.

Hubert A. Sissons
Ronald O. Murray

Preface

The diagnosis of primary bone tumors is often difficult. There are several reasons for this. As primary bone tumors are rare in childhood, practitioners in a number of pediatric subspecialties are not familiar with them. The clinical symptoms and signs are often elusive, the biochemical investigations usually normal and the radiographic features often uncharacteristic. Even the pathologist, who is the final step in arriving at the proper diagnosis and who has all the available clinical, biochemical and radiographic data, may encounter difficulties. A good tissue sample is the basis for microscopic investigation. However, bone tumors often show an extreme variety of structures which confuse even experienced bone pathologists. Therefore, histopathologic analysis must take into account all available clinical, biochemical and radiographic data. The close cooperation of the pathologist with clinicians and, especially, radiologists is of the utmost importance.

This book has been written by a pediatric radiologist from Sydney, Australia and a bone pathologist from Freiburg, Germany. Both members of the International Skeletal Society, we have specialized in the field of skeletal diseases and have exchanged our knowledge many times on difficult cases. At the 1987 Annual Meeting of the International Skeletal Society in Cannes, France, we decided to write this book on *Primary Bone Tumors and Tumorous Conditions in Children*.

During a period of 25 years, more than 10000 primary bone tumors, tumorous conditions and tumor-simulating bone lesions have been diagnosed radiologically and histologically in our institutions. Many cases came from our university hospitals but most of them were sent from elsewhere for consultation. We have studied thousands of radiographs and, in addition, analyzed histologic slides whenever biopsy material was available for investigation. All the material published in this book was critically evaluated, analyzed and documented.

There exists quite a number of books on bone tumors and tumorous conditions that give helpful information concerning clinical symptoms, radiologic appearances and histologic patterns. Nearly all of them cover all bone tumors occurring in all age-groups. In this book, in contrast, we concentrate on bone tumors and tumor-like lesions that primarily affect children and adolescents and, therefore, primarily interest pediatricians, pediatric surgeons and pediatric radiologists. We hope to give help in the recognition of bone lesions as tumors or tumor-like lesions and in the differentiation between benign and malignant tumor growth, as well as providing information on the biologic behavior of tumors and their prognosis.

In this book, we outline the diseases that may be encountered and how the practitioner should deal with them. We include information on the radiologic appearances of these lesions and their pathologic–anatomic features. By referring to the text, the pediatrician should be able to classify a specific bone lesion as a tumorous growth and gain further important information on it, enabling him to decide whether to refer the patient to a specialized pediatric radiologist, who performs a diagnosis, and to the surgeon and pathologist for biopsy and final diagnosis.

In Chapter 1 we outline the approach to diagnosis and list the tumorous lesions most frequently occurring in children and adolescents. In Chapter 2, a detailed description of each bone tumor is undertaken. This starts with a precise definition according to the WHO classification and the essential monographs on bone tumors. The localization of the individual tumor in the skeleton as well as within the involved bone is depicted and the age distribution is recorded. The description starts with those prominent radiologic features that characterize the tumor and must be included in the diagnostic and differential diagnostic considerations by the pathologist when analyzing such a case histologically. Detailed descriptions of macroscopic specimens and, especially, of the histologic pattern are given, and the histology is illustrated. As well as summarizing the features that underlie painful destructive bone lesions, the chapter illustrates for the clinician the extreme difficulties that confront the pathologist in finding the correct diagnosis. In Chapter 3, the most important tumor-like bone lesions are described in the same way and with the same purpose. Chapter 4 takes a regional approach to radiologic diagnosis. The tables provide radiographic checklists and act as reminders of the common tumorous conditions and their differential diagnoses.

This book is not written for experts who are familiar with bone tumors. It is addressed to all "front-line" clinicians who will encounter primary bone tumors – general practitioners, radiologists, orthopedic surgeons and pathologists. They will find in it the basic information required and advice on the best approach to bone tumors. We hope that this book will also be valuable to young doctors specializing in pediatric and related disciplines and to the more keen medical student.

Our hope is that, by facilitating the diagnosis of primary bone tumors in children, this book will ultimately be beneficial to patients.

Acknowledgments

This project could not have been accomplished without the help of many co-workers whom we wish to thank.

Many colleagues at the Reference Center of Bone Disease of the University of Freiburg, Germany were involved in the analysis of many cases, namely Prof Dr W Wenz (radiology), Prof Dr A Reichelt (orthopedic surgery), and Prof Dr E Moser (nuclear medicine). Prof Dr HE Schaefer (pathology) and Mrs M Eckenfels (technical medical assistance), in the Institute of Pathology, have helped in realizing the project.

We are indebted to our Australian and overseas colleagues who provided the illustrations to accompany the text. Without their contribution, Chapter 4 could not have appeared. It is impossible to thank individually all those who have helped, but there are several who should be named: P Sprague, J Masel, L Morris, W MacAlister, A Barylak, J Hoeffel, A Tanconi and, especially, Dr J Campbell who, in helping to collect the necessary material, was most cooperative throughout the years. His contribution went beyond that which any colleague can expect. Other colleagues have supplied illustrations, as indicated in figure legends. Thanks to Dr M de Silva, Dr A Lam and the registrars of the Department of Radiology in the Royal Alexandra Hospital for Children in Sydney, Australia, for continuous help, and thanks to Pixie Moloney who has done most of the photographic work for Chapter 4.

Finally, we acknowledge with pleasure the excellent cooperation of our publishers, especially Mr Michael Jackson who has given us valuable help in arranging this book and has enabled its conversion into correct English, which is not the mother tongue of either author.

We would like to thank Georg Thieme Verlag for permission to reproduce the diagrams in Chapter 2 from *Knochenkrankheiten: Diagnostik makroskopischer, histologischer und radiologischer Strukturveränderungen des Skeletts* (Stuttgart, 1983), by C-P Adler. We are grateful to the publishers and editors to reproduce in Chapter 4 a number of figures from the following journals: *Annales de Radiologie, Australasian Radiology, Fortschitte auf dem Gebiete der Röntgenstrahlen und der neuen bildgebenden Verfahren* (RöFo), *Journal Belge de Radiologie – Belgisch Tijdschrift voor Radiologie, Pediatric Radiology, La Radiologia Medica, British Journal of Radiology*.

Contents

1
INTRODUCTION

The Approach to Diagnosis

The skeleton is the site of several primary benign and malignant tumors and tumorous conditions. Some of these arise from genetic syndromes and others have an unknown origin. Although many arise in children or adolescents, some benign tumors or tumor-like lesions having their origin in childhood may not be detected until adult life. To find the precise diagnosis is crucial to effective management and therapy of these lesions. The general approach to diagnosis is outlined in Fig. 1.1.

The diagnostic procedure starts with the presentation of uncharacteristic symptoms. The pediatrician who sees the child first has to make the first diagnosis, considering acute or chronic disease, such as an osteomyelitis, a skeletal dysplasia, a metabolic disturbance, a traumatic event or a tumorous growth. In cases of joint complaints, a rheumatologist should be consulted. Then the pediatric radiologist is asked to interpret the different bone changes. This is an important step in this diagnostic procedure, for many bone lesions may be recognized and diagnosed radiologically and, in some of them, no biopsy or surgical intervention is required. Indeed, some bone lesions can be called "leave-me-alone-lesions", being harmless and not needing histological analysis or surgery.

The pathologist plays an important role in the diagnosis of most bone lesions, especially bone tumors, for he makes the final and decisive diagnosis on which the appropriate therapy is based (curettage, excision, amputation, radiotherapy or chemotherapy). However, the pediatrician, pediatric surgeon and pediatric radiologist should not merely send the tissue specimens to the pathologist and await news of the diagnosis. The chance of diagnostic error is great because the tissue pattern alone may often be not sufficiently pathognomonic. Therefore, the pathologist needs extensive clinical information on the course of the disease, when it has started, what the symptoms are and what the radiologic features are. He should be informed if the pediatrician or pediatric radiologist thinks that they are dealing with a benign or malignant lesion. Moreover, all radiologic images – plain radiographs, tomograms, computer tomograms (CT), magnetic resonance images (MR), angiograms (DSA) and scintigrams – should be sent to the pathologist together with the tissue specimens. This requires the pathologist who specializes in these diseases to have a great understanding of the radiologic changes and to know how to interpret them in conjunction with the histologic patterns.

There is a paucity of knowledge of bone diseases, especially among physicians (orthopedic surgeons as well as radiologists and pathologists). There are several reasons for this:

1. Bone tumors and tumor-like bone lesions are, compared with other pediatric diseases, relatively rare. This means that medical practitioners do not have extensive experience of them.
2. Bone tumors are very complicated in their clinical appearance and course, their radiologic changes and, especially, their histologic features. The diagnostic analysis is usually extremely difficult and requires a great deal of experience.
3. In complicated cases, it is impossible for a single physician to establish the correct diagnosis of a bone tumor. Pediatricians, radiologists and pathologists have to work together in a "three-dimensional" approach (Fig. 1.2), interpreting the different symptoms and features, and discussing the various aspects, in order to determine the correct diagnosis and plan appropriate therapy.

Pediatricians, pediatric radiologists and pathologists should be aware that, whatever the appearance of a tumor, the lesion might be malignant. In all doubtful cases, the available material (clinical history, biochemical data, imaging data and pathologic material) should be send to one or more reference centers for consultation.

There exist some prominent reference centers, for example:

1. *In the USA*: Mayo Clinic, Rochester, Min.; Montefiore Medical Center, Bronx NY; AFIP, Washington D.C.; Hospital for Joint Diseases (Orthopedic Institute), New York, NY; Memorial Sloan-Kettering Cancer Center, New York, NY; UCLA Medical Center, Los Angeles, CA.

2. *In Germany*: Reference Center of Bone Diseases, University of Freiburg i.Br. and others.

3. *In Austria*: Institute of Pathology, University of Vienna.

4. *In Switzerland*: Institute of Pathology, University of Basle.

5. *In England*: Royal National Orthopaedic Hospital, London and others.

6. *In France*: Institute Gustave Roussy, Villejuif.

7. *In Italy*: Orthopaedic Hospital, Bologna.

8. *In Australia*: Department of Pathology, Prince Alfred Hospital, Sydney.

Prominent specialists may be personally asked for their opinion on an individual case, and the pediatrician should have access to their advice.

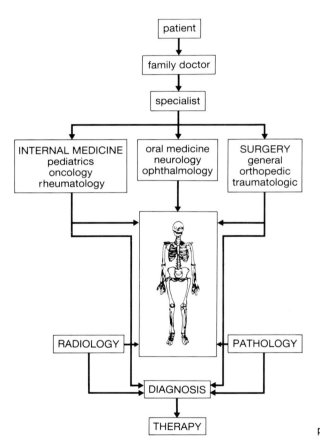

Fig. 1.1. The general approach to diagnosis.

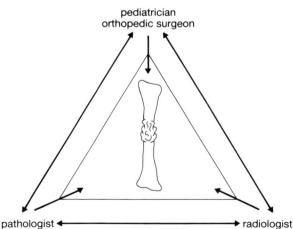

Fig. 1.2. A "three-dimensional" approach to diagnosis and management is required.

Primary Bone Tumors in Children

Almost all primary bone tumors that occur in adults are also seen in children. However, some of them occur so rarely in children that they are not encountered in most medical practices and may be seen only occasionally even in large children's hospitals. The frequency of primary bone tumors in children is not known exactly. Tumor registers, which are now common in developed countries, are relatively recent and do not give reliable statistical data because of the small numbers of cases.

The most trustworthy statistics are those of primary malignant bone tumors treated in hospitals. The statistics for benign primary bone tumors and tumor-like bone lesions are unreliable for several reasons:

1. Many benign bone tumors and tumor-like bone lesions are asymptomatic; a low percentage of them is discovered accidentally on radiographs taken for other reasons.
2. National registers of bone tumors exist in only a few countries, and not all benign bone tumors and tumor-like bone lesions are recorded.
3. Several bone lesions have been diagnosed radiologically as benign primary bone tumors that do not warrant a biopsy. As the diagnosis of these cases is radiological only, it is therefore uncertain and may be inaccurately recorded on registers.
4. Some tumor-like bone lesions (histiocytosis X, aneurysmal bone cyst and others) may be recorded as benign bone tumors, distorting the statistics.
5. We know that some dysplastic bone lesions (osteochondromatosis, enchondromatosis–Ollier's disease, fibrous bone dysplasia, Jaffe–Lichtenstein disease and others) can be classified as both primary benign bone tumors and bone dysplasias. This fact may again distort the statistics.
6. The exact registration of a malignant bone tumor can be a problem if it has developed from a primary benign lesion (chondrosarcoma from primary enchondroma, malignant fibrous histiocytoma from fibrous dysplasia, etc.)
7. New tumorous bone lesions have been reported in recent years (malignant fibrous histiocytoma, osteofibrous dysplasia Campanacci and others) and until recently these were not be analyzed statistically.

There exist some statistics from individual reference centers or hospitals which are of only restricted value because they comprise cases treated in these institutions and are not representative of cases in general. The most reliable statistics are those from institutes of pathology that specialize in bone tumors and so have many cases referred from many hospitals in their country and from all over the world.

We have analyzed 15320 primary bone tumors and 2522 tumor-like bone lesions that have occurred in children, adolescents and adults. These are our statistical findings:

1. *All bone tumors (n = 15320)*
   a) 37.8% are benign and 62.2% are malignant
   b) 42% are detected in children and adolescents (1st and 2nd decade)
   c) 9% occur in children (1st decade)
   d) 33% occur in adolescents (2nd decade)
2. *Benign bone tumors (n = 5786)*
   a) 48% are detected in children and adolescents (1st and 2nd decade)
   b) 12% occur in children (1st decade)
   c) 36% occur in adolescents (2nd decade)
3. *Malignant bone tumors (n = 9534)*
   a) 38% are detected in children and adolescents (1st and 2nd decade)
   b) 7% occur in children (1st decade)
   c) 31% occur in adolescents (2nd decade)
4. *Tumor-like bone lesions (n = 2522)*
   a) 70% are detected in children and adolescents (1st and 2nd decade)
   b) 36% occur in children (1st decade)
   c) 33% occur in adolescents (2nd decade)

These statistics give a general view on the frequency of bone tumors and tumor-like bone lesions in children and adolescents. The most reliable statistics on primary bone tumors in children are those for osteosarcoma and Ewing's sarcoma:

Osteosarcoma is the most frequent primary bone tumor in childhood, with an annual frequency of approximately three cases per million whites younger than 15 years of age, and a slightly lower rate in black children. About 50%–70% of cases occur in the first two decades of life. If secondary osteosarcomas (post-radiation, osteosarcoma in Paget's disease) are excluded, the percentage is even higher.

Ewing's sarcoma is the second most frequent primary bone tumor in children, with an annual frequency of approximately 1.7 cases per million whites younger than 15 years of age. This tumor is rare in Blacks and Asians. It comprises about 6%–9% of all primary malignant bone tumors and occurs in nearly 30% of the cases in the first decade, and in nearly 50% in the second decade of life. It is a rare primary bone tumor in adults, but is observed to the age of 30 years.

Fourteen per cent of *primary bone lymphomas* occur in the first two decades of life. It comprises 7% of all malignant bone tumors. As the initial clinical course of bone lymphoma is silent and the disease is diagnosed when multiple foci are already present, it is often impossible to decide what is the primary site of this tumor.

Chondrosarcoma is, among all bone tumors, the third most common primary bone tumor, after plasmocytoma and osteosarcoma. It constitutes about 11%–16% of all primary bone tumors but is rare in childhood. Only isolated cases have been reported in the first decade of life, but it is more frequent in teenagers.

Fibrosarcoma of bone comprises over 3% of the total number of primary malignant bone tumors. About 15% occur in the two first decades of life. Differentiating this tumor from aggressive fibromatosis or malignant fibrous histiocytoma can be difficult.

Several other primary malignant bone tumors, such as osteoclastoma, malignant fibrous histiocytoma, hemangiosarcoma and liposarcoma, do occur occasionally, but no statistical data are available. Other bone tumors, such as plasmocytoma and chordoma, are almost never seen in children.

The incidence of many common benign bone tumors is unknown. The available statistical data for benign bone tumors and tumor-like bone lesions that provoke clinical symptoms are given in Tables 1.1 and 1.2.

The occurrence of bone metastases in children differs widely from that in adults. In cases of metastatic bone lesions in children, the site and type of the primary tumor is usually already known. The most important metastatic bone disease in children is neuroblastoma. Micrometastases in a bone are probably already present in the early stage of the disease, tumor growth already being advanced. Obviously, the percentage of bone metastases from neuroblastoma is variable, and their detection depends on the imaging methods used in the diagnosis. Plain radiographs and computer

Table 1.1. Incidence of benign bone tumors in children

Tumor	Percentage of all benign bone tumors	Percentage of all bone tumors	Percentage occurring in the first two decades of life	Comments
Osteochondroma	36[a]	8.5[a]	60[a]	Only solitary lesions included
	44[b]	20[b]	70[b]	
Enchondroma	12[a]	3[a]	35[a]	Single and multiple lesions included
Osteoidosteoma	12[a]	3[a]	>70[a,b]	
	11[b]	5[b]		
Osteoblastoma	4[a]	1[a]	>50[a]	
	2.7[b]	1.2[b]	>60[b]	
Chondroblastoma	<1[a]	<4[a]	>60[a]	
	6[b]	2.7[b]	>80[b]	
Chondromyxoid fibroma	2[a]	0.5[a]	40[a]	Most common in the 2nd and 3rd decades of life
	2.3[b]	1[b]	65[b]	
Hemangioma	<4[a]	<1[a]	12[a]	
	2[b]	<1[b]		

[a] Data from Dahlin and Unni (1986).
[b] Data from Schajowicz (1981).

Table 1.2. Incidence of tumor-like bone lesions in children[a]

Lesion	Percentage occurring in the first two decades of life	Comments
Benign cortical defect and nonossifying bone fibroma	>90	Most common tumor-like lesion
Eosinophilic bone granuloma	>70	Only monostotic lesions considered; about 50% occur in the 1st decade of life
Juvenile bone cyst	>90	
Aneurysmal bone cyst	>65	
Fibrous bone dysplasia	55	Only monostotic lesions

[a] Data from Schajowicz (1981).

tomograms are less sensitive than the nuclear scan, the MR and, finally, the bone biopsy that may establish the final diagnosis.

In rare instances, bone metastases may become symptomatic before the primary tumor is detected. Some other extraosseous primary tumors frequently induce bone metastases, for example rhabdomyosarcoma. Occasionally, even primary bone sarcomas (especially osteosarcomas and Ewing's sarcomas) may cause bone metastases that may be diagnosed before the primary tumor is detected.

In summary, primary bone tumors – benign and malignant – may occur in children as well as adults. The specific age distribution has be taken into account in each individual tumor. Most tumor-like bone lesions are seen in children and adolescents. Finally, some tumorous bone lesions definitely have a predilection for younger age-groups and are predominantly seen in children.

LITERATURE

Adler CP. Knochenkrankheiten – Diagnostik makroskopischer, histologischer und radiologischer Strukturveränderungen des Skeletts. Stuttgart: Thieme, 1983.

Adler CP. DNS-Zytophotometrie an Knochentumoren. In: Dietsch P, Keck E, Kruse H-P, Kuhlencordt F. Aktuelle Ergebnisse der Osteologie. Berlin: Walter de Gruyter, 1986;233–9

Adler CP. Pathologie der Wirbelsäulenerkrankungen. Radiologe 1989;29:153–8

Adler CP. Diagnostic problems with semimalignant bone tumors. In: Heuck FHW, Keck E, editors. Fortschritte der Osteologie in Diagnostik und Therapie. Berlin: Springer-Verlag 1988:103–18

Adler CP, Brendle G. Kliniche und morphologische Aspekte von gutartigen Knochentumoren und tumorähnlichen Knochenläsionen. Versicherungsmedizin 1989;4:132–8

Dahlin DC, Unni KK. Bone tumors. General aspects and data on 8542 cases. Springfield: C.C. Thomas, 1986

Dominok GW, Knoch H-G. Knochengeschwülste und geschwulstähnliche Knochenerkrankungen. Stuttgart: Gustav Fischer, 1982

Donath A, Courvoisier B. Bone and tumors. Bern: H. Huber, 1979

Grundmann E. Malignant bone tumors. Berlin: Springer-Verlag 1976

Grundmann E, Roessner A. Moderne Methoden zur histologischen Diagnose von Knochentumoren. GBK-Mitteilungsdienst NF, 1983;H40:13–17

Hudson TM. Radiologic–pathologic correlation of musculoskeletal lesions. Baltimore: Williams & Wilkins, 1987

Huvos AG. Bone tumors. Diagnosis, treatment, and prognosis. Philadelphia: WB Saunders, 1979

Jaffe, HL. Tumors and tumorous conditions of the bones and joints. Philadelphia: Lea & Febiger, 1968

Mirra JM. Bone tumors. Diagnosis and treatment. Philadelphia: JB Lippincott, 1980

Santoro A, Bonadomma G. Soft tissue and bone sarcomas. Cancer Chemother Biol Response Modif 1990;11:544–54

Schajowicz F. Tumors and tumorlike lesions of bone and joints. New York: Springer-Verlag, 1981

Schajowicz F, McGuire MH. Diagnostic difficulties in skeletal pathology. Clin Orthop 1989;240:281–310

Senac MO Jr, Isaacs H, Gwinn J. Primary lesions of bone in the 1st decade of life: retrospective survey of biopsy results. Radiology 1986;160:491–5

Sissons HA, Murray RO, Kemp HBS. Orthopaedic diagnosis. – clinical, radiological and pathological coordinates. Berlin: Springer-Verlag, 1984

Spjut HJ, Dorfman HD, Fechner RE, Ackerman LV. Tumors of bone and cartilage. Washington D.C.: A.F.I.P., 1971

Wenz W, Hofmann E, Schmidt W, Richter G, Adler CP. Knochen- und Weichgewebstumoren – Fortschritt in unserem Jahrzehnt. Langenbecks Arch Chir 1987;372: 289–94

Willich E, Appell RG, Brandeis WE. Skelettmanifestationen von malignen, nichtossären Tumoren im Kindesalter. Radiologe 1985;25:166–76

Wold LE, McLeod RA, Sim FH, Unni KK. Atlas of orthopedic pathology. Philadelphia: WB Saunders, 1990

2
BONE TUMORS

Tumors of Cartilaginous Origin

OSTEOCHONDROMA
(ICD-O-M-9210/0)

Osteochondromas or osteocartilaginous exostoses are by far the most frequent benign bone tumor in childhood. They represent 40% of all benign bone tumors, and 58% of them occur in children or adolescents. *Osteochondroma is a mushroom-shaped bony projection on the external surface of the bone, with a broad cap of cartilage that is most often located at the metaphysis in the juxta-epiphyseal area of the long tubular bones.* This tumor projects in the surrounding soft tissues and has very slow growth. Thus, it is drawn to the attention of the patient by swelling and slight pain together with a mass. Many osteochondromas are, however, asymptomatic and are frequently discovered incidentally in a radiographic study.

Osteochondromas that do not show any clinical symptoms and are found by chance require no therapy. Removal is indicated if the tumor is producing pain or disability or shows an abnormal increase in size. When operating on the lesion, the whole cartilage cap, including the overlying periosteum, must be removed in order to prevent recurrences. Generally, the recurrence rate is 2%. Recurrence suggests the possibility that the original tumor was not removed completely or that it was, right from the beginning, a chondrosarcoma.

Sites (Fig. 2.1)

In most large series there is a predominance of male patients (male:female = 4:2). Osteochondromas may develop in any bone that has derived from enchondral ossification; therefore *osteocartilaginous exostoses* are observed in nearly all bones. The most common locations are the metaphyses of long tubular bone, especially the distal femoral metaphysis (20.5%), the proximal metaphyses of the tibia (11.7%) and the humerus (15.8%). These sites include about one-half (48%) of all osteochondromas. In addition, we have found many of these lesions in the short tubular bones of the feet and hands. All the other locations (skull, ribs, spine, pelvis) are fairly rare.

Age (Fig. 2.2)

Most osteochondromas develop early in skeletal evolution and will be discovered within the first two decades. Forty-six per cent of our patients have been in the second decade. As Fig. 2.2 also shows, many of these lesions may be detected in adult life.

Radiographic Features (Figs 2.3–2.6)

The characteristic radiographic appearance of a solitary osteochondroma is a bony projection of abnormal thickness and longitude that sits on the cortex of a bone in the metaphyseal area. Pedunculated osteochondromas have a stalk and an enlarged distal component with a knobby surface that is orientated in a proximal direction ("hook exostosis") (Fig. 2.3). Usually the lesion has a diameter of 3–4 cm, but lesions over 8 cm may be seen. The exostosis is composed of a cortex and spongiosa continuous with those of the underlying bone. In the overlying cartilaginous cap, irregular zones of calcification may be seen on the radiographs

(Fig. 2.4), but extensive calcifications and irregularities of this area should arouse the suspicion of malignant transformation. Usually the cartilaginous cap is not visible on the radiographs. Some osteochondromas show an extensive overall broadening that often has a cauliflower-like appearance (Fig. 2.5). Sessile osteochondromas have a broad base continuous with the spongiosa and the cortex of the underlying bone (Fig. 2.6). Sometimes, this region of the bone simply appears to be bulged, and the outer contours are sharply delineated. The radiologic diagnosis of an osteochondroma with a broad base (sessile type) is sometimes more difficult, and it may be misdiagnosed as parosteal osteoma or even parosteal osteosarcoma. On the whole, it is usually easy to recognize an osteochondroma from radiographs in two projections, and in these cases no further diagnostic procedures (such as a biopsy) are necessary. In symptomless cases, no treatment in indicated.

Gross Pathologic Features (Figs 2.7–2.9)

Viewed on radiographs, an osteochondroma is a bony protuberance with an enlarged distal component that has a mushroom-like (Fig. 2.7) or often even a cauliflower-like appearance. Osteochondromas of the pedunculated type may show a narrow or broad stalk (Fig. 2.8), which makes it is easy to resect operatively this kind of exostosis. In other cases, the lesion presents as a flat, rounded or plateau-like protuberance (Fig. 2.9). The actual tumor tissue is the cartilaginous cap that covers the entire surface of a sessile tumor or is only present at the rounded end of a stalked exostosis. On the cut surface, this cap is ordinarily 0.1–3.0 cm thick, but it may be broader and irregular in shape in proliferating osteochondromas. This should draw attention to a malignant growth, and it demands, especially in an adult, careful histologic study. In children, the cartilaginous cap usually is broader than in adults. It is covered by a thin, fibrous perichondrium that derives from the adjacent periosteum. The surgeon has to remove completely the whole cartilage cap, including the overlying perichondrium, when excising such an osteochondroma, in order to prevent recurrences.

Occasionally, a bursa may develop on the top of an exostosis that shows an inflammatory reaction. This may cause local pain, and sometimes this is the site of calcified cartilaginous loose bodies.

Histopathologic Features (Figs 2.10–2.13)

An osteochondroma is composed of the bony body and the characteristic cartilaginous cap. These components can easily be seen in a cross-section at low magnification (Fig. 2.10). The only important tissue is that of the cartilaginous cap, because this is the actual tumor tissue. The cartilage cells of this region are usually uniform but may be different in size. They are arranged in parallel clusters, and these linear clusters of chondrocytes mimick normal cartilage growth of the normal epiphysis plate (Fig. 2.11). In children, occasional atypical cells, including binucleate cells, may be seen (Fig. 2.12). There may be some degenerative changes within the cartilage tissue, such as myxoid and cystic degeneration. A very typical histologic pattern is invasion of the cartilage tumor tissue into the subchondral bone trabeculae (Fig. 2.13), so that one can see cartilaginous foci in the center of the bone trabeculae of this region. The focal calcifications of the cartilage tissue that may be seen in such lesions in adults are seldom observed in osteochondromas in children.

The bony component of this tumor shows normal, fully calcified cortical and spongiosal bone tissue, together with a fatty and often active hematopoietic bone marrow. These structures are not part of the actual tumor tissue.

The exostosis is covered by periosteum of fibrous tissue, which is continuous with that of the adjacent bone. In adult life, the cartilaginous cap may involute and, finally, there may be only a bony exostosis without any cartilage tissue.

The pathogenesis of osteochondromas is still the subject of speculation. Some authors regard them as a local malformation of enchondral ossification. Their tendency to proliferate characterizes them as bone tumors; when growing, they may reach a total weight over 5 kg. Less than 1% of solitary osteochondromas undergo malignant transformation later in life.

A special form of this disease is hereditary *multiple osteocartilaginous exostosis* with numerous osteochondromas throughout the skeleton (*osteochondromatosis*). Another entity is the so-called *subungual osteocartilaginous exostosis* in the end of short tubular bones, especially of the first toe. This is a reactive and often exophytic growth of proliferating bone and cartilage due to local pressure, trauma or infection, that may histologically mimic osteochondroma or even chondrosarcoma. The lesion is more often seen in adults than in chidlren.

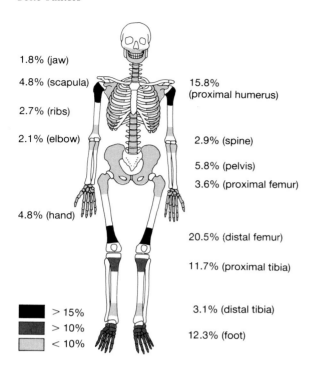

1.8% (jaw)

4.8% (scapula)

2.7% (ribs)

2.1% (elbow)

4.8% (hand)

15.8% (proximal humerus)

2.9% (spine)

5.8% (pelvis)

3.6% (proximal femur)

20.5% (distal femur)

11.7% (proximal tibia)

3.1% (distal tibia)

12.3% (foot)

> 15%
> 10%
< 10%

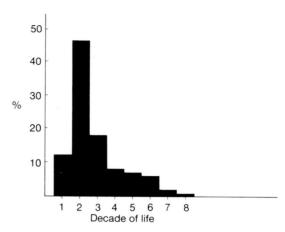

Fig. 2.2. Osteochondroma: age distribution. Most osteochondromas are seen in children and adolescents, mainly in the second decade, but they are also detected in adults.

Fig. 2.1. Osteochondroma: localization. The main sites are the distal femoral metaphysis, the proximal humerus metaphysis, and the proximal tibial metaphysis including the feet bones.

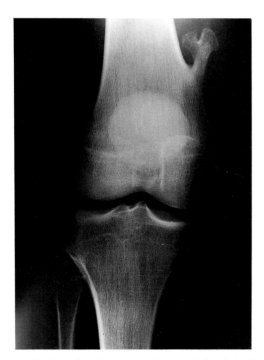

Fig. 2.3. Pedunculated osteochondroma of the right distal femoral metaphysis of a 15-year-old girl, showing a hook-like solitary exostosis attached on the surface of the intact cortex. The lesion consists of a stalk aligned in proximal direction ("hook exostosis") and a mushroom-like expansion on top, bearing the cartilaginous cap.

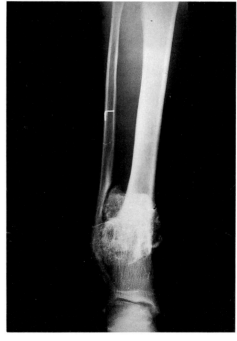

Fig. 2.4. Osteochondroma of the right distal tibial metaphysis of a 15-year-old boy, showing a broad expansion with displacement of the adjacent fibula and local bone atrophy due to impression by the tumor. The overlying cartilaginous cap shows extensive calcification.

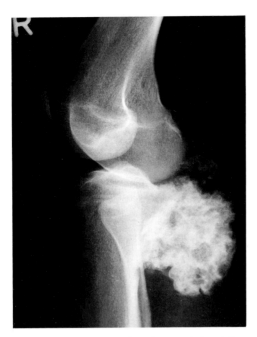

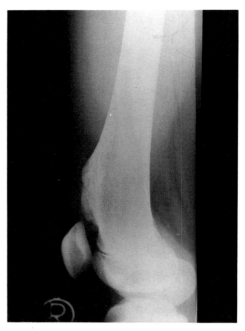

Fig. 2.5. Large sessile osteochondroma of the right proximal tibial metaphysis of a 13-year-old girl, is characterized by a large bony mass with a cauliflower-like appearance and extends far into the posterior soft tissue. The considerable radio-opacity represents large amounts of calcified cartilage.

Fig. 2.6. Osteochondroma with a flat sessile exostosis on the ventral cortex of the right distal femoral metaphysis of a 15-year-old boy. This lesion has a broad base and includes some spotty brightening. The underlying cortex and spongiosa are intact.

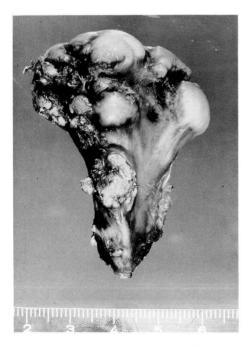

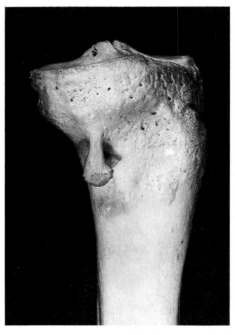

Fig. 2.7. Gross specimen of an osteochondroma that was removed operatively by chiselling from the underlying cortex. The lesion is mushroom-shaped, with many nodular protrusions covered with a layer of cartilage tissue.

Fig. 2.8. Maceration specimen of the left proximal tibia with an osteochondroma of pedunculated type that shows a mushroom-like exostosis attached to the tibial head.

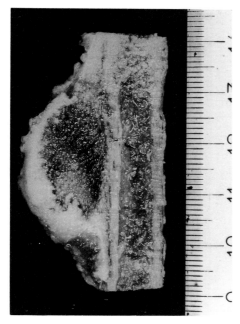

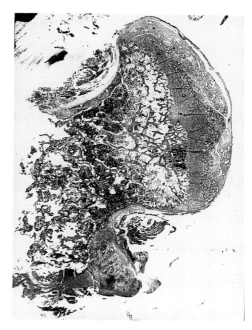

Fig. 2.9. Cut surface of an osteochondroma that shows, macroscopically, the lesion attached to the outer surface of the cortex. In the center of the lesion is a spongy bone area covered by a broad cap of cartilage tissue, which can measure up to 3 cm in thickness.

Fig. 2.10. Histologic section through an osteochondroma at low magnification, showing the typical shape of this lesion: a broad cartilaginous cape covered by a fibrous periosteal layer, with normal spongial bone beneath.

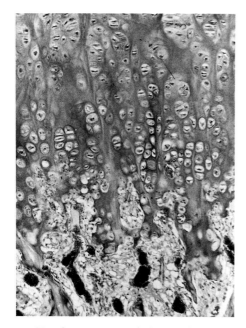

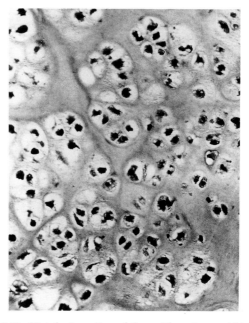

Fig. 2.11. Histologic section of the cartilage cape of an osteochondroma (H&E, ×32) showing many "ballooned", but generally uniform cartilage cells with small, round or elongated nuclei, often arranged in rows simulating the cartilage growth zone of bone. The tumorous cartilage extends diffusely into the subchondral bone, invading the bone trabeculae.

Fig. 2.12. Histologic section of the cartilage tissue at higher magnification (H&E, ×100) showing the polymorphy and hyperchromasy of cartilage cells' nuclei that may be seen in young children but does not imply malignancy.

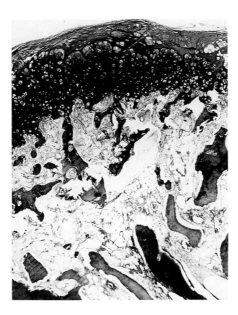

Fig. 2.13. Histologic pattern of an osteochondroma at low magnification (H&E, ×30), showing the typical cartilage cap covered with a layer of fibrous tissue. The subchondral bone trabeculae include cartilage tissue mimicking the growth plate. Further away from the cartilage cap, normal spongy bone tissue interspersed with fat tissue is seen.

ENCHONDROMA
(ICD-O-M-9220/0)

Enchondromas, neoplasms of cartilaginous origin, are the second most frequent benign bone tumor in childhood. They represent 19% of all benign bone tumors, and 24% of them occur in children or adolescents. *An enchondroma is a benign tumor consisting of mature hyaline cartilaginous tissue that arises within the medullary cavity of a bone.* Most of the lesions show a very slow proliferation without any symptoms, and may be detected incidentally on a radiograph. In some cases a pathological fracture may occur in the affected bone, but pain or swelling are seldom found in childhood.

Sites *(Fig. 2.14)*

In our series, we could not find any significant sex predilection in children. More than 60% of the tumors are located in the short tubular bones of the hands and feet, and have an absolutely benign course. In rarer cases, however, enchondromas may be incidentally detected in other sites such as long tubular bones, the ribs or the spine. They are characterized by dense, spotty calcifications and usually show no proliferative activity. In contrast to those in short tubular bones, enchondromas in other sites may start to proliferate in adult life and turn into chondrosarcomas of low-grade malignancy; therefore, they should be followed, especially if they are located in the pelvic bones.

Age *(Fig. 2.15)*

Most enchondromas are discovered in adult life; but nearly a quarter of them are seen in children, mostly in the second decade.

Radiographic Features *(Figs 2.16–2.18)*

Most enchondromas are discovered either incidentally after a pathological fracture or because they produce a local swelling and slight pain. Radiography reveals a centrally localized cystic lesion that often is well-delineated and round or ovoid (Fig. 2.16). This part of the bone may be expanded, and the cortex thinned from the inside but intact and smooth in its outer part. No periosteal reaction is seen, except in cases of pathological fracture. Mottled or stippled calcification is characteristic for all cartilaginous tumors and is usually present in enchondromas (Fig. 2.17). These mineral deposits may show finely stippled foci scattered throughout the lesion, or they may be large, coarse conglomerates. Enchondromas of the long bones and those located in the metaphysis may show a broad expansion of this growing zone, especially in childhood (Fig. 2.18). Within the lesion, some radiolucencies are seen with an irregular sclerosis. In older children or adults, a large lesion of this kind in a long tubular bone that has involved the cortical bone should be suspected of malignant tumor growth and must be histologically analyzed.

Most enchondromas are solitary lesions, but occasionally they may affect several bones (Fig. 2.16). In cases of multiple enchondromas, we are dealing with *Ollier's disease*: in adult life nearly 50% of such patients will develop a chondrosarcoma from one of the cartilaginous lesions.

Gross Pathologic Features *(Fig. 2.19)*

Because most enchondromas are treated by curettage, intact specimens are seldom seen.

The cut surface of the tumor is characteristically composed of confluent masses of bluish, translucent hyaline cartilage that shows a distinctly lobular arrangement (Fig. 2.19). Sometimes the tumor tissue shows some white or yellowish foci of calcification; no spongiosal bone pattern can be seen in this area. The cortex may be attenuated, but in most cases it is intact.

Histopathologic Features *(Figs 2.20, 2.21)*

In this intramedullary lesion, we find a cartilaginous tissue that shows a strongly lobular pattern of nodules of different size (Fig. 2.20). The nodules are surrounded by small septae of fibrous tissue, including some vascular channels. Occasionally some remnants of bone trabeculae may be observed. Usually the cartilage cells are small and of uniform size with one dark round nucleus within a typical lacuna. Occasionally some cells possess two even nuclei, and these may be elongated or stellate. Mitoses are hardly ever found. Between the cartilage cells there is a more or less abundant hyaline ground substance of basophilic appearance and some deposits of calcification may be found. In some enchondromas this ground substance may show myxoid changes, and cartilaginous nodules extremely rich of cells may be encountered (Fig. 2.21), which raises the suspicion of chondrosarcoma. Especially in enchondromas of the long tubular bones, ribs, spine or pelvis, the cytological details of the cartilage cells are of fundamental importance to the diagnosis. Numerous fields need to be examined to ensure that there are no polymorphic and hyperchromatic cell nuclei, no multinucleated cells and no mitoses with sufficient evidence for a chondrosarcoma. Enchondromas of the short tubular bones of the hands and feet are, however, above suspicion of a malignant growth in childhood.

Chondromatous tumors may occur outside the medullary cavity of a bone, in the larynx or the synovial membranes. Such a tumor may grow in the periosteum of a bone (juxtacortical, periosteal chondroma). Multiple chondromas may be associated with angiomas of the soft tissues (*Maffucci's syndrome*).

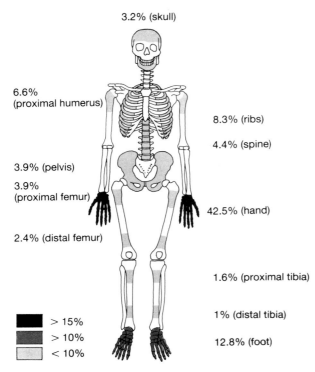

3.2% (skull)

6.6%
(proximal humerus)

8.3% (ribs)

4.4% (spine)

3.9% (pelvis)

3.9%
(proximal femur)

42.5% (hand)

2.4% (distal femur)

1.6% (proximal tibia)

1% (distal tibia)

12.8% (foot)

⬛ > 15%
⬛ > 10%
☐ < 10%

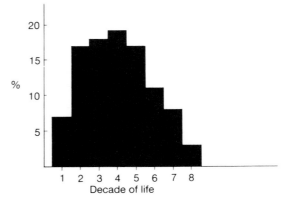

Fig. 2.15. Enchondroma: age distribution. Enchondromas may occur at any age, mainly in adult life. No special preponderance of any age-group can be registered, but many enchondromas are seen in children, especially in the second decade.

Fig. 2.14. Enchondroma: localization. The main sites are the short tubular bones of hands and feet. This bone tumor may occur in other bones, however, such as the long tubular bones, ribs, spine, pelvis or skull, with different prognoses.

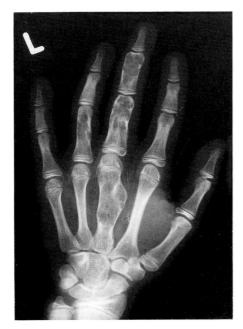

Fig. 2.16. Radiograph of multiple enchondromas of short tubular bones in the phalanges of the third finger of the left hand of a 13-year-old boy. Inside the involved bones, cystic lesions are seen that have eroded the cortex from inside and expanded the bone. The outer cortex is, however, intact and sharply delineated.

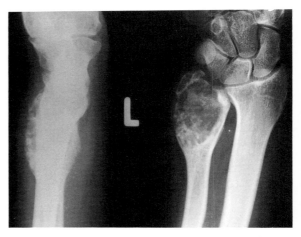

Fig. 2.17. Radiograph of an enchondroma in the left distal ulna of a 14-year-old boy that presented as an expansive, cystic lesion with many stippled calcifications inside. The cortex is extremely rarefied and obviously invaded laterally by the tumor. The adjacent joint surface seems to be interrupted. A malignant tumor growth cannot be excluded by these features alone.

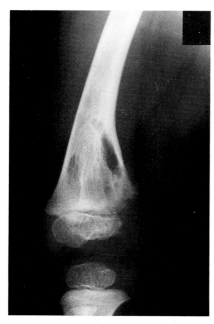

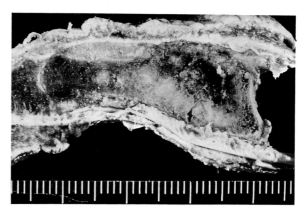

Fig. 2.19. Gross specimen of an enchondroma in a short tubular bone of the finger, showing a translucent (bluish) cartilaginous mass in the medullary cavity where the spongy bone is destroyed. A lobular pattern of the tumor and many nodular foci are characteristic.

Fig. 2.18. Radiograph of an enchondroma located in the distal metaphysis of the right femur of a 2-year-old child, showing a broad expansion of the involved bone and including irregular cystic radiolucencies. The cortex and adjacent growing plate are, however, intact.

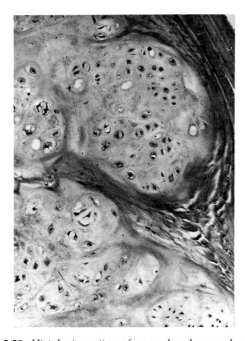

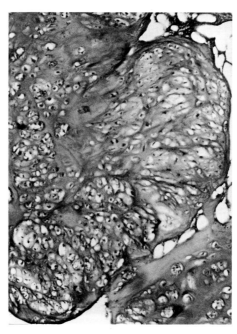

Fig. 2.20. Histologic section of an enchondroma, showing the typical lobular pattern with nodules of different size separated by small septa of fibrous tissue with some small blood vessels (H&E, ×64). The cartilage cells are small and uniform with one dark round nucleus; some binucleate cells can be seen.

Fig. 2.21. Histologic section of an enchondroma with typical lobular pattern and myxoid loosening of the ground substance (H&E, ×30). There are areas extremely rich in "ballooned" cartilage cells, together with some binucleate cells, which make it difficult to exclude a chondrosarcoma.

CHONDROBLASTOMA
(ICD-O-M-9230/0)

This is a fairly rare primary bone tumor that comprises only 1% of all bone tumors. About 62% of these lesions occur in children or adolescents. *Chondroblastoma ("Codman tumor") is considered a benign tumor of cartilaginous origin, which arises from the epiphyses.* In this bony region an osteolytic destruction develops that may expand to the neighboring metaphysis. About 60% of the lesions are found in males.

In most cases the patients have local pain for months or sometimes years but have, at most, only discrete swelling; these symptoms cannot, however, be considered diagnositc. Pathologic fractures are uncommon.

Sites *(Fig. 2.22)*

Chondroblastomas typically arise in the epiphyses, mainly of the long tubular bones. The most frequent sites affected are the epiphysis of the upper end of the humerus (17.4%), the upper tibia (19.6%) and the lower epiphysis of the femur (15.2%). Thus, most have occurred in the region of the knee. Some of them appear in secondary centers of ossification, such as the greater trochanter. Another frequent site is the pelvis (13%), including the upper femur (13%). Involvement of other bones (ribs, spine or short tubular bones) is extremely rare.

Age *(Fig. 2.23)*

Chondroblastoma manifests itself mainly the second decade of life, in which more than half of the patients (58%) have been diagnosed. Four per cent of the patients are children below the age of 10 years. Nevertheless, the tumor may be detected in adulthood.

Radiographic Features *(Figs 2.24, 2.25)*

The most characteristic feature is round or oval osteolysis located eccentrically in the epiphysis. Usually the lesion is sharply limited by a thin marginal sclerosis (Fig. 2.24) but often the border is incomplete and vague. Within the radiolucent zone mottled areas of increased chalky densities may be noted, depending on the degree of calcification within the tumor tissue. The involved bone area may be slightly expanded and the cortex may be broadened, but periosteal bone production is not usually seen. The tumor develops in the epiphysis but may penetrate secondarily into the metaphysis (Fig. 2.25).

Gross Pathologic Features *(Fig. 2.26)*

In accordance with the radiological findings, a roundish area of bone destruction is seen centrally in the epiphysis which, in cases of large tumors, may expand into the metaphysis. Usually, however, the tumor is small. The lesion is sharply demarcated by a sclerotic bony rim. The cut surface is a grayish blue or yellow, partly brown tumor tissue with large zones of hemorrhage and necrosis. There are some white calcium deposits within the tumor substance. Some chondroblastomas may show cystic changes. The tumor tissue may have invaded the cortex, but usually its outer layer is intact and no periosteal reaction is seen. Occasionally, the tumor destroys the bony cortex and produces an extraosseous mass.

Histopathologic Features *(Figs 2.27–2.29)*

Chondroblastomas have a richly cellular tumor tissue in which nodular areas of a chondroid tissue are most obvious (Figs 2.27 and 2.28). The chondroid areas are rather sharply demarcated, and many multinucleate giant cells are seen in association with these tumor components (Fig. 2.28). Within the chondroid areas many chondroblastic cells are seen. These are usually polygonal or roundish, with oval or round nuclei, and have a clearly defined cell membrane and hyperchromatic and even polymorphic nuclei (Fig. 2.29). Some mitotic figures may be detected in these cells. Chondroid substance containing focal areas of calcification is seen. Between these nodular chondroid areas, a cellular connective stroma with many spindle cells is present (Figs 2.27 and 2.28). About 17% of all chondroblastomas show, in addition, the histologic structures of an aneurysmal bone cyst (Fig. 2.27). Because of the pleomorphic cellular pattern, together with mitoses and many multinucleated giant cells and a cellular fibroblastic stroma between the chondroid areas, this lesion is often histologically misdiagnosed as a chondrosarcoma, giant cell tumor or even an osteosarcoma. Another incorrect diagnosis may be aneurysmal bone cyst, in cases in which only cysts have been noted in the biopsy material and radiographs have not been seen.

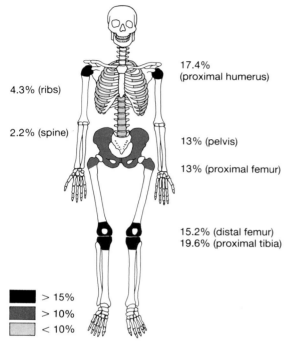

4.3% (ribs)

2.2% (spine)

17.4% (proximal humerus)

13% (pelvis)

13% (proximal femur)

15.2% (distal femur)
19.6% (proximal tibia)

> 15%
> 10%
< 10%

Fig. 2.22. Chondroblastoma: localization. The main sites are the long tubular bones, in which the epiphyses are involved. Most of these tumors are located in the epiphysis of the proximal humerus, the proximal epiphysis of the tibia, the distal and proximal epiphysis of the femur and in the pelvic bones.

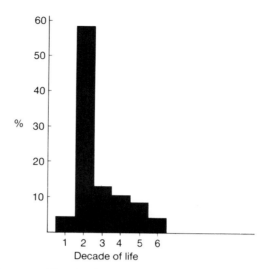

Fig. 2.23. Chondroblastoma: age distribution. Chondroblastomas mainly occur in children and adolescents, in the second decade of life. Some of these tumors may, however, be detected in adults.

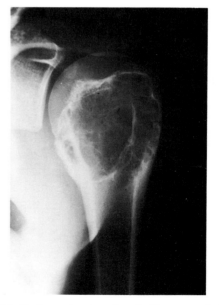

Fig. 2.24. Radiograph of a chondroblastoma of the left humeral head of a 15-year-old boy; it has expanded the bone and there is a cystic lesion with some spotty densities. The lesion is sharply limited, and the thinned cortex is intact and smooth from the outside.

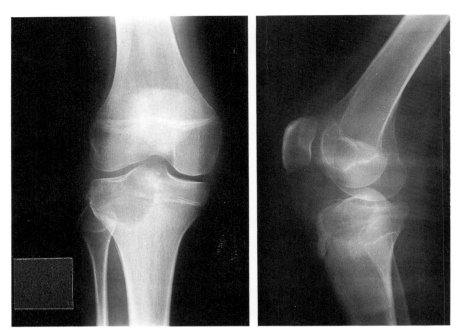

Fig. 2.25. Radiograph of a chondroblastoma located in the right proximal tibial epiphysis of a 14-year-old girl. A lytic lesion is situated primarily in the epiphysis and has expanded secondarily into the adjacent metaphysis. It is demarcated by a thin sclerotic rim.

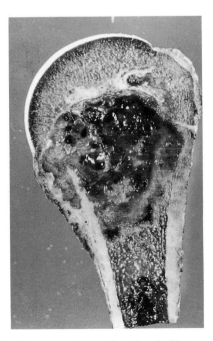

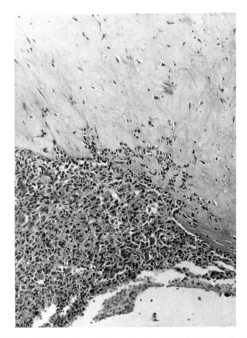

Fig. 2.26. Gross specimen of a chondroblastoma of the proximal humerus, showing a circumscribed destruction of the bone and tumor tissue (grayish blue, partly yellow) with large hemorrhages. At one site, the cortex is partly invaded by the tumor tissue, but the outer cortical layer is intact.

Fig. 2.27. Histologic section of a chondroblastoma showing an area of chondroid substance including small chondro-blasts with small roundish, isomorphic nuclei (H&E, ×40). Adjacent, a cell-rich stroma is seen with many isomorphic fibroblasts, and, in addition, an aneurysmal bone cyst can be identified. Usually, mitoses are very rare in this lesion.

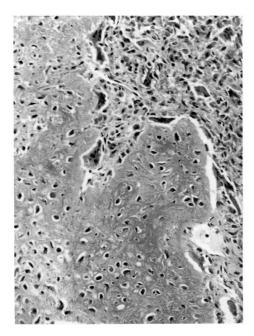

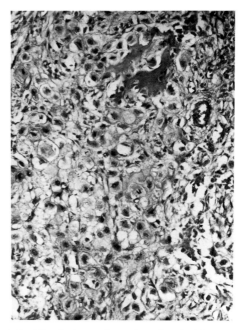

Fig. 2.28. Histologic section of a chondroblastoma that shows the rather sharp margin of a chondroid focus with many attached multinucleate giant cells (H&E, ×64). The chondroblasts are morphologically characterized by a clearly defined cell membrane and a hyperchromatic nucleus that is roundish or polygonal.

Fig. 2.29. Histologic section of a chondroblastoma with sharply delineated chondroblasts that contain hyperchromatic and polygonal nuclei (H&E, ×100). Patches of chondroid substance are laid down amongst the tumor cells.

CHONDROMYXOID FIBROMA
(ICD-O-M-9241/0)

This is a very rare bone tumor which accounts for only 0.5% of all bone tumors. *Chondromyxoid fibroma is a well circumscribed, osteolytic bone tumor consisting of cartilage-forming connective tissue with lobulated areas of spindle-shaped or stellate cells and abundant myxoid or chondroid intercellular material that may show an invasive growth.* This tumor growth usually is benign in character but, because of its locally destructive potential and high recurrence rate, it is a semi-malignant tumor biologically. Metastases are, however, not to be anticipated.

In most cases, the patient complains of local pain, occasionally of long duration, and sometimes a swelling will be noticed. All these symptoms are of little help in diagnosis, and in asymptomatic cases chondromyxoid fibroma may be an incidental finding on radiographs. Rarely, a pathologic fracture draws attention to the tumor growth.

Because of a high recurrence rate after curettage of a chondromyxoid fibroma (12.5%–25.0%), the best treatment is a block excision of the affected area. The tendency for local recurrence after initial curettage seems higher in young children (under the age of 15 years). Radiation therapy is not indicated. After total extirpation of the tumor, the prognosis is good. Sarcomatous change remains a pathologic rarity in this disease.

Sites (Fig. 2.30)

Typical chondromyxoid fibromas are located in the metaphyseal region of the long tubular bones, usually near the epiphyseal plate. Here, they show an eccentric osteolysis and may invade the epiphysis. The upper end of the tibia is the most common site. However, this tumor may be seen in other sites, such as the ribs, the pelvis or even the short tubular bones.

Age (Fig. 2.31)

Most chondromyxoid fibromas are detected in the second decade of life, but they are also found in children between the ages of 5 and 10 years. Thus, the tumor may be seen in all age-groups, children and adults.

Radiographic Features (Figs 2.32 and 2.33)

In typical cases involving the long bones, a large osteolytic defect is seen in the metaphysis, which is eccentric in shape and sharply circumscribed. The adjacent cortex may be expanded, thinned and even partially absent (Fig. 2.32). The internal border is usually well defined by a narrow rim of bone sclerosis (Fig. 2.33). The size of the osteolysis varies from about 1 to 10 cm in greatest dimension, and it can be round or oval, with the long axis parallel to the bone. No internal structures are seen; calcific shadows, although visible histologically, are usually absent on the radiographs. In the small tubular bones, the lesion can produce expansion of its entire contour.

Gross Pathologic Features

Usually chondromyxoid fibromas are curetted, and numerous irregular fragments of the tumor tissue are obtained. In rare cases where a resected specimen is available, an osteolytic lesion of 1.5–10.0 cm in size, usually well circumscribed, is seen in the metaphyseal area of the bone. The cut surface shows a somewhat translucent fibrous mass together with a cartilaginous lobulated texture. Within this area there are solid, gray-white and firm regions and eventually hemorrhages. The cortex may be expanded and partly eroded so that the periosteum is the limiting membrane.

Histopathological Features (Figs 2.34 and 2.35)

Histologically, it can be difficult to distinguish between a benign and malignant tumor growth in many cases of chondromyxoid fibroma. The most striking feature is the nodular and lobulated tissue pattern that is characteristic for all cartilaginous tumors (Fig. 2.34). These nodules are rather sharply demarcated, and an increased concentration of cell nuclei is observed at the periphery of the lobules; this is a highly characteristic feature of chondromyxoid fibroma. The matrix of the chondroid nodules is myxoid in appearance and includes extremely bizarre cells with ovoid, round or polygonal nuclei (Fig. 2.35). Within these spindle-shaped or stellate cells, which lack distinct cytoplasmic borders, no mitoses can be detected. Small foci of calcification are occasionally present within the myxoid and chondroid matrix. In the surrounding cellular areas some dark, nucleated giant cells may be noted. The septa that separate the myxoid areas have a loose collagen stroma with a fair number of fibroblastic elements and some narrow blood capillaries. Because of the presence of large pleomorphic tumor cells with one or more hyperchromatic nuclei and concentrated in the periphery of the nodular foci, the tumor may be misdiagnosed as chondrosarcoma. However, these cells are recognized as only a part of the overall pattern of chondromyxoid fibroma, and the benign nature of the lesion should be firmly established on the basis of the overall radiological and histological pattern. Microscopically, there may be a close resemblance of chondromyxoid fibroma to chondroblastoma, because of small amorphous foci of calcification and cellular areas indistinguishable from those seen in chondroblastoma; but chondroblastoma emerges in the epiphysis and chondromyxoid fibroma in the metaphysis of a long bone.

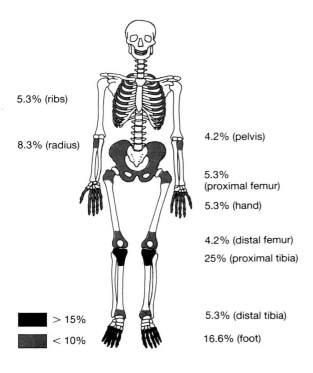

5.3% (ribs)

8.3% (radius)

4.2% (pelvis)

5.3%
(proximal femur)

5.3% (hand)

4.2% (distal femur)

25% (proximal tibia)

5.3% (distal tibia)

16.6% (foot)

■ > 15%

▨ < 10%

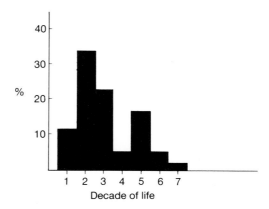

Fig. 2.31. Chondromyxoid fibroma: age distribution. Forty-seven per cent of chondromyxoid fibromas occur in children or adolescents, but they may also be seen in adults, including the older age-groups.

◄─────────────────────────────

Fig. 2.30. Chondromyxoid fibroma: localization. Main sites are the metaphyseal regions of long tubular bones, especially of the proximal tibia. This tumor growth may, however, also be seen in the ribs, pelvis or short tubular bones.

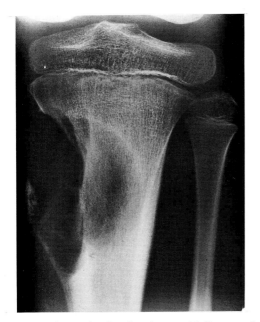

Fig. 2.32. Radiograph of a chondromyxoid fibroma of the left proximal tibial metaphysis of a 10-year-old boy, showing a large osteolytic defect in eccentric location and bulging outward. The adjacent cortex is extremely thin, and the lesion has no internal structures. However, it is demarcated on the inside by a distinct marginal sclerosis.

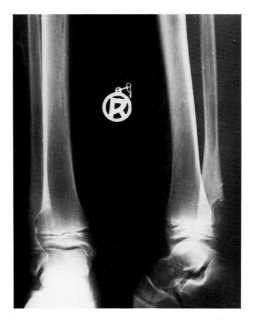

Fig. 2.33. Radiograph of a chondromyxoid fibroma of the right distal fibula metaphysis of a 13-year-old boy, demonstrating a well-defined "bone cyst" that has expanded the bone, with thinning of the cortex.

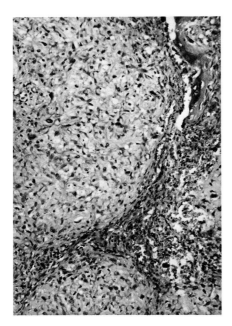

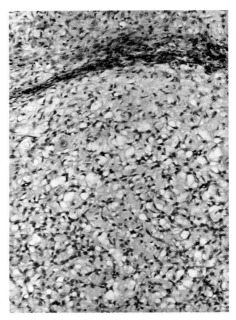

Fig. 2.34. Histologic section of a chondromyxoid fibroma showing a pattern of rather sharply demarcated nodules of chondroid tissue in which a concentration of the cartilage cells is seen in the periphery (H&E, ×50). A strong myxoid loosening of the stroma is obvious.

Fig. 2.35. Histologic section of a chondromyxoid fibroma at higher magnification (H&E, ×100). In the periphery of a tumorous nodule a cell-rich tissue and myxoid stroma is recognizable. The chondroid cells are spindle-shaped without cytoplasmic borders, and have roundish or elongated nuclei. No mitoses are seen.

CHONDROSARCOMA

(ICD-O-M-9220/3)

Chondrosarcoma is a malignant cartilaginous tumor arising from cartilage and is composed of atypical cartilage tissue. *The tumor is characterized by the formation of cartilage, with atypical, pleomorphic cartilage cells and little fibrous tissue, in the absence of new osteoid or bone formation.* The prognosis is distinctly better than for osteosarcomas, and therefore chondrosarcoma should be separated from osteosarcoma.

Primary chondrosarcoma arises de novo centrally within a bone or within the periosteum ("juxtacortical chondrosarcoma"). It may, however, emerge from a pre-existing benign cartilage tumor (e.g. osteochondroma or enchondroma) and is then a *secondary chondrosarcoma*. The tumor is characterized by a slow growth, and therefore patients have a long history in which they exhibit local pain and swelling of the affected part. These symptoms may be present for months and years, and often the tumor is diagnosed and treated far too late.

Typically, there is a tendency for the tumor to invade blood vessels and produce long intravasal tumor bungs that may extend right into the heart and pulmonary arteries. Metastases occur late, initially in the lungs; metastases of the regional lymph nodes occur but are rare. There exists, however, a danger of local implantation metastases when a chondrosarcoma is biopsied or excited operatively. Incomplete tumor excision leads to local recurrences. The only effective therapy for chondrosarcomas is their complete operative removal; the tumor is resistant to radiation or chemotherapy.

Sites (Fig. 2.36)

The majority of central chondrosarcomas involve the trunk (including the pelvic bones and shoulder girdle), the distal ends of the femora and the upper end of the humerus, in which sites we found 78% of all chondrosarcomas. They develop in the epiphyses and extend into the metaphyses secondarily. The pelvis is the most frequent location of chondrosarcomas (28.2%). The next most frequent site is the knee (19.9%). In addition, we have found this tumor in the ribs (12%) and the spine (7.6%). The short tubular bones of hands and feet are, in contrast, very rare locations for this tumor. In rare cases, chondrosarcomas are seen in the maxilla, mandible, nasal septum, larynx, or extraosseously in the soft tissues. They may also develop in the joint capsule.

Age (Fig. 2.37)

Chondrosarcoma occurs more commonly in males than in females (2:1). It is a tumor of adulthood and older age-groups but may be seen in children and adolescents as well (only about 5% of cases). In most cases, it is a secondary chondrosarcoma. Far more often such a malignant growth in children is a chondroblastic osteosarcoma, which is distinct from chondrosarcoma.

Radiographic Features (Figs 2.38–2.40)

In most cases a malignant tumor growth is recognizable on radiographs, showing an osseous destruction in the lesional area that is not sharply demarcated. Characteristically, many mottled dense areas of calcifications are seen within the tumor (Fig. 2.38). Central chondrosarcomas are situated in the metaphysis of a long bone and may extend into the diaphysis along the medullary cavity (Fig. 2.39). They often show a fusiform expansion of the cortex, with elevation and ossification of the periosteum (Fig. 2.40). In cases of cortical destruction the tumor may extend into the soft tissue, and it

exhibits a cloudy tumor shadow with a lobulated mass including spotty calcifications (Fig. 2.39). In these cases, a computerized tomography is helpful in delineating the extent of extraosseous tumor growth. In the periphery, a so-called Codman's triangle of the elevated periosteum may be obvious, indicating malignancy. The extent of calcification is said to be a clue to the degree of differentiation, heavily calcified lesions usually demonstrating the highest degree of differentiation. Central intraosseous chondrosarcomas of long bones with little or no cortical destruction but with characteristic mottled calcifications may cause great difficulties in the differential diagnosis of enchondromas, and even a biopsy out of such a lesion may pose similar difficulties.

Gross Pathologic Features (Fig. 2.41)

The central type of chondrosarcoma in a long bone shows tumor growth that may extend far across the bone margins into the surrounding soft tissue. A smaller tumor may involve only the medullary cave, and the cortex may remain intact. This is also evident on the radiographs. The lesion may have a well-defined border, together with a fibrous capsule. The cut surface shows variably sized nodules of lobulated tumor tissue that has a shiny bluish to gray-white appearance, indicating typical cartilage tissue. In addition, white flecks of calcium deposit are present in the tumor tissue. Focally, the tumor may be myxoid, and in central areas necrotic foci and hemorrhages may be seen. Usually, the original bone within the tumorous region is extensively destroyed. In the periphery the periosteum is elevated, demonstrating a so-called Codman's triangle. Peripheral chondrosarcomas are characterized by a smaller tumor focus, either on the surface of a bone within the periosteum (periosteal chondrosarcoma) or on top of a pre-existing cartilaginous exostosis (secondary chondrosarcoma).

Histopathologic Features (Figs 2.42–2.45)

The histologic diagnosis can be extremely difficult, especially when dealing with a highly differentiated chondrosarcoma. The pathologist has to make the decision whether the tumor is a benign enchondroma or an already well-differentiated chondrosarcoma. Several blocks of tumor tissue should be examined. There are only discrete features indicating malignancy, such as cells with plump and hyperchromatic nuclei or a larger number of cartilage cells with two or more nuclei. Mitoses will not be seen in low-grade chondrosarcomas, and no sarcomatous stroma is present. Therefore clinical data, the location of the tumor and, particularly, radiographic information have to be taken into consideration in diagnosis.

In a high-grade chondrosarcoma the malignant character of the cartilage tissue is obvious. As in all cartilage tumors, the tissue is composed of nodules of different size that are separated by small fibrous strands (Fig. 2.42), and here foci of non-tumorous reactive bone formation may be visible. There are myxomatous changes (Fig. 2.43) and calcium deposits in the cartilage tissue. Cytologic criteria are of decisive importance in the diagnosis of a chondrosarcoma and can be used to classify it into three grades of malignancy. In high-grade tumors a large number of cartilage cells with plump and dark nuclei is conspicuous (Fig. 2.44). Nuclear pleomorphism and hyperchromatism, as well as increased numbers of multinucleated tumor cells, are important features for diagnosis (Fig. 2.45). Mitoses are very rare or even absent. Regarding cellularity, one must take into account that in childhood and adolescence, especially during puberty, tumors of cartilage are often cell-rich and show some cellular atypia even in cases of benign growth such as osteochondroma or enchondroma, especially in Ollier's disease. There may be identical histologic features in a benign enchondroma of the short tubular bones of a growing child and in a central chondrosarcoma of the femur or humerus of an adult. This means that biologic behavior and histologic appearance do not always match, and clinical and radiologic findings have to be taken into consideration in order to make the correct diagnosis. In many cases chondrosarcoma in children runs a rapid course in contrast to its behavior in adults, but these cases are in reality probably chondroblastic osteosarcomas.

There exist some special varieties of chondrosarcoma such as *clear cell chondrosarcoma*, *mesenchymal chondrosarcoma*, or *dedifferentiated chondrosarcoma*. These chondrosarcomas show some differences in histologic pattern and a special biologic behavior, and they have different prognosis. They are, however, very rare in children and adolescents.

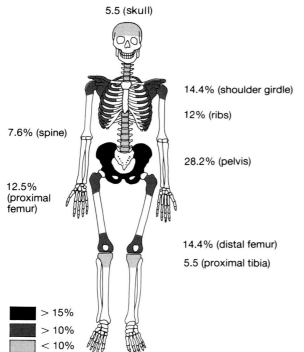

5.5 (skull)

14.4% (shoulder girdle)

12% (ribs)

7.6% (spine)

28.2% (pelvis)

12.5% (proximal femur)

14.4% (distal femur)

5.5 (proximal tibia)

■ > 15%
▨ > 10%
▢ < 10%

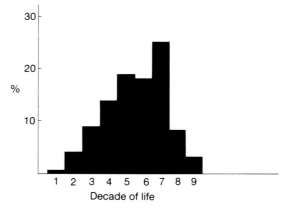

Fig. 2.37. Chondrosarcoma: age distribution. Most chondrosarcomas are seen in adults, mainly of older age. But in rare cases, they may occur in children or adolescents (5%).

◄———————————————————————

Fig. 2.36. Chondrosarcoma: localization. The majority of chondrosarcomas are located in the trunk (pelvis, ribs, spine, shoulder girdle), including the distal ends of long tubular bones (proximal and distal femur, proximal humerus, proximal tibia).

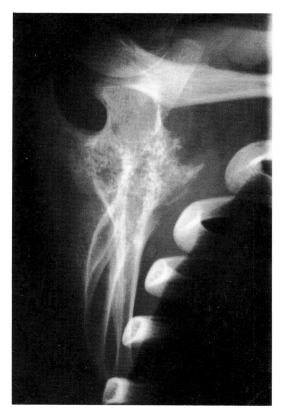

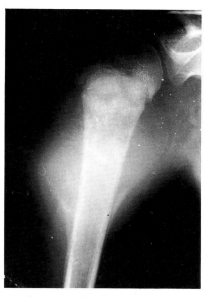

Fig. 2.39. Radiograph of a chondrosarcoma of the right proximal humerus of a 13-year-old boy; it has destroyed the cortex and is expanded into the surrounding soft tissue. The periosteum is elevated, forming a so-called Codman's triangle, which indicates malignancy.

Fig. 2.38. Radiograph of a chondrosarcoma of the right scapula of a 14-year-old girl. There is a large, undefined bone destruction which extends the bony margins and includes many mottled, dense areas of calcification.

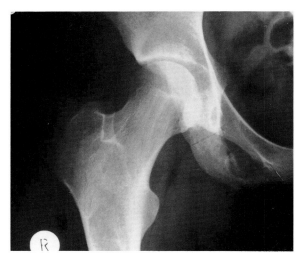

Fig. 2.40. Radiograph of a chondrosarcoma of the right ischial bone of a 16-year-old girl showing a destruction and fusiform expansion of the involved bone. A malignant tumor growth must be diagnosed in such a case.

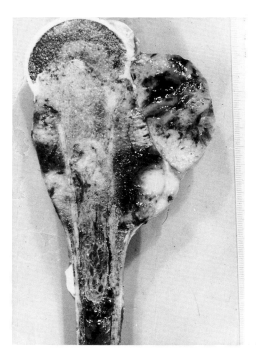

Fig. 2.41. Gross specimen of a chondrosarcoma of the right proximal humerus of a 13-year-old boy showing a large tumor mass inside the bone as well as outside, with protrusion far into the soft tissue. The cut surface of the tumor shows the nodular, shiny (bluish) cartilage tumor tissue and there are large areas of necrosis and hemorrhage.

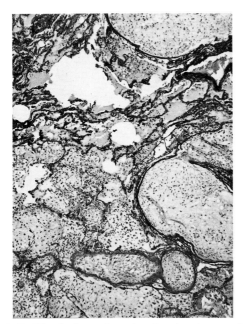

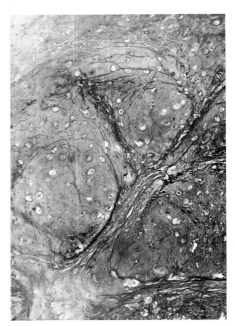

Fig. 2.42. Histologic section of a chondrosarcoma characterized by a nodular cartilaginous tissue in which the nodules of different size are separated by fibrous septa (H&E, ×25). Cellular and nuclear atypism is diagnostic of malignant tumor growth.

Fig. 2.43. Histologic section of a low-grade chondrosarcoma that shows a nodular cartilage tissue with mostly isomorphic tumor cells; some cells may include faintly polymorphic and hyperchromatic or even multiple nuclei (PAS, ×40). Differentiating between this malignant tumor growth and an enchondroma can be extremely difficult.

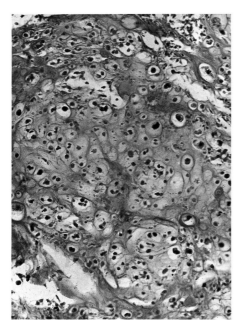

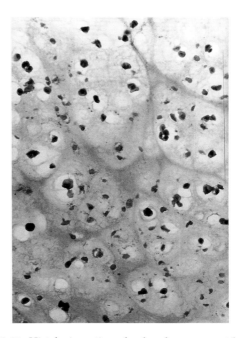

Fig. 2.44. Histologic section of a high-grade chondrosarcoma with clear cellular and nuclear polymorphism, which definitely indicates malignant growth (H&E, ×100).

Fig. 2.45. Histologic section of a chondrosarcoma at higher magnification (H&E, ×125), showing polymorphous, plump and hyperchromatic nuclei, which clearly indicate a highly malignant tumor growth.

LITERATURE
Tumors of Cartilaginous Origin

Adler CP, Klümper A. Röntgenologische und pathologisch-anatomische Aspekte von Knochentumoren. Radiologe 1977;17:355–92

Adler CP. Differential diagnosis of cartilage tumors. Pathol Res Pract 1979;166:45–58

Adler CP, Fringes B. Chondrosarkom der distalen Femurmetaphyse. Med Welt (Stuttg) 1978;29:1511–16

Adler CP, Klümper A, Wenz W. Enchondrome aus radiologische und pathologisch-anatomischer Sicht. Radiologe 1979;19:341–9

Alexander C. Chondroblastoma of the tibia. Case report. Skeletal Radiol 1976;1:63–4

Aprin H, Roseborough EJ, Hall JE. Chondrosarcoma in children and adolescents. Clin Orthop 1982;166:226–32

Batsakis JG, Raymond AK. Chondromyxoid fibroma. Ann Otol Rhinol Laryngol 1989;98:571–2

Bertoni F, Present D, Bacchini P, Picci P, Pignatti G, Gherlinzoni F, et al. Dedifferentiated peripheral chondrosarcomas. A report of seven cases. Cancer 1989;63:2054–9

Dahlin DC, Wells AH. Chondromyxoid fibroma of bone. J Bone Jt Surg 1953;35-A:831–4

Dahlin DC, Ivins JC. Benign chondroblastoma. A study of 125 cases. Cancer (Phil) 1972;30:401–13

Dumontier C, Rigault P, Padovani JP, Touzet P, Finidori G, Mallet JF. Chir Pediatr 1989;30:91–7

Feldmann F, Hecht HL, Johnston AD. Chondromyxoid-fibroma of bone. Radiology 1970;94:249–60

Frassica FJ, Unni KK, Beabout JW, Sim FH. Dedifferential chondrosarcoma. A report of the clinicopathological features and treatment of seventy-eight cases. Bone Jt Surg 1986;68-A:1197–1205

Garrison RC, Unni KK, McLeod RA, Prichard DJ, Dahlin DC. Chondrosarcoma arising in osteochondroma. Cancer 1982;49:1890–7

Henderson ED, Dahlin DC. Chondrosarcoma of bone. A study of two hundred and eighty-eight cases. J Bone Jt Surg 1963;45-A:1450–8

Hermann G, Wagner LD, Klein MJ, Faye-Peterson OM, Lewis MM. Low grade chondrosarcoma (case report). Skeletal Radiol 1989;18:241–4

Huvos AG, Marcove RC, Erlandson RA, Mike V. Chondroblastoma of bone. Cancer 1972;29:760–71

Kuur E, Hansen SL, Lindequist S. Treatment of solitary enchondromas in fingers. J Hand Surg Br 1989;14:109–12

Lichtenstein L, Bernstein D. Unusual benign and malignant chondroid tumors of bone. Cancer (Phil) 1959;12:1142–57

Pope TL Jr, McLaughlin R, Wanebo HJ, Williamson BRJ, Fechner RE. Low-grade cartilaginous tumor with "skip lesion". Skeletal Radiol 1984;12:134–8

Remagen W, Nidecker A, Dolanc B. Enchondroma of the tibia with extensive myxoid degeneration; recurrence with secondary and malignant transformation to highly differentiated chondrosarcoma. Skeletal Radiol 1986;15:330–3

Rosenthal DI, Schiller AL, Mankin HJ. Chondrosarcoma: correlation of radiological and histological grade. Radiology 1984;150:21–6

Salzer M, Salzer-Kuntschik M. Das Chondromyxoidfibrom. Langenbecks Arch Klin Chir 1965;312:216–31

Shives TC, McLeod RA, Unni KK, Schray MF. Chondrosarcoma of the spine. J Bone Jt Surg (Am) 1989;71:1158–65

Ttschernikoff Z, Ditscheva L. A combination of multiple cartilaginous exostses and enchondromaosis of bone in a family. Radiol Diagn Berl 1989;30:53–6

Wilkinson RH, Kirkpatrick JA. Low-grade chondrosarcoma of fermur. Case report. Skeletal Radiol 1976;1:127–8

Young CL, Sim FH, Unni KK, McLeod RA. Chondrosarcoma of proximal humeral epiphysis (case report). Skeletal Radiol 1989;18:403–5

Tumors of Osteoblastic Origin

OSTEOMA
(ICD-O-M-9180/0)

Osteoma is an absolutely benign bone lesion that may arise within a bone or the periosteum. This is a lesion that can grow like a tumor or can be a local reaction, with osseous overgrowth from trauma, infection or an invading tumor such as a meningioma. Therefore osteoma as a true bone tumor is debatable, and some authors have considered it to be a hamartoma of bone or the sclerotized end stage of fibrous bone dysplasia. *In cases of an obviously solitary tumor growth it is a benign lesion consisting of well-differentiated mature bone of compact or spongiosal type, with very slow growth.* This leads to a continuous deformation of the involved bone area and may cause symptoms such as pain or nerval compression. Consequently, the lesions have to be removed operatively.

Sites

Osteomas usually involve the skull and facial bones of desmal origin. They are mostly found in the paranasal sinuses, most commonly the frontal and ethmoid sinuses, and in the jaws. In rarer cases, lesions are seen in bones of the peripheral skeleton, such as the long bones or the vertebra. However, in older patients, many of these probably represent ossified osteochondromas. Skeletal osteomas – predominantly of the skull and jaws – may be associated with intestinal polyps, fibromatous and other connective tissue lesions, and epidermal cysts in Gardner's syndrome. Other bony overgrowth of the jaw includes torus palatinus and torus mandibularis, and hyperostosis cranii (frontalis) can occur in the skull.

Age

Osteomas may occur in children but are more common in adults in their fourth and fifth decades. Juxtacortical osteomas of the long bones are not observed in the first decade, but do occur in the second decade. Twice as many males are afflicted as females.

Radiographic Features (Figs 2.46 and 2.47)

In the frontal sinus an osteoma presents as a circumscribed, dense, radio-opaque and structureless bone mass (Fig. 2.46). This may lead to an expansion of the bone, which is visible on radiographs. In the long bones a well-circumscribed bony lesion is seen within the bone (Fig. 2.47), and the cortex and shape of this region is usually intact. No periosteal reaction is seen.

Gross Pathologic Features

A dense and compact bone focus is seen in the involved bone, which is well-circumscribed and usually adjacent to the underlying cortex. In the periosteum, this appears as a bone focus surrounded by a fibrous membrane.

Histopathologic Features (Figs 2.48 and 2.49)

An *osteoma eburneum* shows a dense bone tissue that is identical with cortical bone (Fig. 2.48), in which narrow Haversian canals are seen.

The bone is fully mineralized. In an *osteoma spongiosum* broad spongiosal trabeculae are seen; they are sharply delineated and lamellarly layered (Fig. 2.49). No osteoblastic or osteoclastic cells are attached. Between these bone trabeculae fat tissue is seen. On the whole this is a mature spongious bone tissue not differing from normal bone tissue. Adjacent to it, the autochthonous cortical bone may be seen.

Osteoma is often asymptomatic and detected accidentally. Characteristic is its slow growth with bone expansion caused by bone deposition.

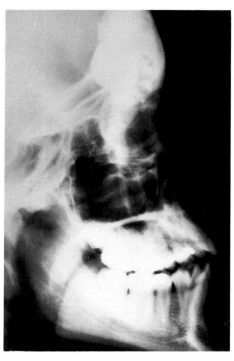

Fig. 2.46. Radiograph of an osteoma of the frontal sinus of a 15-year-old girl showing a dense radio-opaque and structureless bony mass. An expansion of the bone is visible.

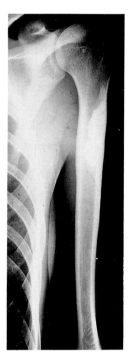

Fig. 2.47. Radiograph of an osteoma of the left proximal humerus of a 16-year-old boy with a well-circumscribed, dense bony mass that extends into the medullary cavity. The cortex of this area is intact and smooth outside.

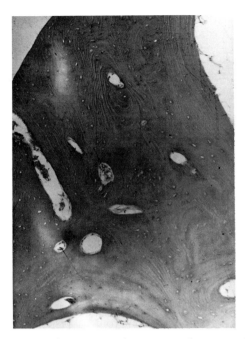

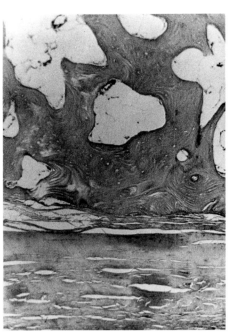

Fig. 2.48. Histologic section of an osteoma eburneum with a fully mineralized and lamellar bone tissue identical with cortical bone (H&E, ×50). Many Haversian channels can be seen.

Fig. 2.49. Histologic section of an osteoma spongiosum, showing broad spongiosal trabeculae that are sharply delineated (H&E, ×50). Fat tissue is present between the trabeculae. The spongiosal tumor tissue borders on the cortex.

OSTEOID OSTEOMA
(ICD-O-M-9191/0)

Among bone tumors of osteoblastic origin, osteoid osteoma shows distinctive symptoms, radiographic findings and pathologic characteristics. *The tumor is characterized by a small intraosseous or intracortical focus of about 1 cm diameter or less which shows osteolysis together with a central density, a "nidus", and severe perifocal osteosclerosis which causes severe pain during the night.* This typical nocturnal pain may be alleviated by giving aspirin. The tumor accounts for 10% of all benign bone tumors, but in many cases the tumor tissue cannot be removed operatively because of the extreme perifocal osteosclerosis; and this has resulted in histological diagnosis of osteoid osteoma being made in only 3% of all benign bone tumors. Therefore all the diagnostic approaches, including radiographs and histology, must be made in order to diagnose the lesion.

On the whole, this is an absolutely benign bone tumor which, while it induces painful symptoms, will not produce a malignant change.

Sites (Fig. 2.50)

The majority of osteoid osteomas are found in the long and short tubular bones, at least half of them in the femur or tibia. The ends of the diaphyses are the most common site. The lesion may occur in the spongiosa as well as in the cortex (cortical osteoid osteoma); in rare cases even periosteal or extraosseous osteoid osteomas have been described. When it occurs in the vertebrae, the arch is most commonly involved. Here, the tumor may give rise to painful scoliosis or sciatica in adolescents. Nearly all bones of the skeleton may be the site of an osteoid osteoma, though it is never seen in the skull, sternum, clavicula, vertebral bodies or distal phalanges of hands or feet.

Age (Fig. 2.51)

Osteoid osteoma occurs mainly in children and adolescents, more than 80% of cases being between the fifth and 25th year of life. Most cases are detected in the second decade. Osteoid osteoma is thus a tumor of the young.

Radiographic Features (Figs 2.52 and 2.53)

The lesion is characterized by an intensive osteosclerosis that may involve the most of the affected bone. In a cortical osteoid osteoma a large part of the cortex is broadened and expanded, but a discrete radiolucent focus is usually found centrally in the osteosclerotic area – at least in CTs – and this so-called "nidus" is the tumor (Fig. 2.52). However, in cases of severe perifocal osteosclerosis, it may be extremely difficult to detect this nidus and to excise it operatively. In plain radiographs and CTs, the nidus appears as a small radiolucent zone with a central round density, surrounded by extremely osteosclerotic bone tissue (Fig. 2.53). This lesion has to be removed operatively to effect a cure.

Gross Pathologic Features (Fig. 2.54)

The features seen on radiographs are similarly seen in macroscopic cross-sections. There is a round focus in the middle of the sclerotic zone; it appears loose and cloudy and is a gray-red color. This nidus rarely exceeds 1 cm in greatest dimension.

Histopathologic Features (Figs 2.55–2.57)

Histologically, osteoid osteoma presents as a circumscribed focus of osteoid trabeculae that is clearly separated from the surrounding spongy or cortical bone (Fig. 2.55). Within the nidus, an irregular network of interlacing osteoid trabeculae is the prominent feature (Fig. 2.56). Between the trabeculae there is a loose fibrous stroma with many vascular blood-filled channels. The osteoid trabeculae are usually thin and of differing width (Fig. 2.57), and many activated osteoblasts and osteoclasts are accompanied. Cartilage is not present in this tumor tissue.

A malignant transformation is not to be expected.

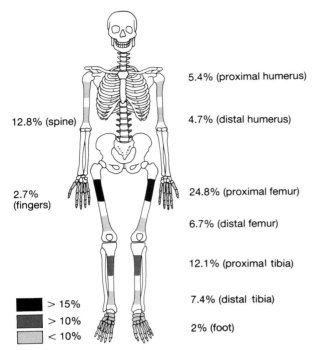

5.4% (proximal humerus)

4.7% (distal humerus)

12.8% (spine)

2.7%
(fingers)

24.8% (proximal femur)

6.7% (distal femur)

12.1% (proximal tibia)

7.4% (distal tibia)

2% (foot)

> 15%
> 10%
< 10%

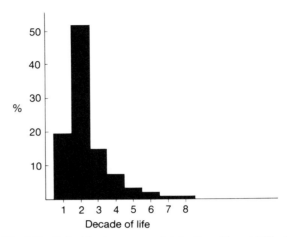

Fig. 2.50. Osteoid osteoma: localization. The majority of osteoid osteomas (66%) are located in the long and short tubular bones. Most often, the proximal femur and proximal tibia are involved. All bones may be involved, with the exception of the vertebral bodies, sternum, clavicles and skull, in which osteoid osteomas are extremely rare.

Fig. 2.51. Osteoid osteoma: age distribution. Almost 80% of these tumors are seen in children and adolescents, with a peak in the second decade. In rarer cases, the lesion may be found in adults.

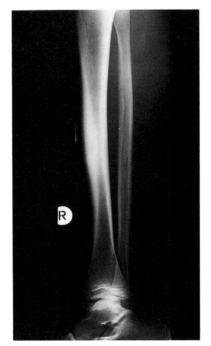

Fig. 2.52. Radiograph of an osteoid osteoma in the cortex of the right tibial shaft of a 14-year-old boy. An extensive broadening and sclerotic density of the ventral cortex, together with a bowing protrusion, are the most impressive radiologic symptoms. In the center of the osteosclerosis a faint radiolucent "nidus" is visible.

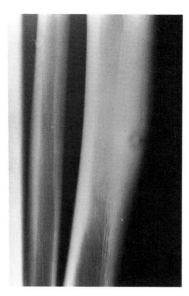

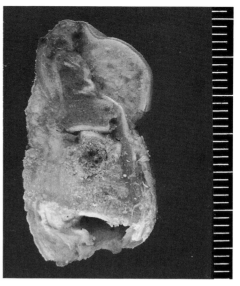

Fig. 2.53. Radiograph of a cortical osteoid osteoma of the left tibial shaft of a 7-year-old boy shows a typical "nidus" that includes the tumor tissue in the cortex. The "nidus" presents as a round focus with a central dense nucleus surrounded by a light halo. The adjacent cortex is broadened and shows a dense osteosclerosis.

Fig. 2.54. Gross specimen of an osteoid osteoma of the middle phalanx of the third right toe of a 14-year-old girl. In the center of the short tubular bone a round focus (gray-red color) is seen, with a dense bony center and surrounding osteosclerosis. This "nidus" is the tumor.

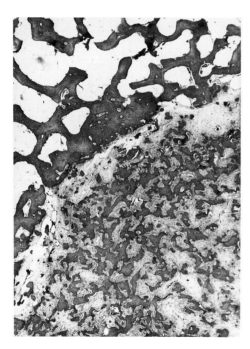

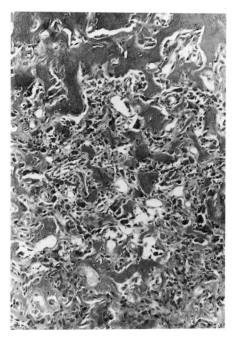

Fig. 2.55. Histologic section of an osteoid osteoma, demonstrating the "nidus" and the adjacent spongy bone (H&E, ×20). A clear morphologic difference can be seen between the lamellar bone trabeculae of the normal spongiosa and the small osteoid depositions of the tumor. Both patterns are sharply delineated.

Fig. 2.56. Histologic section of an osteoid osteoma at higher magnification (H&E, ×55). The "nidus" consists of a dense network of irregular osteoid trabeculae attached by prominent osteoblasts. Between these, a loose highly vascularized stroma is obvious.

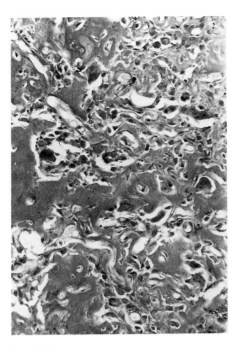

Fig. 2.57. Histologic section of an osteoid osteoma that shows the irregular osteoid deposits and many activated osteoblasts and osteoclasts in a loose stroma rich in blood capillaries (H&E, ×100).

OSTEOBLASTOMA

(ICD-O-M-9200/0)

Osteoblastoma has a close similarity to osteoid osteoma, and the two may sometimes be difficult to separate radiologically and histologically. Differences between the two include size, the degree of perifocal osteosclerosis and the clinical symptoms. *Osteoblastoma is an unusual benign osteoblastic bone tumor which develops in the bony spongiosa and consists of broad and long osteoid trabeculae within a vascular stroma, accompanied by many activated osteoblasts but without severe surrounding osteosclerosis.* In contrast to osteoid osteoma, it may reach a size of 2–10 cm in diameter, and perifocal sclerosis is scant or even absent. Benign osteoblastoma causes slight, inconstant pain, but there is none of the severe

nocturnal pain characteristic of osteoid osteoma. The symptoms may be present for anything from a few weeks to as long as 5 years. In the spine, an osteoblastoma may induce severe neurological symptoms. This solitary benign neoplasm is fairly rare and comprises about 12% of all benign and less than 1% of all bone tumors. A pronounced predominance in males (4:1) can be noted.

Sites *(Fig. 2.58)*

The main location is the vertebral column, where more than 40% of osteoblastomas are found. Here, they develop mostly in the vertebral arch or processus. About 30% of these lesions involve the femur, tibia and humerus, and 15% the short tubular bones of the hands and feet. In the long tubular bones, the metaphyses or diaphyses may be affected.

Age (Fig. 2.59)

Osteoblastoma is a tumor of younger people, and more than 50% of the patients are children or adolescents. Most cases are detected between the tenth and 25th year of life.

Radiographic Features (Figs 2.60–2.62)

The radiographic features of this tumor are not as characteristic as those of osteoid osteoma and may be misinterpreted as aneurysmal bone cyst or even osteosarcoma or chondrosarcoma. In the spine, the involved vertebral arch is expanded, but the outer contours are still preserved (Fig. 2.60). Inside, some cystic radiolucencies may be seen, but no real "nidus" is visible. It is worth noting that, in a child or an adolescent, an unusual destructive lesion of the spine having a benign radiologic appearance should be considered a benign osteoblastoma until another diagnosis has been established histologically. In the long bones, such as the tibial head (Fig. 2.61), the lesion is a large, well-circumscribed, lytic lesion, often without perifocal osteosclerosis. In other sites, such as the right iliac bone (Fig. 2.62), the lesion may be surrounded by a dense sclerotic zone similar to that seen in an ordinary osteoid osteoma, and only the larger size of the osteolytic focus ("nidus") characterizes the lesion as osteoblastoma.

Histopathologic Features (Figs 2.63–2.65)

Osteoblastomas have a severe variable histological pattern that consists of a loose connective tissue stroma with many blood vessels.

Within this cellular tissue, many irregular strands of osteoid and primitive bone with uneven outlines are visible; these are clearly larger than those seen in osteoid osteomas (Fig. 2.63). They are, additionally, more orderly than osteoid deposits in osteosarcoma. Between the osteoid deposits, an extremely cell-rich stroma is seen that is very loose – in contrast to the solid stroma of osteosarcoma – and consists of many prominent fibroblasts, osteoblasts and also multinucleated osteoclasts (Fig. 2.64). These giant cells are much smaller than the osteoclasts found in an osteoclastoma and have fewer nuclei. Connective tissue cells with hyperchromatic nuclei and even mitoses may be found, but atypical mitoses are not seen. Besides numerous large blood vessels in the stroma, many layers of prominent osteoblasts attached to the tumor osteoid or tumorous bone are typical features (Fig. 2.65).

When such cell-rich tumor tissue is observed, osteosarcoma must be considered in the differential diagnosis; it can be extremely difficult to classify such a tumor as benign osteoblastoma or osteosarcoma. In some cases, the tumor shows clinically an aggressive and destructive local growth with frequent recurrences but without metastases. In such instances we are dealing with a so-called *aggressive osteoblastoma*. In the radiographs we see an osteolytic and highly destructive lesion without any of the delineation that indicates a malignant lesion (Fig. 2.66). Sometimes severe destruction of many bones may even be observed (Fig. 2.67). Histologically, the pattern typical of an osteoblastoma is seen, but together with foci of broad calcified osteoid deposits ("spiculated blue bone") and adjacent prominent "epithelioid" osteoblasts that show polymorphic and hyperchromatic nuclei and even some atypical mitoses (Figs 2.68 and 2.69). These features are very similar to low malignancy osteosarcoma; to date, aggressive osteoblastomas are of unpredictable course.

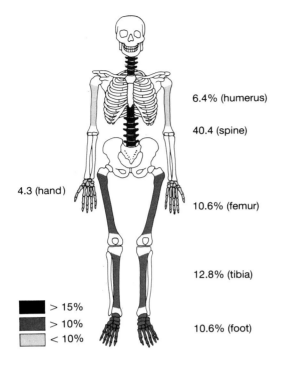

6.4% (humerus)

40.4 (spine)

4.3 (hand)

10.6% (femur)

12.8% (tibia)

10.6% (foot)

> 15%
> 10%
< 10%

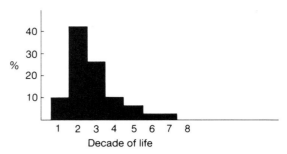

Fig. 2.59. Osteoblastoma: age distribution. More than 50% of osteoblastomas occur in children and adolescents, with a peak in the second decade. However, adults are also affected.

Fig. 2.58. Osteoblastoma: localization. The main site is the spine (more than 40% of osteoblastomas). The lesion is also frequently seen in the long tubular bones (tibia, femur, humerus) and in the short bones of the feet and hands. In other bones, it is relatively rare.

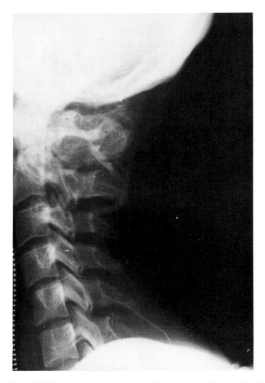

Fig. 2.60. Radiograph of an osteoblastoma of the left atlas arch in a 19-year-old male. The involved bone is expanded, showing a spongy appearance, but the outer contours are still preserved.

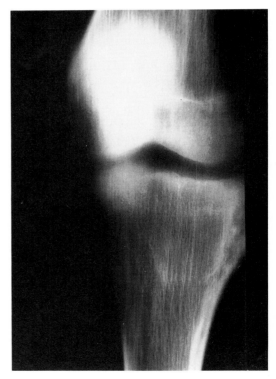

Fig. 2.61. Tomogram of an osteoblastoma of the tibial head of a 16-year-old girl, showing a large well-circumscribed osteolysis with little perifocal osteosclerosis.

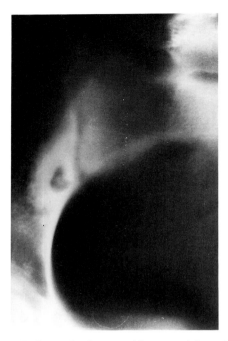

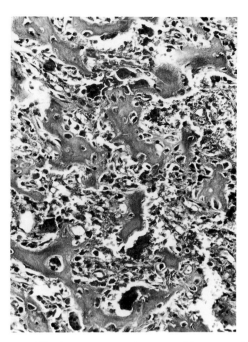

Fig. 2.62. Radiograph of an osteoblastoma of the right iliac bone, near the iliosacral joint, in a 14-year-old girl, showing a small osteolytic focus surrounded by dense sclerotic bone. This lesion could be an osteoid osteoma, but the larger size indicates an osteoblastoma.

Fig. 2.63. Histologic section of an osteoblastoma with a cell-rich tumor pattern that includes a highly vascularized stroma and many very long and broad osteoid trabeculae attached by extremely prominent osteoblasts and multinucleated osteoclasts (H&E, ×82).

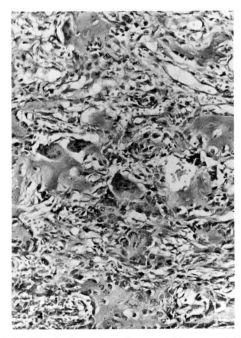

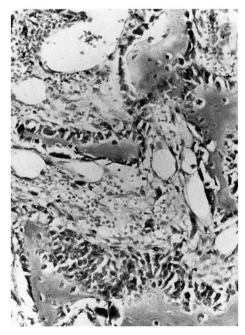

Fig. 2.64. Histologic section of an osteoblastoma at higher magnification shows the high cellularity of the tumor tissue, with many activated osteoblasts and some multinucleated osteoclasts (H&E, ×100).

Fig. 2.65. Histologic section of an osteoblastoma with broad trabecular or patchy osteoid deposits aligned with activated osteoblasts, often in rows (H&E, ×160).

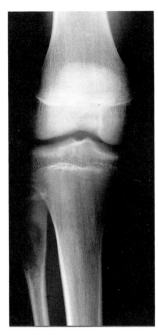

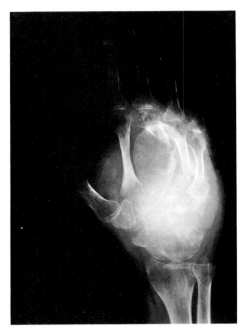

Fig. 2.66. Radiograph of an aggressive osteoblastoma of the right proximal fibular metaphysis of a 15-year-old boy, showing an osteolytic destruction and some mottled densities.

Fig. 2.67. Radiograph of an aggressive osteoblastoma of the right wrist of a 12-year-old boy; there is severe destruction of several bones, but the radiograph does not permit the primary location of the tumor to be determined. A malignant tumor is obvious.

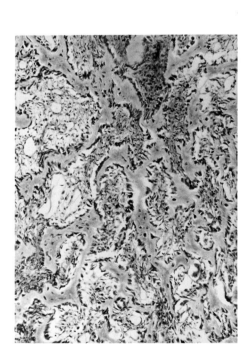

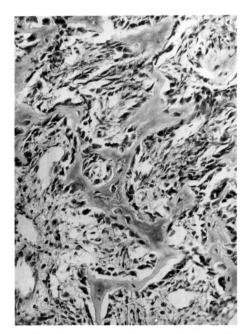

Fig. 2.68. Histologic section of an aggressive osteoblastoma demonstrating deposits of "spiculated blue bone", i.e. broad calcified osteoid deposits (PAS, ×64). Many prominent osteoblasts are attached to the osteoid trabeculae, and between them there is a loose, vascularized stroma.

Fig. 2.69. Histologic section of an aggressive osteoblastoma at higher magnification (PAS, ×100), showing prominent "epithelioid" osteoblasts with polymorphic and hyperchromatic nuclei and some atypical mitoses adjacent to the osteoid deposits.

OSTEOSARCOMA
(ICD-O-M-9180/3)

Among the malignant tumors of the skeleton in children and adolescents, osteosarcomas are particularly important because of their high incidence and because there is a great chance of successful treatment using chemotherapy in combination with surgery. *Osteosarcoma derives directly from the bone tissue, with atypical osteoblasts – the malignant tumor cells – producing atypical osteoid or bone within a sarcomatous fibroblastic stroma.* The lesion is characterized by a great variety of different malignant tissues scattered irregularly within the tumor tissue. Thus, malignant cartilage, fibrosarcoma tissue or even the pattern of an osteoclastoma or malignant fibrous histiocytoma may be seen in large areas. This gives rise to problems in obtaining a representative tissue biopsy that includes tumor osteoid, which is histologically the decisive element in classifying the tumor as osteosarcoma. Nevertheless, even small foci of tumor osteoid within a predominantly chondroblastic, fibroblastic, histiocytic or osteoclastic tumor gives the diagnosis of osteosarcoma. Therefore osteosarcoma is characterized by the direct formation of bone or osteoid tissue by tumor cells (WHO definition).

Osteosarcoma is the most common malignant bone tumor in children, about 15% of the total, and occurs in more males (60%) than females (40%). Pain and swelling are the most common symptoms. Metastases are to be expected first in the lungs and may occur early on during the highly malignant growth of the tumor. Regional metastases in lymph nodes are extremely rare.

Nowadays, the most successful therapy can be achieved using the COSS-study (cooperative osteosarcoma study) therapy. After achieving a definite diagnosis by biopsy, combined chemotherapy will be applied during about 3 months and the tumor is later excised operatively (en-bloc resection or amputation). The pathologist has to check the effect of the chemotherapy by quantitatively estimating the degree of necrosis within the tumor tissue as a whole. By this method it can be determined whether the individual tumor is a "responder" or "non-responder". In case of a "responder", the chemotherapy regimen will be continued; in case of "non-responder", the chemotherapy has to be modified in order to prevent metastases.

Since the introduction of this approach, the prognosis of osteosarcoma has greatly improved and survival time is significantly longer.

Sites (Fig. 2.70)

Usually an osteosarcoma develops in a metaphysis of a long bone, and most cases are in the region of the knee (distal femur, proximal tibia: 60%). Other main sites are the metaphyses of the femur, tibia and humerus, as well as pelvic and spinal bones. Any bone may be affected.

Age (Fig. 2.71)

About 10% of all osteosarcomas are found in children in the first decade of life, but most cases occur in the second decade (about 38%). In our experience, nowadays more osteosarcomas are occurring in older age-group (third and fourth decade); most of these are secondary osteosarcomas (i.e. osteosarcoma in Paget's disease, post-radiation osteosarcoma, low-grade intramedullary osteosarcoma, dedifferentiated chondrosarcoma, among others).

Radiographic Features (Figs 2.72–2.75)

This malignant bone tumor generally shows an osteolytic or osteoblastic destruction of the involved bone, which indicates a malignant growth. The involved metaphysis may be completely destroyed and the tumor may have expanded into the surrounding soft tissue (Fig. 2.72). The tumor is mainly sclerotic, but spotty osteolyses occur between scleroses. In addition, a bony periosteal reaction is seen, either as a sclerotic broadening (Fig. 2.72) or as so-called spicules (Fig. 2.73). An osteolytic osteosarcoma is characterized by a diffuse and partly spotty destruction of the bone, which may include the cortex (Fig. 2.74). In cases of osteoblastic osteosarcomas there is an extremely dense lesion within the whole metaphysis, involving the cortex together with "spicules" of the periosteum (Figs 2.73 and 2.75). The so-called Codman's triangle (a zone of dense reactive bone production on the margin of the tumor growth, but without actual tumor tissue) indicates malignancy (Fig. 2.75). Usually the tumor is sharply demarcated at the cartilaginous epiphyseal growth plate. In all cases, the expansion of an osteosarcoma is indistinct, and no marginal sclerosis is present.

Gross Pathologic Features (*Figs 2.76 and 2.77*)

In accordance with the radiographic features, macroscopic specimens of osteosarcomas show a tumorous destruction of the metaphysis (including the cortex), sharply separated from the cartilaginous epiphyseal growth plate but diffuse towards the proximal end. In an osteoblastic osteosarcoma, an extremely dense mass of tumorous bone is seen (Fig. 2.76), and in an osteolytic osteosarcoma a soft grayish-red tissue replaces the original bone (Fig. 2.77). When the tumor penetrates the cortical bone, the periosteum is elevated, infiltrated by tumor tissue, and shows reactive bone production (Fig. 2.77).

Histopathologic Features (*Figs 2.78–2.83*)

Characteristic histological features of osteosarcoma are the presence of tumorous osteoid, bone and cartilage scattered in a checkered pattern within a sarcomatous fibrous stroma. In addition, several other tissue components may be included in this tumor, such as patterns of osteoclastoma, hemangiopericytoma, hemangiosarcoma, malignant histiocytoma, and aneurysmal bone cyst. Consequently, an osteosarcoma can pose severe difficulties in diagnosis, especially when interpreting a biopsy specimen.

The decisive feature in diagnosis of osteosarcoma is the proof of tumorous osteoid within the tumor tissue. This is abundant in an *osteoblastic osteosarcoma* and may show irregular broad trabeculae attached by polymorphous osteoblasts (Figs 2.78 and 2.79). In many cases, there is a loose, highly vascularized sarcomatous stroma interspersed with many small osteoid deposits (Figs 2.80 and 2.81). In cases of *fibroblastic osteosarcomas*, the fibrosarcomatous tissue prevails and inbetween more or less tumorous osteoid deposits are seen (Fig. 2.82). In a *chondroblastic osteosarcoma* chondroid tumor tissue is dominant, together with some deposits of tumor osteoid (Fig. 2.83). The prevailing tumor pattern within an osteosarcoma should be analyzed by the pathologist because a chondroblastic osteosarcoma has a better prognosis (i.e. longer survival time) than an osteoblastic one, though chondroblastic tumors

are much more resistant towards chemotherapy and most cases are "non-responders".

Types of Osteosarcoma

There exist several special types of osteosarcoma that also occur in children and have to be taken into account:

1. *Telangiectatic osteosarcoma*. This osteolytic tumor has an even worse prognosis than conventional osteosarcomas, with early pulmonary metastases and short survival time. Chemotherapy, nevertheless, is mostly effective. On the radiographs we see a highly destructive lesion, and *angiograms* demonstrate hypervascularity, with many pathologic vessels (Fig. 2.84). *Histologically*, the tumor tissue is characterized by a loose sarcomatous stroma, with septa and spaces as in aneurysmal bone cyst, together with many ectatic blood vessels (Fig. 2.85). There are many highly anaplastic tumor cells, including malignant giant cells, with many pathologic mitoses, but osteoid production is minimal or sometimes even absent.

2. *Parosteal osteosarcoma*. This special type of osteosarcoma develops on the surface of a bone, mainly of the distal posterior portion of the shaft of the femur (fossa poplitea). Here, a bony mass has encircled the shaft, expanding into the soft tissue, which can be demonstrated in *radiographs* (Fig. 2.86) or even better in computer tomograms. The medullary cavity is usually not involved, but bony invasion may occur in advanced stages. *Histologically*, well-formed osseous trabeculae are seen in an actively proliferating fibroblastic tissue which generally appears to be benign (Fig. 2.87). The osseous trabeculae are regularly arranged, and in the intermingled stroma only slightly atypical, proliferating spindle cells are found. Mitotic figures are rare. Chondroid areas are frequent, in which chondrocytes show atypia. On the whole, this is a highly differentiated osseous tissue that histologically may be classified as a simple parosteal bone reaction or, in cases of chondroid differentiation, as osteochondroma. Therefore, the radiographic features have to taken into consideration in diagnosis. A parosteal osteosarcoma shows the best prognosis of all osteosarcomas (grade 1), metastases being rare and late, and there is a chance of complete healing after complete removal.

3. *Periosteal osteosarcoma*. This special osteosarcoma may occur in children. It arises from

the periosteum and grows outward from the bone, forming a large tumor mass that extends into the surrounding soft tissue. This becomes obvious on radiographs as well as in *macroscopic specimens* (Fig. 2.88). Usually, no infiltration of the tumor tissue into the medullary cavity of the bone can be found. All bones and sites within individual bone may be involved. *Histologically*, this tumor is characterized by a predominantly chondroblastic differentiation, which itself indicates periosteal chondrosarcoma, but together with a combination of cartilage, tumorous bone and osteoid and fibrosarcomatous

tissue (Fig. 2.89). This type of osteosarcoma has slightly better prognosis than medullary osteosarcomas (grade 2 malignancy) but a significantly worse prognosis than parosteal osteosarcoma. Therefore, radical therapy has to be performed.

A series of other types of osteosarcomas can be distinguished, such as *high-grade surface osteosarcoma*, *low-grade central osteosarcoma*, *postradiation osteosarcoma* or *Paget-osteosarcoma*, and others are known, but they are usually extremely rare and do not occur in children or adolescents.

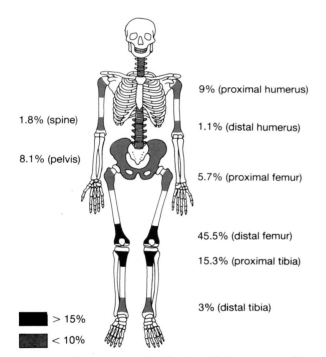

Fig. 2.70. Osteosarcoma: localization. This tumor usually develops in the metaphyses of long bones, especially in the region of the knee (distal femur, proximal tibia; it may also occur in the distal metaphyses of these bones as well as in the proximal and distal humerus). Some osteosarcomas are even found in the pelvis and the spine.

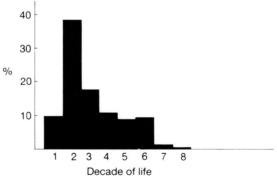

Fig. 2.71. Osteosarcoma: age distribution. About half of all osteosarcomas are diagnosed in children and adolescents (10% in the first decade, 38% in the second). This malignant tumor may, however, also occur in adults. In older age-groups, secondary osteosarcoma is predominant.

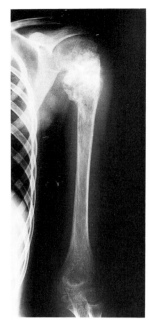

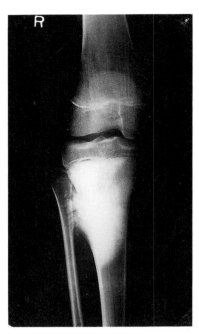

Fig. 2.72. Radiograph of an osteosarcoma of the left proximal humerus of a 9-year-old girl, showing a severe destruction of the metaphysis with expansion of the tumor into the surrounding tissue.

Fig. 2.73. Radiograph of an osteoblastic osteosarcoma of the right proximal tibia of a 14-year-old girl. Here a large osteosclerosis that includes the spongiosa as well as the cortex is seen, and, in addition, "spicules" of periosteal bone reaction are obvious, indicating malignancy.

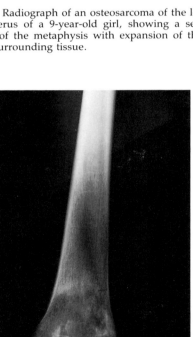

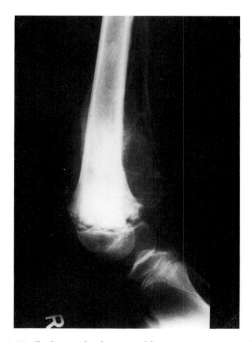

Fig. 2.74. Radiograph of an osteolytic osteosarcoma of the left distal femoral metaphysis of a 15-year-old boy; there is an undefined destructive osteolysis with some densities.

Fig. 2.75. Radiograph of an osteoblastic osteosarcoma of the right distal femoral metaphysis of a 10-year-old boy; there is a large dense osteosclerosis that is "blurred", reaching down to the epiphyseal growth plate. In the periosteum, a "Codman's triangle' is visible, indicating malignancy.

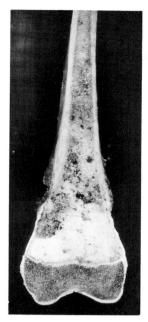

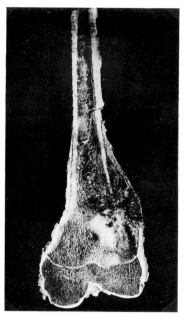

Fig. 2.76. Gross specimen of an osteoblastic osteosarcoma of the distal femoral metaphysis of a 15-year-old boy, showing a mass of tumorous bone that is sharply separated from the cartilagineous epiphyseal growth plate. The tumor is not sharply defined towards the proximal medullary cavity.

Fig. 2.77. Gross specimen of an osteolytic osteosarcoma of the distal femoral metaphysis in a 12-year-old boy, showing bone destruction by tumor tissue (soft grayish-red) that has penetrated the cortex and invaded the adjacent periosteum. The epiphyseal growth plate is, however, intact.

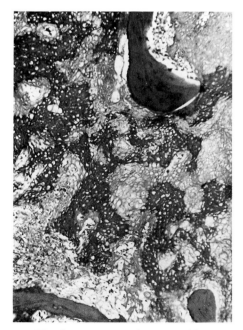

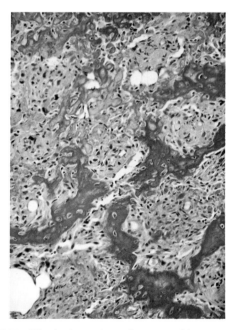

Fig. 2.78. Histologic section of an osteoblastic osteosarcoma, which is characterized by a sarcomatous stroma with broad deposits of tumorous osteoid between the original bone trabeculae (H&E, ×50).

Fig. 2.79. Histologic section of an osteoblastic osteosarcoma, consisting of broad deposits of tumorous osteoid and tumorous bone, including many osteoblasts with polymorphic and hyperchromatic nuclei (van Gieson's, ×82).

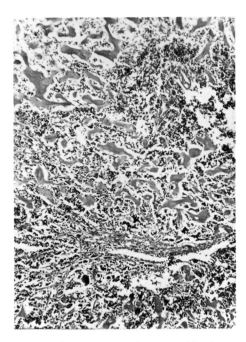

Fig. 2.80. Histologic section of an osteoblastic osteosarcoma; there is a loose, cell-rich stroma including numerous slender tumorous osteoid trabeculae (H&E, ×50). The sarcomatous stroma cells are characterized by their varied size and hyperchromasia and polymorphy of their nuclei, together with atypical mitoses.

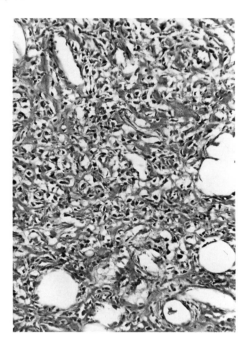

Fig. 2.81. Histologic section of an osteoblastic osteosarcoma showing a loose, highly vascularized stroma that includes many polymorphous osteoblasts and a dense lacework of tumorous osteoid (H&E, ×82).

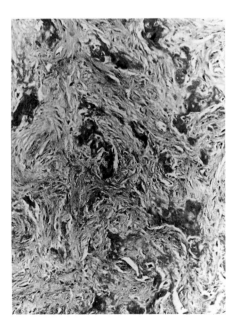

Fig. 2.82. Histologic section of a fibroblastic osteosarcoma in which the fibrous sarcomatous stroma with polymorphic spindle cells predominates, including more discrete tumorous osteoid deposits (PAS, ×64).

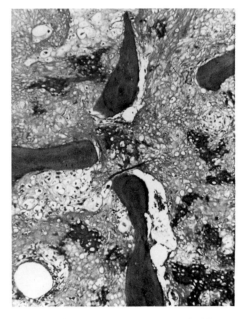

Fig. 2.83. Histologic section of a chondroblastic osteosarcoma in which a sarcomatous cartilage tissue is seen between the original bone trabeculae (H&E, ×40). However, trabecular deposits of tumorous osteoid are also visible, leading to the diagnosis of osteosarcoma.

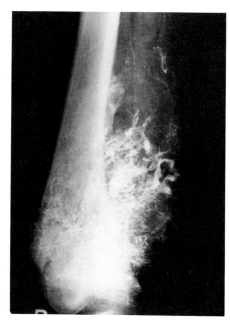

Fig. 2.84. Radiograph of a telangiectatic osteosarcoma of the right distal femur of a 15-year-old boy, showing numerous atypical blood vessels within the tumor. The extraosseous part, particularly, of this sarcoma demonstrates a malignant tumor.

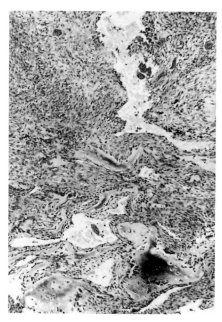

Fig. 2.85. Histologic section of a telangiectatic osteosarcoma with a cell-rich sarcomatous stroma, including spindle cells with polymorphous and hyperchromatic nuclei and only a little in the way of tumorous osteoid deposit (PAS, ×32). The presence of many ectatic blood vessels is characteristic of this type of osteosarcoma.

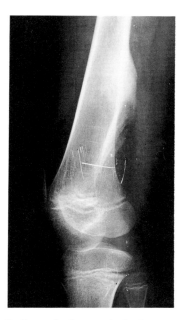

Fig. 2.86. Radiograph of a parosteal osteosarcoma of the left distal femoral metaphysis of a 10-year-old boy, showing a bony mass that seems to be laid down at the rear cortex (fossa poplitea) and extends into the soft tissue. No intra-osseous tumor growth can be seen.

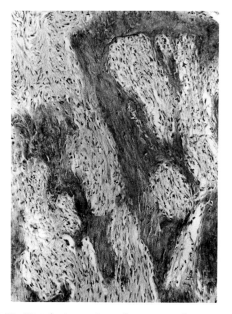

Fig. 2.87. Histologic section of a parosteal osteosarcoma showing well-formed, woven bone trabeculae in a fibrous stroma which includes many spindle cells having only slight polymorphy and hyperchromasy of the nuclei and only scant mitoses (H&E, ×50). It can be difficult to recognize these histologic features as malignant tumor growth.

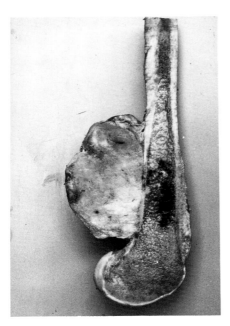

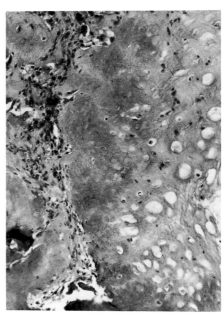

Fig. 2.88. Gross specimen of a periosteal osteosarcoma of the right distal femur, showing a large extraosseous tumor mass attached to the back of metaphyseal bone and no intraosseous infiltration.

Fig. 2.89. Histologic section of a periosteal osteosarcoma with predominating areas of a nodular, chondrosarcomatous cartilage tumor tissue including polymorphous cartilage cells; between these is a sarcomatous stroma with tumorous osteoid deposits, which is characteristic (H&E, ×50).

LITERATURE
Tumors of Osteoblastic Origin

Adler CP. Parosteal (juxtacortical) osteosarcoma of the distal femur. Pathol Res Pract 1980;169:388–95

Adler CP, Schmidt A. Aneurysmale Knochenzyste des Femurs mit malignem Verlauf. Verh Dtsch Ges Pathol 1978;62:487

Adler CP, Uehlinger E. Grenzfälle bei ·Knochentumoren. Präneoplatische Veränderungen und Geschwülste fraglicher Dignität. Verh Dtsch Ges Pathol 1979;63:352–8

Atik OS, Caglar M, Bölükbase S, Gögüs S, Gögüs MT. Osteogenic sarcoma of the distal femur in a young child. Hum Pathol 1982;13:766

Ayala AG, Raymond AK, Jaffe N. The pathologist's role in the diagnosis and treatment of osteosarcomas in children. Human Pathol 1984;15:258–66

Baum PA, Nelson MC, Lack EE, Bogumill GP. Parosteal osteoma of the tibia. Skeletal Radiol 1989;18:406–9

Bertoni F, Unni KK, McLeod RA, Dahlin DC. Osteosarcoma resembling osteoblastoma. Cancer 1985;55:416–26

Bilbao JI, Martin Algarra S, Martinez de Negri J, Lecumberri F, Longo J, Sierrasesumaga L, et al. Osteosarcoma: correlation · between radiological and histological changes after intra-arterial chemotherapy. Eur J Radiol 1990;11: 98–103

Brodeur GM, Caces J, Williams DL, Look TA, Pratt CB. Osteosarcoma, fibrous dysplasia, and a chromasomal abnormality in a 3-year-old child. Cancer 1980;46: 1197–1201

Campanacci M, Picci P, Gherlinzoni F, Guerra A, Bertoni F, Neff JR. Parosteal osteosarcoma. J Bone Jt Surg 1984; 66-B:313–21

Camuzard JF, Vaille G, Santini J, Raspaldo H, Demard F. Gardner's syndrome. Review of the literature. Report of a familial form. Ann Otolaryngol Chir Cervicofac 1990; 107:509–13

Carter TR. Osteoid osteoma of the hip: an alternate method of excision. Orthop Rev 1990;19:903–5

Carter JR, Abdul-Karim FW. Pathology of childhood osteosarcoma. Perspect Pediatr Pathol 1987;9:133–70

Crim JR, Mirra JM, Eckardt JJ, Seeger LL. Widespread inflammatory response to osteoblastoma: the flare phenomenon. Radiology 1990;177:835–6

Dahlin DC, Unni KK. Osteosarcoma of bone and its important recognizable varieties. Am J Surg Pathol 1977; 1:61–72

Delling G, Pompesius-Kempa M, Welkerling H, Dreyer T, Maas R, Heise U, Winkler K. Morphological investigation of tumor growth and distribution of viable tumor areas in osteosarcomas after chemotherapy. Chir Organi Mov 1990;75:45–47

Dorfman HD, Weiss SW. Borderline osteoblastic tumors: problems in the differential diagnosis of aggressive osteoblastoma and low-grade osteosarcoma. Semin Diagn Pathol 1984;1:215–234

Dowell JK, Edgar MA. A case report of recurrent osteoblastoma of the rib presenting as painless progressive scoliosis. Spine 1990;15:141–2

Enneking WF, Kagan A. "Skip" metastases in osteosarcoma. Cancer 1975;36:2192–205

Enneking WF, Spanier SS, Goodman MA. The surgery of musculoskeletal sarcoma. J Bone Jt Surg 1980;62-A: 1027–30

Giangaspero F, Stracca V, Visona A, Eusebi V. Small-cell osteosarcoma of the mandible. Case report. Appl Pathol 1984;2:28–31

Goorin AM, Abelson HT, Frei III E. Osteosarcoma: fifteen years later. N Engl J Med 1985;313:1637–43

Grigo B, Blau HJ. Neuroblastoma, nephroblastoma and osteosarcoma in patients at 2 pediatric oncologic centers. A 15-year report. Arch Geschwulstforsch 1990;60:365–72

Hall RB, Robinson LH, Malawar MM, Dunham WK. Periosteal osteosarcoma. Cancer 1985;55:165–71

Haug RH, Hauer C, Camillo AJ, Araneta M. Benign osteoblastoma of the mandible: report of a case. J Oral Maxillofac Surg 1990;48:743–8

Heymer B, Kreidler J, Adler CP. Strahleninduziertes Osteosarkom des Unterkiefers. Dtsch Z Mund Kiefer Gesichtschir 1988;12:113–19

Hochstetter von AR. Spontaneous necrosis in osteosarcomas. Chir Organi Mov 1990;75:32–5

Hopper KD, Haseman DB, Moser RP Jr, Sweet DE, Madewell JE. Osteosarcomatosis (Case report). Skeletal Radiol 1990;19:535–7

Huvos AG. Clinicopathologic spectrum of osteogenic sarcoma. – Recent observations. Pathol Anat 1979;14: 123–44

Huvos AG, Rosen G, Bretsky SS, Butler A. Teleangiectatic osteogenic sarcoma. – A clinicopathologic study of 124 patients. Cancer 1982;49:1679–89

Irnberger TH. Infantiles Osteoid-Osteom der Tibia. – Röntgenologische und computertomographische Diagnose und Differentialdiagnose. Wien Med Wochenschr 1983;3:67–71

Jackson JR, Bell MEA. Spurious "benign osteoblastoma". J Bone Jt Surg 1977;59-A:397–401

Kavanagh TG, Cannon SR, Pringle J, Stoker DJ, Kemp HB. Parosteal osteosarcoma. Treatment by wide resection and prosthetic replacement. J Bone Jt Surg 1990;B-72:959–65

Kozakewich H, Perez-Atayde AR, Goorin AM, Wilkinson RH, Gebhardt MC, Vawter GF. Osteosarcoma in young children. Cancer 1991;67:638–42

Kroon HM, Schurmans J. Osteoblastoma: clinical and radiologic findings in 98 new cases. Radiology 1990; 175:783–90

Lacheretz M, Herbaux B, Hossein-Foucher C, Lecouffe P, Richir M. Détection isotopique pré-operatoire dans le traitement de l'osteome ostéoide chez l'enfant. Chirurgie 1989;115:413–16

Levine E, DeSmet AA, Huntrakoon M. Juxtacortical osteosarcoma. A radiologic and histologic spectrum. Skeletal Radiol 1985;14:38–46

Levy ML, Jaffe N. Osteosarcoma in early childhood. Pediatrics 1982;70:302–3

López-Barea F, Contreras F, Sanchez-Herrera S. Grade III conventional sclerosing osteosarcoma of the calcaneus. Skeletal Radiol 1989;18:237–40

Lowbeer L. Multifocal osteosarcomatosis – a rare entity. Bull Pathol 1968;9:52–3

Marin SF, Dwyer A, Kissane JM, Costa J. Small-cell osteosarcoma. Cancer 1982;50:990–6

Marsh BW, Bonfiglio M, Brady LP, Enneking WF. Benign osteoblastoma: Range of manifestations. J Bone Jt Surg 1975;57-A:1–9

Matsuno T, Unni KK, McLeod RA, Dahlin DC. Teleangiectatic osteogenic sarcoma. Cancer (Phil) 1976; 38:2538–47

McCarthy EF, Matsuno T, Dorfman HD. Malignant fibrous histiocytoma of bone: a study of 35 cases. Human Pathol 1979;10:57–70

McLeod RA, Dahlin DC, Beabout JW. The spectrum of osteoblastoma. Am J Roentgenol 1976;126:321–35

Mirra JM, Kendrick RA, Kendrick RE. Pseudomalignant osteoblastoma versus arrested osteosarcoma: a case report. Cancer (Phil) 1976;37:2005–14

Mitchell ML, Ackerman LV. Metastatic and pseudomalignant osteoblastoma: a report of two unusual cases. Skeletal Radiol 1986;15:213–18

Mohr VD, Bauer T, Schmitt B. Osteoid osteoma at the end of the phalanx of the big toe. Dtsch Med Wochenschr 1990; 115:1470–4

Moss CS, Williams C, Burton IE, Gaba AR. Osteoblastic osteosarcoma of the navicular. Skeletal Radiol 1989;18: 70–4

Parham DM, Pratt CB, Parvey LS, Webber BL, Champion J. Childhood multifocal osteosarcoma. Clinicopathologic and radiologic correlates. Cancer 1985;55:2653–8

Penman HG, Ring PA. Osteosarcoma in association with total hip replacement. J Bone Jt Surg 1984;B-66:632–4

Picci P, Bacci G, Campanacci M, Gasparini M, Pilotti S, Cerasoli S, et al. Histologic evaluation of necrosis in osteosarcoma included by chemotherapy. Regional mapping of viable and nonviable tumor. Cancer 1985; 56:1515–21

Revell PA, Scholtz CL. Aggressive osteoblastoma. J Pathol 1979;127:195–8

Roberts P, Davies AM, Starkie CM, Grimer RJ. The nidus of an osteoid osteoma mimicking an os supratrochleare dorsale. Br J Radiol 1990;63:899–902

Roessner A, Metze K, Heymer B. Aggressive osteoblastoma. Pathol Res Pract 1985;179:433–6

Ruiter DJ, Cornelisse CJ, van Rijssel TG, van der Velde EA. Aneurysmal bone cyst and teleangiectatic osteosarcoma. A histo-pathological and morphometric study. Virchows Arch [A] 1977;373:311–25

Ryan J, Baker L, Benjamin R, Murphy W, Balcerzak S, Gottlieb J. Long-term followup in the cure of osteogenic sarcoma. The Southwest oncology group. Chir Organi Mov 1990;75:48–9

Sanerkin NG. Definitions of osteosarcoma, chondrosarcoma, and fibrosarcoma of bone. Cancer 1980;46:178–85

Schajowicz F, Lemos D. Malignant osteoblastoma. J Bone Jt Surg 1976;58-B:202–11

Seki T, Fukuda H, Ishii Y, Hanaoka H, Yatabe S,

Takano M, et al. Malignant transformation of benign osteoblastoma. J Bone Jt Surg 1975;57-A:424–6

Semer LC, Drossner B, Fleming WC, Levin R. Osteoblastoma of the distal phalanx of the hallux. J Foot Surg 1990;29:357–60

Siegal GP, Dahlin DC, Sim FH. Osteoblastic osteogenic sarcoma in a 35-month old girl. Am J Clin Pathol 1975;63:886–90

Sim FH, Unni KK, Beabout JW, Dahlin DC. Osteosarcoma with small cells simulating Ewing's tumor. J Bone Surg (Am) 1979;61:207–15

Sim FH, Kurt AM, McLeod RA, Unni KK. Low-grade central osteosarcoma. (Case report). Skeletal Radiol 1990;19:457–60

Simon MA. Causes of increased survival of patients with osteosarcoma: current controversies. J Bone Jt Surg 1984;66-A:306–10

Simon MA, Bos GD. Epiphyseal extension of metaphyseal osteosarcoma in skeletally immature individuals. J Bone Jt Surg 1980;62-A:195–204

Stutch R. Osteoblastoma – a benign entity? Orthop Rev 1975;4:27–33

Tonai M, Campbell CJ, Ahn GH, Schiller AL, Mankin HJ. Osteoblastoma. Classification and report of 16 patients. Clin Orthop Rel Res 1982;167:222–35

Triebel HJ, Spielmann RP, Maas R. Unusually localized osteosarcoma. RöFo 1989;150:615–16

Tsuchiya H, Morikawa S, Tomita K. Osteosarcoma arising from a multiple exostoses lesion: case report. Jpn J Clin Oncol 1990;20:296–8

Unni KK, Dahlin DC, Beabout JW, Ivins JC. Parosteal osteogenic sarcoma. Cancer (Phil) 1976;37:2466–75

Unni KK, Dahlin DC, Beabout JW. Periosteal osteogenic sarcoma. Cancer (Phil) 1976;37:2476–2485

Unni KK, Dahlin DC, McCloud RA, Pritchard DJ. Intraosseous well-differentiated osteosarcoma. Cancer 1977;40:1337–47

Uribe-Botero G, Russell WO, Sutoro WW, Martin RG. Primary osteosarcoma of bone: a clinicopathologic investigation of 243 cases, with necropsystudies in 54. Am J Clin Pathol 1977;67:427–35

Wang NH, Ma HL, Lo WH, Yang DJ. Osteoid osteoma: clinical and investigative features. Taiwan I Hsueh Hui Tsa Chih 1990;89:366–72

Williams J, Barret G, Pratt C. Osteosarcoma in 2 very young children. Clin Pediatr (Phil) 1977;16:548–51

Wold LE, Beabout JW, Unni KK, Prichard DJ. High-grade surface osteosarcomas. Am J Surg Pathol 1984;8:181–6

Wuisman P, Enneking WF. Prognosis of osteosarcoma with "skip" metastasis. Chir Organi Mov 1990;75:60–4

Yoshikawa H, Takaoka K, Hamada H, Ono K. Clinical significance of bone morphogenetic activity in osteosarcoma. A study of 20 cases. Cancer 1985;56:1682–7

Zappia JJ, LaRouere MJ, Telian SA. Massive ossifying fibroma of the temporal bone. Otolaryngol Head–Neck Surg 1990;103:480–3

Tumors of Fibrous Tissue Origin

NONOSSIFYING FIBROMA
(ICD-O-M-7494/0)

Among all primary bone tumors nonossifying fibroma is the most frequently occurring one in children and adolescents. It is questionable whether it is a true neoplasm because it usually undergoes a spontaneous resolution later in life. *The lesion is fibrous and appears as an osteolytic, cystic defect in the metaphysis of a bone and is well delimited by a grape-like marginal sclerosis consisting of fibrous tissue in a whorled pattern and including histiocytes, foam cells and multinucleated giant cells.* No bone formation is seen within the lesion. It develops eccentrically in a bone and, in contrast to metaphyseal fibrous cortical defect, expands towards the cortex from the inside which will be rarefied. Many nonossifying bone fibromas are detected accidentally, i.e. they are symptomless. Multiple lesions simultaneously in different bones do occur.

This absolutely benign bone tumor can in most cases be diagnosed radiologically with adequate accuracy, and no therapy is necessary. Only in cases of pathologic bone fracture should the tumor tissue be removed operatively.

Sites (*Fig. 2.90*)

The metaphyseal portion of the long bones is the site of most nonossifying bone fibromas, though they may be seen in other bones (jaws, clavicle or ribs). Most of the lesions develop in the metaphyses of the femur, tibia or fibula.

Age (*Fig. 2.91*)

Eighty-two per cent of all nonossifying bone fibromas are detected in children. In rare cases, a lesion may be found in an older patient, in whom it has existed since early youth but has not given clinical symptoms until adult life.

Radiographic Features (*Figs 2.92–2.94*)

In a metaphysis of the involved long bone there is an eccentrically located cystic lesion defined by slim marginal sclerosis, giving a 'grapefruit' appearance (Fig. 2.92). On its inner side the lesion is attached to the cortex, which is narrowed and slightly bulged, but its outside is smooth. Sometimes trabecular or diffuse densities (Fig. 2.93) may be seen inside the lesion. Often, a pathologic fracture may occur in such a lesion (Fig. 2.94), but the underlying lesion is still visible.

Histopathologic Features (*Figs 2.95–2.97*)

The typical histological appearance of nonossifying bone fibroma is a cell-rich fibroblastic tissue disposed in whorled bundles and without any bone formation (Fig. 2.95). The fibroma contains many isomorphic fibroblasts and histiocytes in which there are no mitoses. The cortex is clearly rarefied from the inside but is not penetrated. Within the lesion there are some giant cells, containing fewer nuclei than do those of giant cell tumor, in uneven distribution (Fig. 2.96). In many lesions, nests of foam cells with broad and light cytoplasm can be found (Fig. 2.97). In cases in which the tumor includes mainly lipophages it may be called "xanthofibroma".

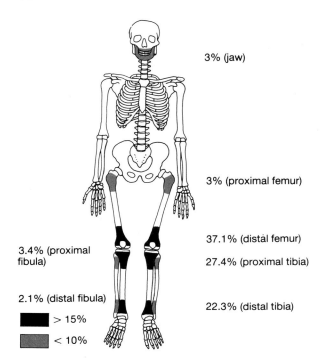

3% (jaw)

3% (proximal femur)

3.4% (proximal fibula)

37.1% (distal femur)

27.4% (proximal tibia)

2.1% (distal fibula)

22.3% (distal tibia)

■ > 15%

▨ < 10%

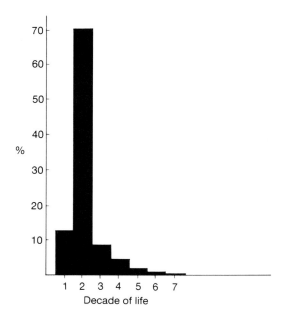

Fig. 2.90. Nonossifying fibroma: localization. In most cases the proximal or distal metaphyses of the femur and tibia are involved, where about 90% of these lesions are found. However, other bones, especially the jaw bones, can also be sites of a nonossifying fibroma.

Fig. 2.91. Nonossifying fibroma: age distribution. This is a bone tumor of childhood: 82% of all such lesions occur in children or adolescents, with a high age peak in the second decade. However, lesions are also detected in adults.

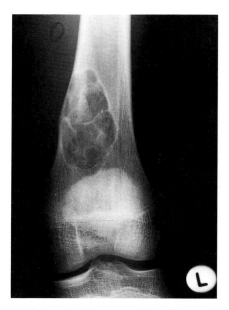

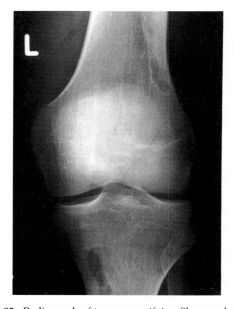

Fig. 2.92. Radiograph of a nonossifying fibroma of the left distal femoral metaphysis of a 14-year-old girl, demonstrating a large, eccentrically located "bone cyst" sharply demarcated by a small sclerotic rim to form a grapefruit shape. The adjacent cortex is slightly bulged, but intact.

Fig. 2.93. Radiograph of two nonossifying fibromas located in the left distal femoral metaphysis and in the left proximal tibial metaphysis of a 16-year-old boy. Both cystic lesions, with grapefruit-like appearance, are eccentrically attached to the intact cortex and are sharply delineated towards the inside of the bone by a small sclerotic rim.

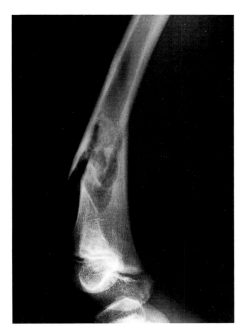

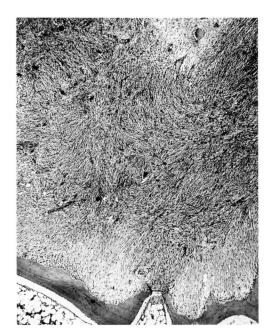

Fig. 2.94. Radiograph of a nonossifying fibroma of the distal femoral metaphysis of a 6-year-old child with a pathologic fracture. The typical lesion, showing an eccentric "bone cyst" with marginal sclerosis, is clearly visible.

Fig. 2.95. Histologic section of a nonossifying fibroma, showing a cell-rich fibroblastic tissue in whorled bundles, including some multinucleated giant cells; no new bone formation is seen (H&E, ×25).

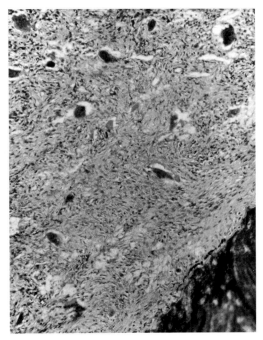

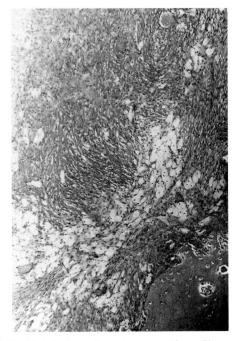

Fig. 2.96. Histologic section of a nonossifying fibroma at higher magnification (Goldner, ×64), showing uniform fibrous tissue, including isomorphic fibroblasts and histiocytes and dispersed multinucleated giant cells. In this tumorous area, no bone formation is seen.

Fig. 2.97. Histologic section of a nonossifying fibroma that shows many histiocytic foam cells within the fibrohistiocytic tumor tissue (H&E, ×32).

BENIGN FIBROUS HISTIOCYTOMA
(ICD-O-M-8832/0)

This is an absolutely benign and rare bone lesion that occurs in children or adolescents; it develops in the medullary cavity of a bone. From a histomorphologic standpoint, a close relationship to nonossifying fibroma or fibrous cortical defect can be noted. *A benign fibrous histiocytoma is a primary bone tumor that develops in the center of a bone and produces a fibrous tissue in a storiform pattern including many histiocytes.* The lesion shows a slowly progressive tumor growth with local bone destruction.

Sites

Benign fibrous histiocytoma often develops in soft tissues; when it occurs in bone the diaphyses of femur and tibia are most frequent sites. The lesion may occur in any bone of the skeleton.

Age

The tumor is detected at all ages, and children and adolescents are equally involved.

Radiographic Features (*Fig. 2.98*)

A well-circumscribed osteolytic lesion in a bone without internal scleroses is typical of a benign fibrous histiocytoma. A special marginal sclerosis, as found in nonossifying bone fibroma, is absent. The lesions are usually located in the shaft of a bone and not without exception in a metaphysis, as is the case for nonossifying fibroma. The adjacent cortex usually is rarefied, but has an intact exterior. Bulging of the cortex may be seen.

Histopathologic Features (*Fig. 2.99*)

The tumor shows a cell-rich tissue with numerous cells that can be identified as typical histiocytes, including focal aggregations of foam cells which show a broad, faint cytoplasm. Benign giant cells are present in variable numbers, but they are sparse and small in size. All cells are isomorphic, as are their nuclei, and mitoses are absent. Focally, in more fibrogenic zones, a storiform pattern with a woven or matted arrangement of collagen fibres is seen.

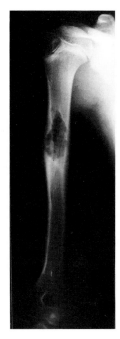

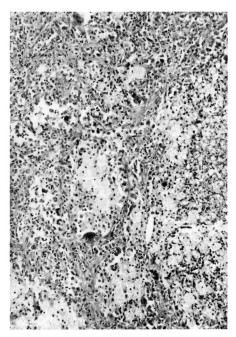

Fig. 2.98. Radiograph of a benign fibrous histiocytoma of the right proximal humerus of a 13-year-old boy, showing a well circumscribed osteolytic lesion lacking a marginal sclerosis and expanding into the cortical bone, the exterior of which is nevertheless intact.

Fig. 2.99. Histologic section of a benign fibrous histiocytoma; there is a cell-rich tissue consisting exclusively of isomorphic histiocytes and foam cells (PAS, ×64). Some small histiocytic giant cells are intermingled.

METAPHYSEAL FIBROUS CORTICAL DEFECT
(ICD-O-M-7491/0)

Metaphyseal fibrous cortical defect occurs in children, but is also detected in adolescents and younger adults. *It is a harmless proliferation of fibrous tissue of the periosteum that locally invades the cortex, inducing a bony defect from the outside.* Usually no symptoms are noted. Probably this is not a true tumor.

Sites

The metaphyseal portion of a long bone is the only site of this lesion. The femur, tibia or fibula are most frequently involved.

Age

The lesion develops almost exclusively in childhood and adolescence.

Radiographic Features (*Fig. 2.100*)

There is a broad impression of the cortex from the outside that is demarcated by a sclerotic rim towards the inner bone. Such a radiographic appearance is virtually pathognomonic.

Histopathologic Features (Fig. 2.101)

A proliferating fibrous tissue with a storiform pattern, including some multinucleated giant cells, is found in this lesion. The tissue contains isomorphic fibroblasts and histiocytes, and no mitotic activity can be seen. However, there is erosion of the cortical bone, which shows resorption cavities.

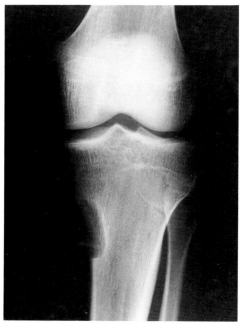

Fig. 2.100. Radiograph of a metaphyseal fibrous cortical defect of the left proximal tibial metaphysis of a 17-year-old boy. The prominent osteolytic defect has impressed the cortex from outside and is sharply delineated by a sclerotic rim inside.

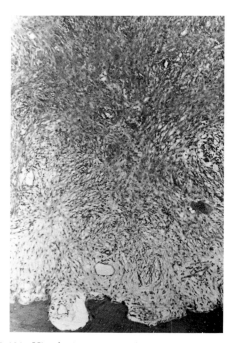

Fig. 2.101. Histologic section of a metaphyseal fibrous cortical defect, showing a fibrous tissue – with storiform pattern and isomorphic spindle cells – that invades the cortex from the outside (H&E, ×40).

FIBROBLASTIC PERIOSTEAL REACTION
(ICD-O-M-4900/0)

A fibrous proliferation of the periosteum can appear radiologically to be a bone tumor but actually may merely be a reactive growth. *Such a fibroblastic periosteal reaction occurs in the distal femoral metaphysis of adolescents; there is fibrous widening of the periosteum on the posterior aspect of the femur.*

The patient complains of knee pain, but this harmless lesion, frequent in teenagers, should not provoke any operative intervention.

Sites

The distal metaphysis of the femur is the only site of this lesion.

Age

Most cases are adolescents of about 15 years of age who are active in sports (cyclists, footballers, etc).

Radiographic Features (*Fig. 2.102*)

A lateral view of the knee region reveals widening of the periosteum adjacent to the cortex, but no cortical destruction is seen.

Histopathologic Features (*Fig. 2.103*)

Adjacent to the cortex, there is proliferating fibroblastic tissue containing isomorphic fibroblasts without any mitoses. The cortex, however, may be irregularly delimited, and some resorption lacunae or even splintering of the outer part may be observed.

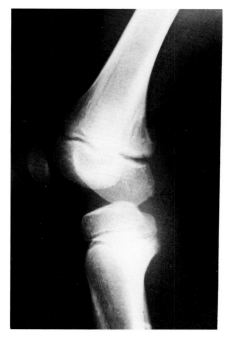

Fig. 2.102. Radiograph of a fibroblastic periosteal reaction in the distal femoral metaphysis of a 7-year-old boy, with a broadening of the periosteum on the intact posterior cortex.

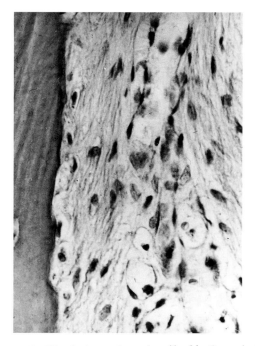

Fig. 2.103. Histologic section of a fibroblastic periosteal reaction in the distal femoral metaphysis, in which an isomorphic fibroplastic tissue erodes the exterior of the cortex (H&E, ×160).

OSSIFYING BONE FIBROMA
(ICD-O-M-9262/0)

A fibrous tumorous lesion of bone may be accompanied by a severe bone proliferation within the tumor tissue. *An ossifying bone fibroma is a circumscribed, central bone lesion characterized by a severe proliferation of fibrous tissue, together with differentiation of many woven bone trabeculae accompanied by activated osteoblasts.* This benign lesion is almost exclusive to the jaw bones and shows a continuously expansive growth which is symptomless for a long time. The tumor mainly affects adults but is occasionally found in children. It has to be excised operatively, after which a complete healing can be expected. Rarely, a histologically similar lesion is seen in the long bones (tibia, fibula, humerus), but this is now classified as "osteofibrous dysplasia".

Sites

The jaw bones, especially the mandibles, are almost the only sites.

Age

Most ossifying bone fibromas of the jaw occur in adults, but they are encountered in children and adolescents.

Radiographic Features (*Fig. 2.104*)

An ossifying fibroma is seen as a well-circumscribed focus of dense bone located centrally in a jaw bone that may be expanded. Sometimes this lesion is adjacent to a mislocated tooth.

Histopathologic Features (*Fig. 2.105*)

The lesion consists of a loose fibrous stroma and a dense network of woven bone trabeculae rimmed by activated osteoblasts. In addition, some osteoclasts may be seen. This histologic feature differentiates ossifying bone fibroma from fibrous dysplasia. However, there are histologic similarities between these two lesions, especially in the jaw bones. No polymorphic cells or atypical mitoses are found in the stromal fibroblasts. The lesion is well circumscribed.

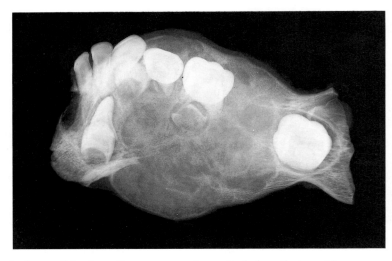

Fig. 2.104. Radiograph of an ossifying bone fibroma removed operatively from the jaw. A large osseous tumor mass is seen, driving out the teeth. The tumor is well circumbscribed.

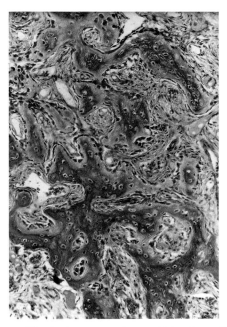

Fig. 2.105. Histologic section of an ossifying bone fibroma showing a dense network of woven bone trabeculae attached by prominent osteoblasts, between these there is a loose, vascularized fibrous stroma visible (H&E, ×64).

FIBROUS BONE DYSPLASIA (Jaffe-Lichtenstein)
(ICD-O-M-7491/0)

A fibrous tumor-like bone lesion, in reality a local malformation but giving the impression of a bone tumor, may be seen in one or more bones. *Fibrous bone dysplasia is a common osteolytic bone lesion in which the bone is replaced by fibrous tissue intermingled with slim and long woven bone trabeculae, without adjacent osteoblasts, that directly emerge from the fibrous tissue.* Thus, transformation into lamellar bone does not take place. In children and adolescents, fibrous bone dysplasia is a very common bone lesion that may occur as monostotic or polyostotic abnormality. It develops in the center of a bone and may give rise to a pathologic bone fracture. In weight-bearing bones, such as the femoral neck or tibia, a local bending of the bone may occur. In many cases, however, the lesion is detected by chance, the patient having had no symptoms. Often no therapy is necessary. Usually, growth of the lesion continues during skeletal growth but ceases in adult life. Rarely, unilateral polyostotic fibrous dysplasia is associated with precocious puberty, neurologic symptoms, endocrine dysfunctions (acromegaly, hyperparathyroidism, Cushing's syndrome), and abnormal skin pigmentation, known as

Albright's syndrome (predominantly found in young girls). A spontaneous malignant transformation of fibrous dysplasia is unlikely.

Sites (*Fig. 2.106*)

Fibrous dysplasia is the most common benign tumor of the ribs, where it is mostly a monostotic process. Another prominent localization is the proximal femur, especially the femoral neck. Lesions are also found in the skull and jaw bones and in long tubular bones (metaphyses and shaft).

Age (*Fig. 2.107*)

This is a disease of childhood, but only about 40% of the cases are diagnosed in children or adolescents. Frequently, fibrous dysplasia is first diagnosed in adult life.

Radiographic Features (*Fig. 2.108*)

In the femoral neck a fibrous dysplasia leads to expansion of the bone, including some broad osteolyses that may extend into the adjacent diaphysis. There is a diffuse shadow within the cystic osteolysis, and the adjacent cortex is narrowed from the inside. Especially in the ribs, such a lesion may appear as a bone cyst with local bone expansion. A pathologic bone fracture may occur in such a defect (Fig. 2.109).

Gross Pathologic Features (*Fig. 2.110*)

A fibrous bone dysplasia is morphologically characterized by a broad expansion of the whole of the involved bone compartment, with osteolytic cavities. In the femoral neck severe bending, like a bishop's crook, occurs; similar deformities may be seen in other weight-bearing bones. The spongiosa is replaced by a soft, grayish tissue and the cortex is extremely thinned, though it remains intact. Some cysts may be seen in the lesion; in the ribs, especially, the lesion is often predominantly cystic.

Histopathologic Features (*Figs 2.111–2.114*)

The soft intraosseous tissue consists of a dense collagenous matrix, with isomorphic fibroblasts and focally a storiform or cartwheel arrangement. Inside, many long and slender fibrous bone trabeculae are evenly distributed, forming a distinctive pattern (Fig. 2.111). The trabeculae usually have a woven appearance, including many prominent osteocytes, and seem to emerge directly from the fibrous ground tissue. Characteristically no osteoblasts are attached to the trabeculae (Fig. 2.112). In older lesions, the slender and bent trabeculae may be more or less calcified, and they are separated by cellular fibrous tissue (Fig. 2.113); again, no adjacent osteoblasts are seen. Even in older lesions, the bone appears woven and has a prominent distorted outline with irregular formations (Fig. 2.114). No regular lamellar bone trabeculae are found within such a lesion; reactive new bone trabeculae rimmed by activated osteoblasts may be seen in the surrounding bone but do not belong to the lesion itself. Foci of cartilage may occur in fibrous dysplasia in young age-groups, but this is a rare feature. On the whole, no histologic sign of malignancy is observed in such a lesion.

Fig. 2.108. Radiograph of a fibrous bone dysplasia of the right proximal femur of a 7-year-old girl. The femoral neck and the whole proximal femur are expanded, and broad osteolyses with dull appearance is seen inside the bone. The cortex is narrowed from the interior.

Fig. 2.109. Radiograph of a fibrous bone dysplasia of the left proximal femoral shaft, with cystic expansion of the involved bone and a pathologic fracture right in this area.

Fig. 2.110. Gross specimen of a fibrous bone dysplasia of the proximal femur, including the femoral neck and shaft. All of the involved bone is expanded, and the spongiosa is replaced by a soft, grayish tissue, with cystic cavities. The femoral neck is bent like a bishop's crook.

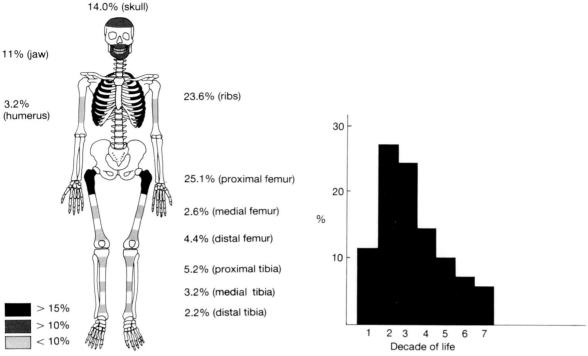

14.0% (skull)

11% (jaw)

3.2%
(humerus)

23.6% (ribs)

25.1% (proximal femur)

2.6% (medial femur)

4.4% (distal femur)

5.2% (proximal tibia)

3.2% (medial tibia)

2.2% (distal tibia)

■ > 15%
▨ > 10%
▦ < 10%

Fig. 2.106. Fibrous bone dysplasia: localization. The most frequent sites are the femoral neck and the ribs, where nearly 50% of the lesions are found. The jaw bones and the skull are other frequent sites, but fibrous dysplasia may also emerge in any part of the skeleton, especially in the long tubular bones.

Fig. 2.107. Fibrous bone dysplasia: age distribution. About 40% of the lesions are detected in children or adolescents. In many cases, fibrous dysplasia is found in adult life, mainly by chance, but in reality, the lesion has in fact developed in early childhood.

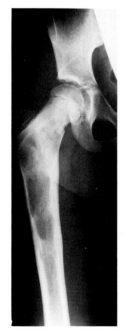

Fig. 2.108

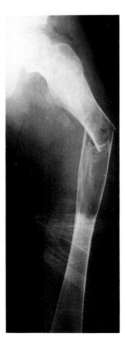

Fig. 2.109

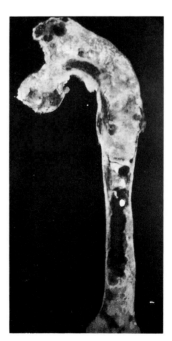

Fig. 2.110

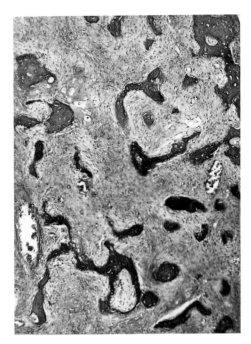

Fig. 2.111. Histologic section of a fibrous bone dysplasia, characterized by a dense collagenous tissue with evenly distributed, slender, fibrous, often bowed, bone trabeculae (van Gieson's, ×50).

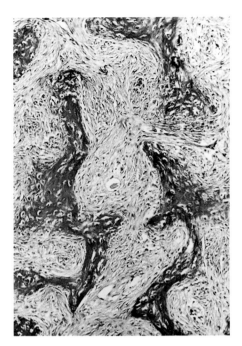

Fig. 2.112. Histologic section of a fibrous bone dysplasia at higher magnification, showing woven bone trabeculae that emerge directly out of the basic fibrous tissue without any adjacent osteoblasts (Goldner, ×82).

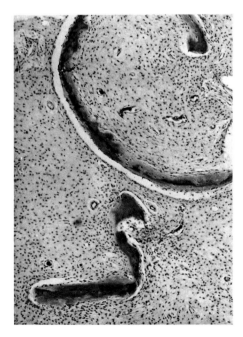

Fig. 2.113. Histologic section of a fibrous bone dysplasia in an older lesion in which the slender and bowed bone trabeculae are unevenly calcified (H&E, ×82). No adjacent osteoblasts are seen, and the fibrous tissue dominates.

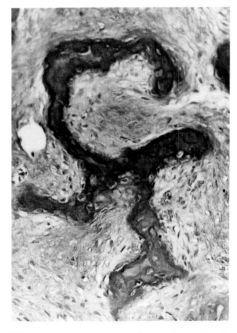

Fig. 2.114. Histologic section of a fibrous bone dysplasia at a high magnification (van Gieson's, ×132), showing a woven bone trabecula, with a distorted outline, that has emerged directly from the fibrous tissue without involvement of osteoblasts. The trabecula is irregularly bent.

OSTEOFIBROUS BONE DYSPLASIA (Campanacci)

In this lesion there is structural transition from fibrous bone dysplasia to ossifying bone fibroma. *The lesion is very similar histologically to ossifying bone fibroma, with a large area of bone destruction and osteosclerotic bone remodelling within a long tubular bone, especially in the tibial shaft.* On the whole, this is a rare disease. In some cases, an "adamantinoma of the long bones" is accompanied by osteofibrous dysplasia, and this has to be carefully excluded by histological investigations.

Sites

This lesion occurs only in the shafts of long tubular bones (tibia, fibula, femur, humerus). The tibial shaft is the most frequent site.

Age

Children and adolescents are affected mainly. Most lesions are found in children below the age of 10 years.

Radiographic Features (Fig. 2.115)

Typically the lesion is located in the middle of the tibial shaft, which is expanded and shows small and large osteolytic foci within a dense, sclerotic area. The osteolyses include some faint inner densities. The protruding cortical bone remains intact and appears smooth on the outside. No periosteal reaction is seen.

Histopathologic Features (Fig. 2.116)

There is an irregular network of broad woven bone trabeculae, to which are attached rows of activated osteoblasts (similar to ossifying bone fibroma). The attached osteoblasts distinguish osteofibrous dysplasia from fibrous dysplasia. Between the trabeculae there is a fibrous stroma with isomorphic fibroblasts showing no mitoses. Within this stroma there may be seen discrete infiltrations of an epithelioid tumor, and therefore "adamantinoma of the long bones" has to be excluded. An osteofibrous bone dysplasia alone is a harmless local bone lesion that merely leads to a misshapen bone, eventually accompanied by slight dysfunction and pain.

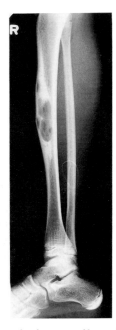

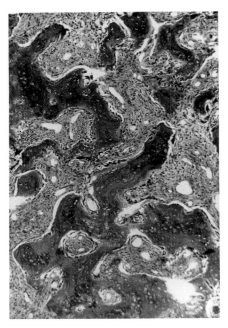

Fig. 2.115. Radiograph of an osteofibrous bone dysplasia of the right tibial shaft of a 16-year-old girl, showing a multicystic lesion surrounded by a sclerotic bone. The involved bone area is clearly expanded, but the cortex is intact.

Fig. 2.116. Histologic section of an osteofibrous bone dysplasia; there is an irregular network of broad woven bone trabeculae, to which are attached rows of activated osteoblasts (H&E, ×64). Between the trabeculae there is a fibrous stroma rich in fibroblasts. This pattern is similar to that seen in an ossifying bone fibroma.

DESMOPLASTIC BONE FIBROMA
(ICD-O-M-8823/1)

This rare fibrous tumor is listed by the WHO as a benign condition, but it does show a locally aggressive and infiltrative growth, together with local destruction and high recurrence rate, which put it in a "borderline" position with regard to malignancy. *Desmoplastic bone fibroma is a semi-malignant bone tumor characterized by abundant collagen fibers, with sparse isomorphic spindle cells lacking mitoses; it destructively invades the bone and leads to recurrences, but no metastases are to be expected.* All of the tumor tissue has to be removed operatively in order to avoid recurrences.

Pain and local swelling are the main symptoms of this tumor growth. Functional disability or even pathologic bone fracture may occur in some cases.

Sites

The majority of desmoplastic bone fibromas are seen in the long tubular bones (humerus, femur, tibia) or flat bones (ilium, scapula, mandible); they are mostly located in the bone ends.

Age

The great majority of the patients are children, adolescents and young adults under the age of 30 years.

Radiographic Features *(Fig. 2.117)*

There is a more or less large osteolytic defect, centrally located in the bone, that may be reasonably well demarcated, expanding the thinned cortex. The outline may be partly fuzzy, and the cortex may be destroyed, with extension into the adjacent soft tissues. In such cases, the radiographs may indicate malignancy.

Gross Pathologic Features

The tumor tissue consists of a dense, grayish white fibrous tissue of firm elastic consistency. The adjacent bone is severely destroyed.

Histopathologic Features *(Fig. 2.118)*

The tumor is characterized by a dense collagenous tissue in which are bundles of broad collagen fibers and sparse fibroblasts. The nuclei of the fibroblasts are small and elongated or ovoid; hyperchromatic, polymorphic nuclei are rare. No mitoses are seen. This histologic pattern differentiates desmoplastic fibroma from fibrosarcoma. Neither multinucleated giant cells nor osteoid or bone formation are seen in this lesion. On the whole, the tumor tissue appears relatively harmless, histologically, but radiographic features identify it as a semimalignant tumor.

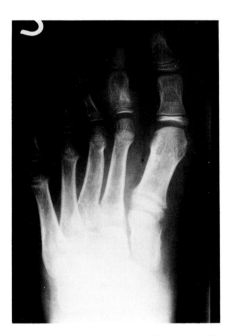

Fig. 2.117. Radiograph of a desmoplastic bone fibroma of the proximal phalanx of the second toe in a 13-year-old boy, showing a centrally located osteolytic defect that is well demarcated. The bone is slightly expanded.

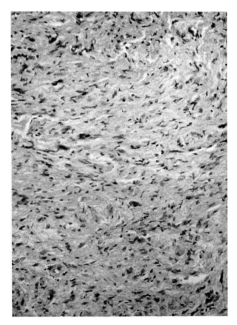

Fig. 2.118. Histologic section of a desmoplastic bone fibroma. The fibroma consists of a dense collagenous tissue with bundles of broad collagen fibers and fibroblasts; in the latter are small, elongated and often polymorphic and hyperchromatic nuclei (H&E, ×100). No mitoses are seen.

OSTEOCLASTOMA (Giant Cell Tumor)
(ICD-O-M-9250/1)

This is a primary bone tumor that gives rise to many clinical and diagnostic problems. *It is a locally aggressive tumor growth of questionable biologic behavior; it is characterized by a large, expanding osteolysis and includes masses of multinucleated giant cells, supposed to be osteoclasts, within a highly vascularized, spindle-cell stroma.* Although the giant cells are the dominating histologic feature, they are not the actual tumor cells but rather the spindle cells of the stroma. Histologically, "benign" osteoclastoma may be separated from "malignant" osteoclastoma, but both may have a malignant course. Therefore, this aggressive tumor must be regarded as bone sarcoma; right from the beginning of therapy, the whole tumor tissue has to be completely removed.

Sites *(Fig. 2.119)*

Osteoclastomas develop in the epiphyses of bones, and the metaphyses may be involved secondarily. Most of these tumors are found in the long bones, the knee region (distal femur, proximal tibia) being the main location. However, other bones may be implicated.

Age *(Fig. 2.120)*

Osteoclastoma rarely affects patients under the age of 15 years and is rare in adolescents. Most cases are females around 30 years of age.

Radiographic Features *(Fig. 2.121)*

Usually, a large, "soap-bubble" osteolysis is seen in the epiphysis of a bone; it may extend considerably into the metaphysis, and metaphyseal extension may be the main portion of the tumor. Generally, no special structures are seen inside the lesion, but there may be some sclerotic densities in some cases. The defect is usually not defined by a sclerotic rim, but it may be circumscribed. The adjacent cortex is thinned and, in progressive cases, it may be destroyed. This indicates malignant tumor growth.

Gross Pathologic Features

In section, a gray or red fleshy tumor is eccentrically located in the involved epiphysis, extending into the adjacent metaphysis. The involved bone region is expanded, and the cortex is destroyed from the inside or penetrated by the tumor tissue.

Histopathologic Features *(Figs 2.122–2.124)*

The most impressive histologic feature of the tumor tissue is a fibrous stroma containing many multinucleated giant cells presumed to be osteoclasts. No bone tissue – authochthonous or newly and reactively produced – is seen in the lesion. Recent investigations, however, have ascertained that the osteoclasts are not true tumor cells but rather are accompanying cells, and that the stroma cells are in fact the tumor cells of osteoclastomas. In either case, osteoclastoma is malignant: different grades of malignancy may be deduced, according to the individual tissue pattern:

Grade 1: many multinucleated giant cells are distributed evenly in a fibrous stroma that includes isomorphic stromal spindle cells with oval or round nuclei. No pathologic mitoses occur (Fig. 2.122).

Grade 2: the giant cells are fewer in number and smaller in size. The stromal tissue is predominant, showing polymorphic spindle cells with some hyperchromatic nuclei and more mitoses than in grade 1 (Fig. 2.123).

Grade 3: there is a clearly sarcomatous stroma with polymorphic spindle cells, including polymorphic and hyperchromatic nuclei together with many pathological mitoses (Fig. 2.124). Giant cells are rare and small in size, with only a few polymorphic and hyperchromatic nuclei.

Grade 3 osteoclastoma is obviously a malignant tumor growth, but the other osteoclastomas, histologically of lower grade of malignancy, also have malignant potential. Therefore all osteoclastomas have to be considered as malignant bone tumors. They are, however, rare in children.

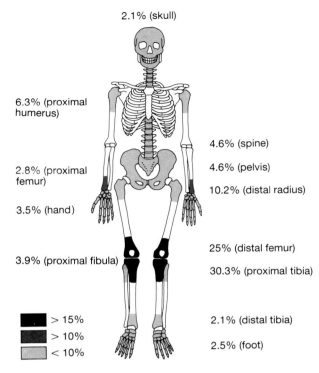

2.1% (skull)

6.3% (proximal humerus)

2.8% (proximal femur)

3.5% (hand)

3.9% (proximal fibula)

4.6% (spine)

4.6% (pelvis)

10.2% (distal radius)

25% (distal femur)

30.3% (proximal tibia)

2.1% (distal tibia)

2.5% (foot)

■ > 15%
■ > 10%
■ < 10%

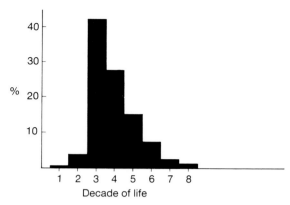

Fig. 2.120. Osteoclastoma: age distribution. Below the age of 15 years, this tumor is extremely rare. It is a tumor of adults and is rarely found in adolescents.

◄───────────────────────────

Fig. 2.119. Osteoclastoma: localization. Most osteoclastomas are found in the distal femoral and proximal tibial epiphyses; the distal radial epiphyses are also frequent sites. Other locations are involved but are rare.

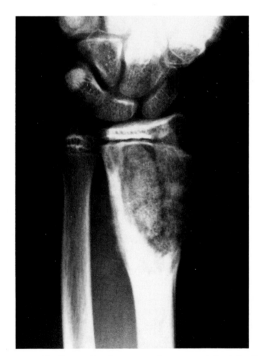

Fig. 2.121. Radiograph of an osteoclastoma of the left distal radius of a 14-year-old boy, involving the epiphysis as well as the metaphysis. It is an undefined cystic lesion without marginal sclerosis and containing some sclerotic densities. Part of the growth plate is destroyed by this tumor growth.

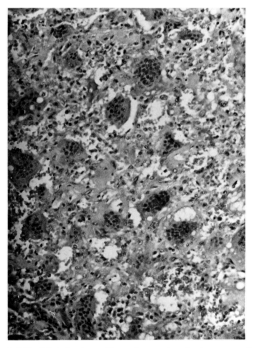

Fig. 2.122. Histologic section of an osteoclastoma, grade 1, characterized by a loose, highly vascularized stroma with isomorphic spindle cells and many evenly distributed multinucleated osteoclastic giant cells (H&E, ×82). No nuclear atypism and no pathologic mitoses are seen.

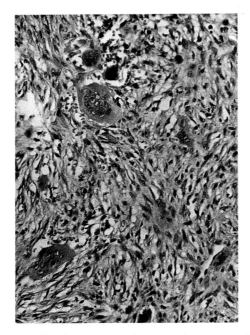

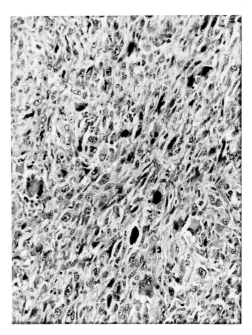

Fig. 2.123. Histologic section of an osteoclastoma, grade 2, in which the number and sizes of the prominent giant cells are less than in grade 1; the fibrous stroma predominates, with many polymorphic spindle cells, including hyperchromatic nuclei and some mitoses (H&E, ×100). No bone formation is seen in such a lesion.

Fig. 2.124. Histologic section of an osteoclastoma, grade 3, in which a sarcomatous stroma with highly polymorphic spindle cells dominates and giant cells are rare and small (H&E, ×100). The tumor cells have polymorphic and hyperchromatic nuclei, and pathologic mitoses are abundant.

MALIGNANT FIBROUS HISTIOCYTOMA
(ICD-O-M-8830/3)

In this tumor, a fibrogenic differentiation and areas of histiocytes are the characteristic features. This pattern may be seen in other malignant bone tumors, such as osteosarcoma or dedifferentiated chondrosarcoma, and they have to be distinguished from fibrosarcoma. *Malignant fibrous histiocytoma is a malignant neoplasm that arises primarily in the medullary cavity of a bone and consists of fibrous stroma in a storiform pattern; there are polymorphic fibroblasts and mostly atypical histiocytes with nuclear abnormalities and pathologic mitoses.* Malignant histiocytes may prevail, and fibrous tissue may be scant, i.e. the lesion can be a pure, non-fibrous histiocytoma. This sarcoma may also develop in soft tissues.

Pain and swelling are the most frequent symptoms and a pathological bone fracture may occur. Among primary malignant bone tumors, malignant fibrous histiocytoma is not rare.

Surgical excision or amputation is the treatment of choice; irradiation is only recommended in inoperable cases, providing some alleviation. Prognosis is poor, with a short survival time.

Sites (*Fig. 2.125*)

Most malignant fibrous histiocytomas are encountered in the knee region (distal femur, proximal tibia and fibula); however, other bones, especially in the pelvic girdle, may be involved. The tumor may also occur in the shaft or epiphysis and extend into the joint.

Age (*Fig. 2.126*)

The tumor is rare in children but is sometimes seen in adolescents. However, most patients are adults.

Radiographic Features (*Fig. 2.127*)

An obviously malignant osteolysis with ill-defined margins is seen in the involved bone; there is severe local destruction of bone, including cortical bone. Inside, irregular densities are usually visible. Periosteal bone formation is almost always absent. Radiographic features indicate a malignant tumor growth but are not specific to malignant fibrous histiocytoma. Therefore, the diagnosis has to be made by biopsy and histology.

Gross Pathologic Features (*Fig. 2.128*)

In an amputation specimen, the medullary cavity is found to be filled by a yellowish, brownish or hemorrhagic tissue of soft consistency. The cortex is usually infiltrated and destroyed, and the tumor may extend into the soft tissues.

Histopathologic Features (*Figs 2.129 and 2.130*)

The overall histologic image may be confusing. The most characteristic pattern is a storiform arrangement of collagen fibers (Fig. 2.129). Two populations of tumor cells predominate: (a) there are many histiocytes with large polymorphic and hyperchromatic nuclei, which frequently have atypical mitoses (Fig. 2.130); (b) in addition, polymorphic fibroblasts are seen between these, producing a sarcomatous stroma. Multinucleated giant cells are frequent; these are malignant tumor cells. The bone trabeculae in the area of growth are destroyed and eroded at the periphery. Within such tumor tissue there may be areas of heavy collagenization and hyalinization, or often prominent lymphocytic inflammation. Differential diagnoses by histologic features, include fibrosarcoma, osteoclastoma or osteosarcoma.

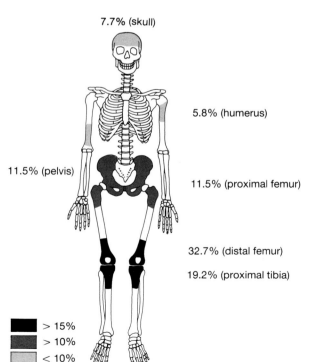

7.7% (skull)

5.8% (humerus)

11.5% (pelvis)

11.5% (proximal femur)

32.7% (distal femur)

19.2% (proximal tibia)

■ > 15%
▨ > 10%
▨ < 10%

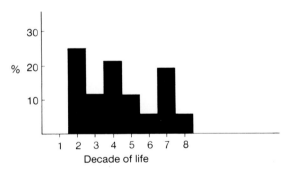

Fig. 2.126. Malignant fibrous histiocytoma: age distribution. This tumor is seen in adults of any age; however, 25% of cases occur in adolescents.

Fig. 2.125. Malignant fibrous histiocytoma: localization. About 52% of these lesions are seen in the knee area (distal femur, proximal tibia). Other frequent sites are the proximal femur and pelvic bones. However, this tumor may occur in any bone.

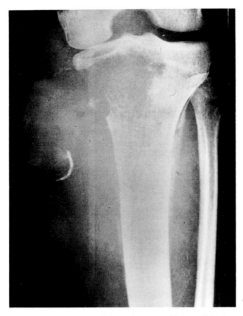

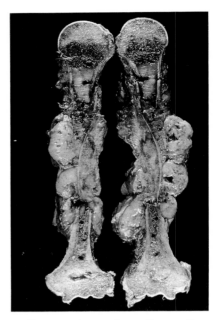

Fig. 2.127. Radiograph of a malignant fibrous histiocytoma of the left proximal tibia of a 16-year-old boy, showing a large indistinct osteolysis in the metaphysis, where the cortex is destroyed. It is obvious that the tumor has already infiltrated the soft tissue.

Fig. 2.128. Gross specimen of a malignant fibrous histiocytoma of the right shaft of the humerus, showing broad expansion into the surrounding area. The tumor tissue fills the medullary cavity and has destroyed the bone.

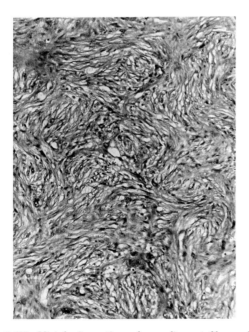

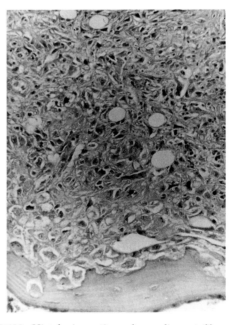

Fig. 2.129. Histologic section of a malignant fibrous histiocytoma that has a typical storiform pattern in which the collagen fibers are arranged in whorls and bundles (H&E, ×64). Atypical histiocytes and fibroblasts with polymorphic and hyperchromatic nuclei are visible.

Fig. 2.130. Histologic section of a malignant fibrous histiocytoma at higher magnification (PAS, ×100) shows the histiocytic and fibroblastic tumor cells, with polymorphic and hyperchromatic cell nuclei and numerous atypical mitoses. In addition, destruction of bone by the tumor is seen.

FIBROSARCOMA OF BONE
(ICD-O-M-8810/3)

Similar to corresponding tumor growth in soft tissues, fibrosarcoma can develop in the medullary cavity of a bone. *It is a primary bone tumor that has its origin in fibrous elements of the medullary cavity; it is accompanied by severe local bone destruction.* Fibrosarcoma may also arise in the periosteum. Since malignant fibrous histiocytoma was first identified, fibrosarcomas have become rare though they are seen once a while. It shows a slow progressive growth, and metastases occur late, so prognosis is rather good.

Swelling and pain of short duration are the main symptoms. Surgical removal of the tumor is the only helpful therapy because it is resistant to radiation or chemotherapy.

Sites (Fig. 2.131)

Nearly 50% of all fibrosarcomas are located in the knee region (distal femur, proximal tibia), but lesions may also be found in other tubular bones, mostly in the metaphyses. Another frequent site is the skull, and the spine, ribs or pelvic bones may also be involved.

Age (Fig. 2.132)

Fibrosarcomas are rather evenly distributed throughout life. Most of these tumors are seen in adults, but about 20% of these lesions are seen in children and adolescents.

Radiographic Features (Fig. 2.133)

Fibrosarcoma does not have any radiological features that differentiate it from other malig-nant growths. There is a permeative or mottled osteolysis, with ill-defined borders and, eventually, cortical destruction, indicating malignant growth. Rarely, a slightly sclerotic marginal border may be observed.

Gross Pathologic Features (Fig. 2.134)

A firm mass of fibrous tissue is seen that has destroyed the bone and mostly has penetrated into the adjacent cortex. This tumor tissue has a grayish-white appearance, with red hemorrhages. Areas of necrosis exhibit a jelly-like substance. Often, the tumor expands into the adjacent soft tissue, forming a nodular tumor mass.

Histopathologic Features (Figs 2.135 and 2.136)

The histologic pattern is the same as that in fibrosarcomas of soft tissue. It consists of a fibrous tissue with mature-appearing collagen fibers arranged in streams or whorls. An outstanding feature is the ''herring-bone'' arrangement of fibrous tumor cells, which is seen in parts of the tumor tissue (Fig. 2.135). The tumor-cells are spindle-shaped with ovoid or elongated, but clearly polymorphic and hyperchromatic, nuclei (Fig. 2.136) in which atypical mitoses may be observed. No tumoral osteoid depositions or bone formation can be seen in the lesion. The degree of differentiation and dedifferentiation can be deduced from the cellular pleomorphism.

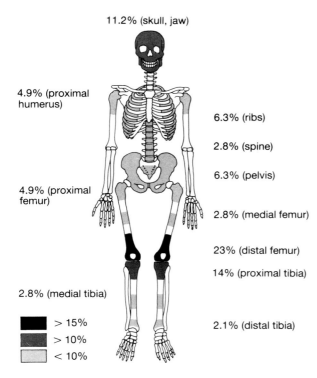

11.2% (skull, jaw)

4.9% (proximal humerus)

6.3% (ribs)

2.8% (spine)

6.3% (pelvis)

4.9% (proximal femur)

2.8% (medial femur)

23% (distal femur)

14% (proximal tibia)

2.8% (medial tibia)

> 15%
> 10%
< 10%

2.1% (distal tibia)

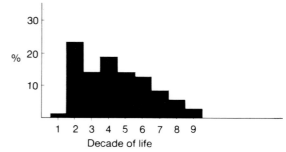

Fig. 2.132. Fibrosarcoma of bone: age distribution. Most osseous fibrosarcomas develop in adult life, but about 20% of them are seen in children and adolescents.

Fig. 2.131. Fibrosarcoma of bone: localization. Most of these tumors are seen in the knee region (distal femur, proximal tibia) and in the skull. However, the tumor may occur in any bone.

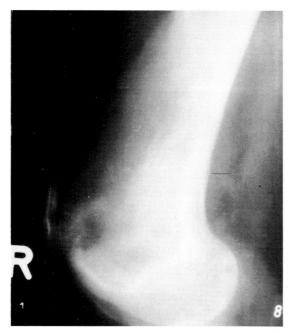

Fig. 2.133. Radiograph of a bone fibrosarcoma of the right distal femur of a 16-year-old, showing a malignant bone destruction of the frontal part of the bone, including the cortex. The area of tumorous destruction is ill-defined, and some osteolyses are visible.

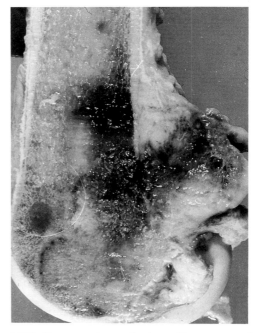

Fig. 2.134. Gross specimen of a bone fibrosarcoma of the distal femur, showing a firm fibrous tumor tissue in the medullary cavity, with areas of hemorrhage. The spongiosa and cortical bone in this area is severely destroyed, and the tumor has expanded through the cortex into the soft tissue.

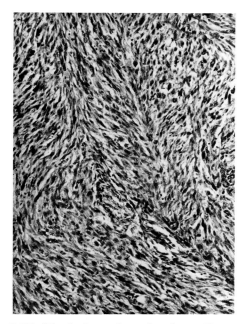

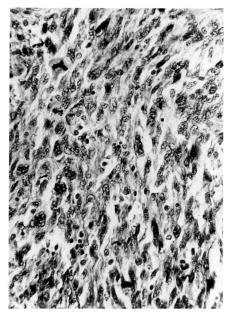

Fig. 2.135. Histologic section of a bone fibrosarcoma. Streams and whorls of collagen fibers form a "herring-bone" pattern (H&E, ×82). Many spindle cells with polymorphous and hyperchromatic nuclei are seen. The original bone, in the area shown, is completely destroyed.

Fig. 2.136. Histologic section of a bone fibrosarcoma at higher magnification (H&E, ×140), showing the extremely pleomorphic cell nuclei with many atypical mitoses.

LITERATURE
Tumors of Fibrous Tissue Origin

Adler CP. Klassifikation der Knochentumoren und Pathologie der gutartigen und semimalignen Knochentumoren. In: Frommhold W, Gerhardt P. Knochentumoren. Klinisch-radiologisches Seminar, vol. X. Stuttgart: Thieme, 1980

Adler CP. Fibromyxoma of bone within the femoral neck and the tibial head. J Cancer Res Clin Oncol 1981;101: 183–9

Adler CP, Reinartz H. Fleckige Osteosklerose des Tibaischaftes: Osteofibröse Knochendysplasie Campanacci der linken Tibia. Radiologe 1988;28:591–2

Adler CP, Uehlinger E. Grenzfälle bei Knochentumoren. Präneoplastische Veränderungen und Geschwülste fraglicher Dignität. Verh Dtsch Ges Pathol 1979;63:352–8

Bagò-Granell J, Aquirre-Canyadell M, Nardi J, Tallada N. Malignant fibrous histiocytoma of bone at the site of a total hip arthroplasty: a case report. J Bone Jt Surg 1984; B-66:38–40

Bullough PG, Walley J. Fibrous cortical defect and non-ossifying fibroma. Postgrad Med J 1965;41:672–6

Caballes RL. The mechanism of metastasis in so-called "benign giant cell tumors of bone". Hum Pathol 1981; 12:762–7

Caffey J. On fibrous defects in cortical walls of growing tubular bones. Adv Pediat 1955;7:13–51

Campanacci M, Giunti A, Olmi R. Giant-cell tumors of bone: a study of 209 cases with long-term follow-up in 130. Ital J Orthop Traumatol 1975;1:249–77

Cohen DM, Dahlin DC, Pugh DG. Fibrous dysplasia associated with adamantinoma of the long bones. Cancer (Phil) 1962;15:515–21

Cunningham JB, Ackerman LV. Metaphyseal fibrous defects. J Bone Jt Surg 1956;A-38:797–808

Dahlin DC, Ivins JC. Fibrosarcoma of bone: a study of 114 cases. Cancer (Phil) 1969;23:35–41

Dahlin DC, Unni KK, Matsuno T. Malignant (fibrous)

histiocytoma of bone – fact or fancy? Cancer (Phil) 1977; 39:1508–16

Feldman F, Lattes R. Primary malignant fibrous histiocytoma (fibrous xanthoma) of bone. Skeletal Radiol 1977;1:145–60

Frazer AK, Hannah RH, Buxton PH. Fibrous dysplasia of the ethmoid presenting with proptosis. Br J Surg 1969; 56:300–5

Goldenberg RR, Campbell CJ, Bonfiglio M. Giant-cell tumor of bone: an analysis of two hundred and eighteen cases. J Bone Jt Surg 1970;A-52:619–63

Gunterberg B, Kindblom LG, Laurin S. Giant-cell tumor of bone and aneurysmal bone cyst. A correlated histologic and angiographic study. Skeletal Radiol 1977;2:65–74

Haag M, Alder CP. Malignant fibrous histiocytoma in association with hip replacement. J Bone Jt Surg 1989; B-71:701

Henry A. Monostotic fibrous dysplasia. J Bone Jt Surg 1969; B-51:300–6

Huvos AG. Primary malignant fibrous histiocytoma of bone. Clinicopathologic study of 18 patients. NY St J Med 1976; 76:552–9

Huvos AG. Heilweil M, Bretsky SS. The pathology of malignant fibrous histiocytoma of bone. A study of 130 patients. Am J Surg Pathol 1985;9:853–71

Jaffe HL, Lichtenstein L, Portis RB. Giant cell tumor of bone. Its pathologic appearance, grading, supposed variants and treatment. Arch Pathol 1940;30:993–1031

Johnston J. Giant cell tumor of bone. The role of the giant cell in orthopedic pathology. Orthop Clin N Am 1977;8: 751–70

Kasahara K, Yamamuro T, Kasahara A. Giant cell tumour of bone: cytological studies. Br J Cancer 1979;40:201–9

Kempson RL. Ossifying fibroma of the long bones. A light and electron microscopic study. Arch Pathol 1966;82: 218–33

Kumar R, Madewell JE, Lindell MM, Swischuk LE. Fibrous lesions of bones. Radiographics 1990;10:237–56

Lichtenstein L. Giant-cell tumor of bone. Current status of problems in diagnosis and treatment. J Bone Jt Surg 1951;A-33:143–50

McCarthy EF, Matsuno T, Dorfman HD. Malignant fibrous histiocytoma of bone: A study of 35 cases. Hum Pathol 1979;10:57–70

McGrath PJ. Giant cell tumor of bone. An analysis of 52 cases. J Bone Jt Surg 1972;B-54:216–19

Meister P, Finsterer H. Der Riesenzelltumor des Knochens und seine Problematik. Münch Med Wschr 1972;114: 55–60

Meister P, Konrad E, Engert J. Polyostotische fibröse kortikale Defekte (bzw. nicht ossifizierende Knochenfibrome). Arch Orthop Trauma Surg 1977; 89:315–18

Mellin W, Roessner A, Grundmann E, Wörmann B, Hiddemann W, Immenkamp M. Biological characterization of human bone tumors. VII. Detection of malignancy in a giant cell tumor of bone by flow cytometric DNA-analysis. Pathol Res Pract 1985;180:619–25

Michael RH, Dorfman HD. Malignant fibrous histiocytoma associated with bone infarcts. Report of a case. Clin Orthop 1976;118:180–3

Mirra JM, Ulich T, Magidson J, Kaiser L, Eckardt J, Gold R. A case of probable benign pulmonary "metastases" of implants arising from a giant cell tumor of bone. Clin Orthop 1980;162:245–54

Rock MG, Pritchard DJ, Unni KK. Metastases from histologically benign giant cell tumor of bone. J Bone Jt Surg 1984;A-66:263–73

Roessner A, v. Bassewitz DB, Schlake W, Thorwesten G, Grundmann E. Biologic characterization of human bone tumors. III. Giant cell tumor of bone. A combined electron microscopical, histochemical, and autoradiographical study. Pathol Res Pract 1978;178:431–40

Scaglietti O, Stringa G. Myxoma of bone in childhood. J Bone Jt Surg 1961;A-43:67–80

Schajowicz F. Giant-cell tumors of bone (osteoclastoma). A pathological and histochemical study. J Bone Jt Surg 1961;A-43:1–29

Selby S. Metaphyseal cortical defects in the tubular bones of growing children. J Bone Jt Surg 1961;A-43:395–400

Spanier SS. Malignant fibrous histiocytoma of bone. Orthop Clin N Am 1977;8:947–61

Steiner GC. Fibrous cortical defect and nonossifying fibroma of bone. Arch Pathol 1974;97:205–10

Uehlinger E. Osteofibrosis deformans juvenilis (Polyostotische fibröse Dysplasie Jaffe-Lichtenstein). Virchows Arch [A] 1940;306:255–99

Yoshida H, Akeho M, Yumoto T. Giant cell tumor of bone. Enzyme histochemical, biochemical and tissue culture studies. Virchows Arch [A] 1982;395:319–30

Tumors of Marrow Origin

LIPOMA OF BONE
(ICD-O-M-8850/0)

This benign bone tumor, arising from the medullary fat tissue is, on the whole, a very rare bone lesion, but it does occur in children. *Lipoma is an absolutely benign lesion that develops slowly in the medullary cavity of a bone, with proliferation of the marrow fat tissue and usually inducing a clearly demarcated "bone cyst".* No clinical symptoms result, and mostly the lesion is detected by chance.

Unless problems of stability are evident, this is a "leave-me-alone-lesion", no operative intervention being necessary.

Sites

The tumor may occur in any bone, but is most frequent in the calcaneus.

Age

Lipoma occurs in all age-groups, including children.

Radiographic Features *(Fig. 2.137)*

Usually, the bone cyst is sharply circumscribed by marginal sclerosis. There may be some sclerotic densities in the center consequent to dystrophic calcification.

Histopathologic Features *(Fig. 2.138)*

In the medullary cavity there is a circumscribed focus of proliferating fat tissue, together with some fibrous septa and thin blood capillaries. This proliferating fat tissue is difficult to differentiate from normal medullary fat tissue, but no bone trabeculae are seen in the former. There are no obvious signs of a proliferative tumor growth. Therefore, in most cases, no operative intervention is indicated.

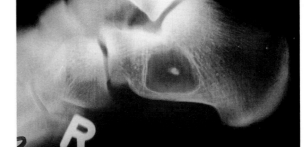

Fig. 2.137. Radiograph of a bone lipoma in the right calcaneus in a 14-year-old boy, demonstrating a well-circumscribed bone cyst with marginal sclerosis and a central spotty density.

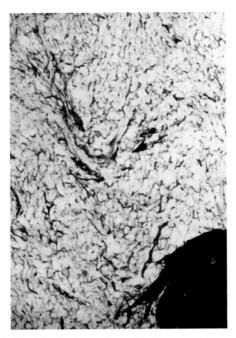

Fig. 2.138. Histologic section of a lipoma of bone, with replacement of the spongy bone by a slightly nodular fat tissue in which no bone trabeculae are present (van Gieson's, ×40).

LIPOSARCOMA OF BONE
(ICD-O-M-8850/3)

This is a rare malignant primary bone tumor of the medullary fat tissue. It is a locally destructive growth and may induce metastases. It is not seen in children.

HISTIOCYTOSIS X

(ICD-O-M-4405/0)

EOSINOPHILIC BONE GRANULOMA

Eosinophilic bone granuloma is a nontumorous intraosseous lesion that may give the impression that it is a malignant tumor growth. *This non-neoplastic lesion, which produces a local osteolysis in a bone, is characterized by a proliferation of a reticulohistiocytic granulation tissue, with numerous eosinophilic leukocytes of unknown etiology; it belongs to the disease complex of histiocytosis X.* It is found mainly in children and adolescents (about 75% of the cases) but may also be detected in adults. An eosinophilic bone granuloma is usually a solitary lesion that may, however, show an extremely rapid and destructive growth similar to a malignant tumor. In reality, though, it is a harmless lesion that may even disappear spontaneously.

It may cause local pain or swelling and even pathologic fracture, but in many cases it is detected by chance.

Sites

The most frequent sites are the skull (predominantly the frontal and parietal bones and mandibles), the ribs and, especially, the long bones. Other sites, for instance vertebrae and the ilium, may be involved.

Age

Eosinophilic bone granuloma mostly occurs in children (57%) or adolescents (20%). In adults, histiocytosis X must be considered, including Hand–Schüller–Christian's disease or even malignant histiocytosis.

Radiographic Features (Figs 2.139 and 2.140)

The lesion appears as a local osteolysis within a bone. It may image as a well-circumscribed "bone cyst" but often is ill-defined, showing a severe destruction of the spongiosa and often even the cortical bone (Fig. 2.139). In the long bones, most lesions are located in the diaphysis, but the metaphyses can also be affected. Periosteal new bone formation may be seen and, if the "onion-skin" type of periosteal reaction occurs, osteomyelitis or Ewing's sarcoma must be considered in differential diagnosis. In other cases, the involved bone is expanded, including several large and small osteolyses, but the cortex is intact (Fig. 2.140). In the spine, a vertebral body can be completely collapsed producing a "vertebra plana". In the skull or mandible, lesions usually have a sharply defined, punched-out appearance and are of variable size, without dense inner regions.

Histopathologic Features (Figs 2.141–2.144)

An eosinophilic bone granuloma is histologically characterized by a cell-rich granulation tissue mainly including reticulum cells and histiocytes that contain rounded, vesicular and often indented nuclei. In addition, large groups or diffuse infiltrations of eosinophilic leukocytes, together with some lymphocytes, plasma cells, neutrophil granulocytes and fibroblasts, are visible in the "proliferative" phase (Fig. 2.141). In the second, "granulomatous" phase, a loose granulation tissue with many capillaries and infiltrations of histiocytes and eosinophilic leukocytes is the typical pattern. Here, "eosinophilic microabscesses" can be seen. The third, "xanthomatous" phase is characterized by many large histiocytes and foam cells with small, isomorphic nuclei, and eosinophilic leukocytes are scarce (Fig. 2.142). Sometimes multinucleated giant cells with phagocytic activity are seen. Finally, there is a fourth, "scar" phase in which proliferating fibroblasts forming collagen fibers are predominant; this pattern indicates spontaneous healing.

HAND–SCHÜLLER–CHRISTIAN DISEASE

Other histiocytoses show a close relationship to eosinophilic bone granuloma, especially Hand–Schüller–Christian disease. This is clinically characterized by map-like skull, exophthalmos and diabetes insipidus. On radiographs, one or several osteolytic foci identical to those in eosinophilic bone granuloma are seen. The skull is the most common site. The *histologic pattern* is almost identical to that in the "xanthomatous" phase of eosinophilic granuloma (Fig. 2.142).

Histiocytes of different sizes and with roundish, indented vesicular nuclei and many histiocytic multinuclear giant cells, are the predominant constituent (Fig. 2.143). It is often impossible to decide, from the histology, whether the lesion is a *benign proliferate* or a *malignant histiocytosis* in which the histiocytes show some nuclear polymorphism together with numerous mitoses (Fig. 2.144), and in which severe bone destruction is obvious.

ABT–LETTERER–SIWE DISEASE

A special form of histiocytosis is Abt–Letterer–Siwe disease, which is a rare malignant lesion with multiple foci throughout the skeleton. This develops exclusively in young children under the age of 2 years.

DIFFERENTIATING BETWEEN HISTIOCYTOSES

The three lesions described show a quite similar, or even identical histologic pattern. They are all included under the term "histiocytosis X" as we are unable to differentiate, histologically, between them. Their clinical course cannot be predicted.

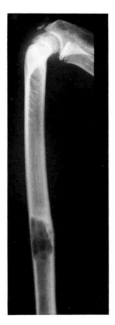

Fig. 2.139. Radiograph of an eosinophilic bone granuloma (histiocytosis X) of the shaft of the left humerus of a 9-year-old boy, showing a large well-defined osteolysis that has thinned the cortical bone from the inside but remains intraosseous.

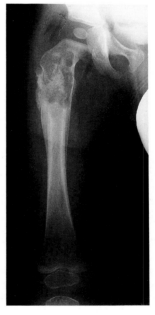

Fig. 2.140. Radiograph of an eosinophilic bone granuloma (histiocytosis X) of the right proximal femur of a 1-year-old child. The involved bone is expanded by the multicystic lesion, but the cortex is still intact. Distal to the lesion, a broad periosteal reaction is visible.

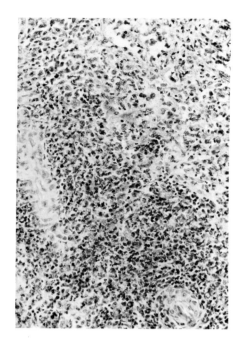

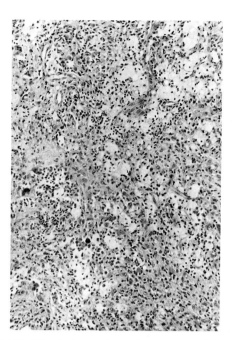

Fig. 2.141. Histologic section of an eosinophilic bone granuloma in its "proliferative" phase, with a cell-rich granulation tissue, including reticulum cells and histiocytes with isomorphic, roundish nuclei (H&E, ×82). Eosinophilic leukocytes are fairly rare but predominate in the second "granulomatous" phase when eosinophilic microabscesses may be observed.

Fig. 2.142. Histologic section of an eosinophilic bone granuloma in its "xanthomatous" phase, in which large histiocytes and foam cells predominate; many eosinophilic leukocytes are scattered between these (H&E, ×50). An identical histologic pattern is seen in Hand–Schüller–Christian disease.

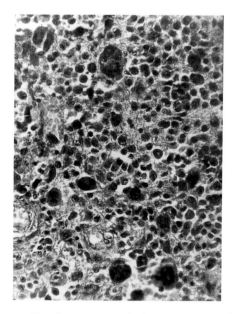

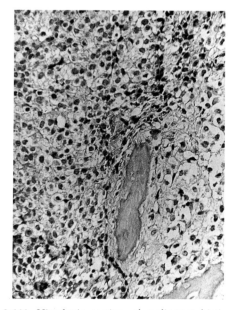

Fig. 2.143. Histologic section of a histiocytosis X at higher magnification shows histiocytes of different sizes and with roundish, indented nuclei (PAS, ×160). Many histiocytic giant cells are obvious.

Fig. 2.144. Histologic section of malignant histiocytosis, with histiocytes that have polymorphous and hyperchromatic nuclei and numerous mitoses (H&E, ×110).

EWING'S SARCOMA
(ICD-O-M-9260/3)

Ewing's sarcoma is a primary bone tumor that is almost entirely confined to children and adolescents; it is hardly ever seen in adults of more than 30 years. *It is a highly malignant tumor, consisting of densely-packed, small, uniform cells with round nuclei but without prominent nuclei or distinct cytoplasmic outlines; a prominent feature of the cells is that they contain glycogen granules.* In contrast to reticulosarcoma, no intercellular network of reticulin fibers is present. The pathogenesis of Ewing's sarcoma remains unknown. This highly anaplastic, small, round cell sarcoma of unknown histogenesis often cannot be differentiated in a biopsy from a metastatic malignant tumor such as neuroblastoma, small cell cancer of the lung or even leukemia.

The tumor causes severe local bone destruction of non-specific appearance, and local pain and swelling are the most common symptoms. The disease often imitates an acute osteomyelitis, with fever, leukocytosis, anemia and increased sedimentation and, in such cases, can only be diagnosed by bone biopsy. Ewing's sarcoma has a bad prognosis. Nowadays, it is treated with radiotherapy, multiagent chemotherapy and amputation, which has improved 5-year survival from less than 10% to about 40%.

Sites *(Fig. 2.145)*

Most Ewing's sarcomas develop in the marrow of the long tubular bones (femur, tibia, humerus) and the pelvis, but any bone may be involved, including the ribs, short tubular bones or jaw bones. The diaphyseal region is the most common location.

Age *(Fig. 2.146)*

Of all Ewing's sarcomas, 90% develop in children (32%) or adolescents (58%), and only 10% of the patients are older than 20 years. In the patient older than 30 years, metastatic carcinoma must be excluded.

Radiographic Features *(Figs 2.147–2.149)*

First, it must be emphasized that Ewing's sarcoma does not produce a characteristic radiologic picture. It may show a bone destruction similar to osteomyelitis or eosinophilic granuloma or another malignant tumor (e.g. osteosarcoma, lymphoma, central chondrosarcoma). Often, the involved bone shows a mottled destruction of the medullary bone, including the cortex (Fig. 2.147). A bone sclerosis, accompanied by circumscribed, irregular central areas of bone destruction (including the cortex), is a common feature of Ewing's sarcoma (Fig. 2.148). An irregular area of bone destruction together with sclerotic densities in a tubular or flat bone of a child should arouse suspicion of Ewing's sarcoma (Fig. 2.149). The lesion is ill-defined, and severe cortical destruction is typical. In addition, several periosteal bone reactions may be seen and some of these have an "onion-skin" appearance. On the whole, Ewing's sarcoma cannot be diagnosed radiologically with sufficient certainty, and in all cases a bone biopsy has to be performed.

Gross Pathologic Features *(Fig. 2.150)*

In the gross specimen, a grayish-white, translucent and glistening tumor tissue is seen in the involved bone, and there are areas of hemorrhage. The original bone, spongy and cortical, is severely destroyed, and the tumor may expand into the adjacent soft tissue. A prominent broadening of the periosteum is present, often in an "onion-skin" fashion. The neoplastic tissue may be admixed with the proliferating bony and fibrous periosteal tissue.

Histopathologic Features *(Figs 2.151 and 2.152)*

This is an extremely cellular tumor with many small rounded cells that are closely packed in dense sheets, cords or nests, between which large areas of necroses are prominent (Fig. 2.151). There is a rich vascular background; the tumor cells are best preserved around the numerous vessels, forming a rosette-like pattern. A fibrous stroma is scant, and the tumor tissue is extremely vulnerable, so that squeezing artifacts may very easily occur when performing a biopsy; this can make a histological diagnosis impossible. Tumor bone or cartilage formation is absent, and the original bone is completely destroyed. At higher magnification, the cells show round, hyperchromatic nuclei of rather uniform size, and mitoses are rare (Fig. 2.152). The tumor cells are about two or three times the size of lymphocytes, without distinctive cytoplasm. No reticulin fibers are demonstrated between the tumor cells. Using PAS stain, glycogen granules can be demonstrated within the cytoplasm, provided that specimens have

been properly decalcified (using EDTA), fixed (e.g. in 80% alcohol) and stained. This, together with the absence of reticulin fibers, enables differential diagnosis from reticulum cell sarcoma. On the whole, Ewing's sarcoma is a completely undifferentiated malignant tumor comprised of uncertain "round cells" and without any differentiated features. Other "round-cell" tumors (e.g. neuroblastoma, lymphoma, or primitive neuroectodermal tumor) must be considered in differential diagnosis.

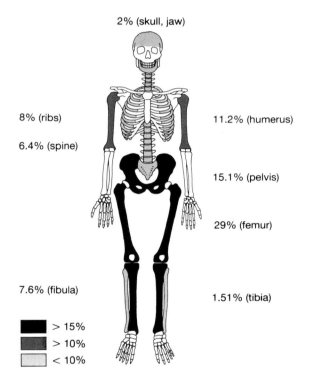

2% (skull, jaw)

8% (ribs)

6.4% (spine)

11.2% (humerus)

15.1% (pelvis)

29% (femur)

7.6% (fibula)

1.51% (tibia)

> 15%
> 10%
< 10%

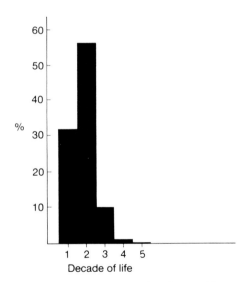

Fig. 2.145. Ewing's sarcoma: localization. Most of the tumors develop in the long tubular bones of the femur, tibia and humerus and the pelvic bone. However, other bones may also be involved.

Fig. 2.146. Ewing's sarcoma: age distribution. This sarcoma occurs mostly in children or adolescents and seldom in young adult life. In patients over 30 years of age it is extremely rare.

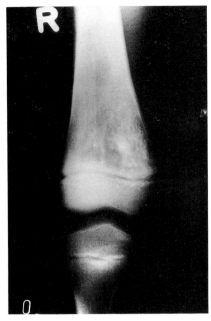

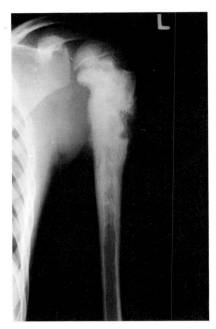

Fig. 2.147. Radiograph of a Ewing's sarcoma of the right distal femur of a 5-year-old child, showing a zone of mottled destructive osteolyses and sclerotic densities. These changes include the spongiosa as well as the cortex. The lesion is sharply demarcated by the epiphyseal plate, but is ill-defined towards the proximal bone.

Fig. 2.148. Radiograph of a Ewing's sarcoma of the left proximal humerus of an 11-year-old child. Bone sclerosis involves the total tumorous area, together with some small osteolyses. The tumor has penetrated the cortex, showing a severe expansion of the proximal humerus into the soft tissue.

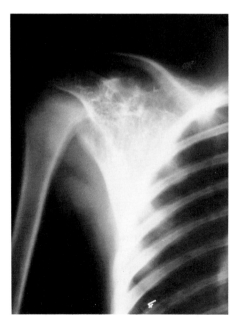

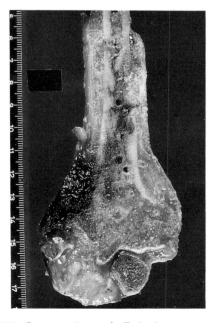

Fig. 2.149. Radiograph of a Ewing's sarcoma of the right scapula of a 10-year-old child. There is irregular bone destruction with sclerotic densities and spotty osteolyses. The cortex is also involved by the destructive process, indicating malignancy.

Fig. 2.150. Gross specimen of a Ewing's sarcoma of the left distal humerus of a 13-year-old child. The bone is completely destroyed and replaced by a grayish-white tumor tissue that has infiltrated the periosteum.

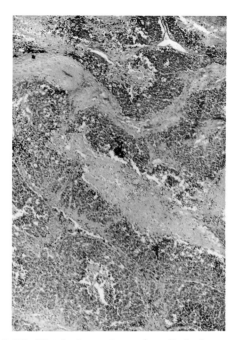

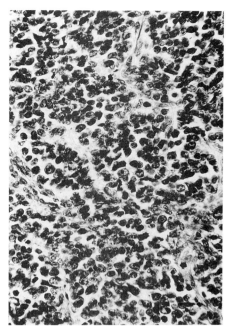

Fig. 2.151. Histologic section of a Ewing's sarcoma, showing a cellular tumor tissue with masses of small rounded cells that are closely packed in sheets, cords or nests, without any specific differentiation (H&E, ×40). Large areas of necrosis are seen in the tumor tissue, and the tumor cells are best preserved around the blood vessels.

Fig. 2.152. Histologic section of a Ewing's sarcoma at high magnification, showing the small, round tumor cells with polymorphic and hyperchromatic nuclei in loose distribution, without any special differentiation (PAS, ×140). In the scant cytoplasm of the tumor cells, glycogen granules, very characteristic of this tumor, can be demonstrated by PAS staining.

MALIGNANT LYMPHOMA OF BONE
(Reticulum Cell Sarcoma)
(ICD-O-M-9640/3)

Among other "round cell" sarcomas of bone, this tumor shows a remarkably better prognosis than Ewing's sarcoma. *It is a primary bone tumor that develops in the medullary cavity of a bone and derives from the reticular cells of the lymphatic system.* Therefore, this tumor is one of malignant lymphomas that occurs in the lymphatic tissues (lymph nodes, spleen, etc.) but, in some cases, starts in a bone. While most "reticulosarcomas" of the extraosseous system (lymph nodes) have proved to be immunoblastic sarcomas, reticulum cell sarcoma of the bone has not. In spite of the fact that other malignant lymphomas, such as Hodgkin's lymphomas, non-Hodgkin's lymphomas and leukemia, may primarily develop in a bone and may hardly be separable from reticulum cell sarcoma, the latter is sufficiently different, clinically and morphologically, to be considered a separate entity among bone marrow tumors.

This malignant tumor has a fairly good prognosis. It may be treated with chemotherapy or radiation therapy, but metastases can occur in regional lymph nodes (22%), lungs (10%) and other organs (47%).

Sites (Fig. 2.153)

Any bone may be involved, but most of the lesions are seen in the diaphyses of long bones (femur, tibia, humerus), and the knee region is the most frequently involved. Other frequent sites are the spine, pelvis, ribs and jaws.

Age (Fig. 2.154)

Most cases of malignant lymphomas of the skeleton are adults of higher age-groups; but this disease may also occur in children and adolescents (about 20%). In children, though, this is a fairly rare tumor (5%).

Radiographic Features (Fig. 2.155)

Reticulum cell sarcoma appears as a destructive lesion that may only reveal a faint loosening of the spongiosa and cortex which is ill-defined; in some cases, however real osteolytic defects may

even be seen, indicating malignant growth. In the early stage, little cortical destruction and periosteal reaction is recognized; later, however, the cortex is disrupted and an adjacent soft tissue mass can be seen.

Histopathologic Features (Fig. 2.156)

A diffuse pattern of reticulum cells fills the marrow space between the original bone trabeculae, which show some destruction. Necrotic areas are rare. The tumor cells have indistinct boundaries and little cytoplasm, with processes adjoining neighboring cells. Their nuclei are larger than those in Ewing's sarcoma, varying in size and shape; but they are hyperchromatic, indented, polymorphous, and irregular in shape. Mitoses are rare. Fields of lymphocytes and lymphoblasts may be seen within the tumor pattern. Most reticulum cell sarcomas have a mixed cell population, including some multinucleated giant cells. A miscellaneous fibrous stroma is present, but the prominent feature is the dense network of reticulin fibers, which distinguishes the lesion from Ewing's sarcoma. In addition, and in contrast to Ewing's sarcoma, no PAS-positive granules (glycogen) are seen in the cytoplasm in reticulum cell sarcoma.

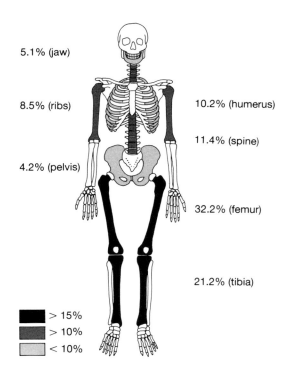

5.1% (jaw)

8.5% (ribs)

4.2% (pelvis)

10.2% (humerus)

11.4% (spine)

32.2% (femur)

21.2% (tibia)

■ > 15%
■ > 10%
□ < 10%

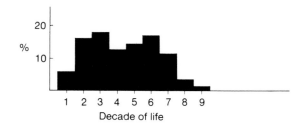

Fig. 2.154. Reticulum cell sarcoma: age distribution. There is an even distribution throughout life; children and adolescents account for 20% of the cases.

Fig. 2.153. Reticulum cell sarcoma: localization. The diaphyses of long bones (femur, tibia, humerus) are the most frequent sites of this medullary bone tumor; other bones, especially the spine, may also be involved.

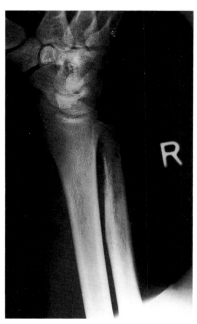

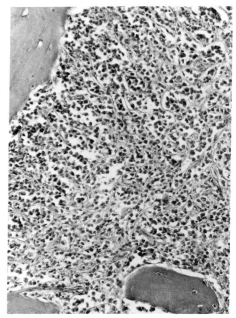

Fig. 2.155. Radiograph of a reticulum cell sarcoma of the right distal ulna of a 15-year-old boy, showing an undefined destructive lesion with a faint loosening of the spongiosa and cortex, with small osteolyses.

Fig. 2.156. Histologic section of a reticulum cell sarcoma of bone, with a diffuse pattern of atypical reticulum cells that fills the whole narrow space (H&E, ×100). The tumor cells have indistinct boundaries and little cytoplasm; they have polymorphous and hyperchromatic nuclei, but mitoses are rare. Within this miscellaneous small cell tumor tissue, including various lymphoid cells, exists a dense network of reticulin fibers that can be demonstrated histologically.

MEDULLARY PLASMOCYTOMA
(Plasma Cell Myeloma)
(ICD-O-M-9730/3)

This is a frequent malignant primary bone tumor deriving from the bone marrow. However, it never occurs in children or adolescents.

LITERATURE
Tumors of Marrow Origin

Adkins KF, Marinez MG, Hartley MW. Ultrastructure of giant-cell lesions. A peripheral giant-cell reparative granuloma. Oral Surg 1969;28:713–23

Adler CP. Granulomatöse Erkrankungen im Knochen. Verh Dtsch Ges Pathol 1980;64:359–65

Adler CP, Härle F. Zur Differentialdiagnose osteofibröser Kiefererkrankungen. Verh Dtsch Ges Pathol 1974;58: 308–14

Adler CP, Schaefer HE. Histiocytosis X of the left femur – proximal segment. Case report. Skeletal Radiol 1988; 17:531–5

Augerau B, Thuilleux G, Moinet Ph. Eosinophil granuloma of bones. Report of 15 cases including 10 survivals with an average follow up of 4 years. J Chir (Paris) 1977;113: 159–70

Austin LT Jr, Dahlin DC, Royer EQ. Giant-cell reparative granuloma and related conditions affecting the jawbones. Oral Surg 1959;12:1285–95

Bauer FHC, Mirra JM, Urist MR. Bone induction by Ewing's sarcoma. Arch Pathol Lab Med 1981;105:322–4

Beckstead JH, Wood GS, Turner RR. Histiocytosis X cells and Langerhans cells: enzyme histochemical and immunologic similarities. Hum Pathol 1984;15:826–33

Bergholz M, Schauer A, Poppe H. Diagnostic and differential diagnostic aspects in histiocytosis X diseases. Pathol Res Pract 1979;166:59–71

Catto M, Stevens J. Liposarcoma of bone. J Pathol Bacteriol 1963;86:248–53

Cheyne C. Histiocytosis X. J Bone Jt Surg 1971;B-53:366–82

Child PL. Lipoma of the os calcis. Report of a case. Am J Clin Pathol 1955;25:1050–2

Cuvelier A, L'Her P, Schill H, Jancovici R, Bassoulet J, Vauterin G, et al. Ewing's sarcoma and peripheral neuroectodermal tumors. Report of a case with laterothoracic localization. Rev Pneumol Clin 1990;46:116–22

Dawson EK. Liposarcoma of bone. J Pathol Bacteriol 1955; 70:513–20

Dickman PS, Liotta LA, Triche TJ. Ewing's sarcoma: characterization in established culture and evidence of its histogenesis. Lab Invest 1982;47:375–82

Estes DN, Magill HL, Thompson EI, Hayes FA. Primary Ewing sarcoma: follow-up with Ga-67 scintigraphy. Radiology 1990;177:449–53

Evans JE. Ewing's tumour: uncommon presentation of an uncommon tumour. Med J Aust 1977;1:590–1

Favara BE, McCarthy RC, Mierau GW. Histiocytosis X. Hum Pathol 1983;14:663–76

Fiche M, Le-Tourneau A, Audouin J, Touzard RC, Diebold J. A case of primary osseous malignant immunoblastic B-cell lymphoma with intracytoplasmic mu lambda immunglobulin inclusions. Histopathology 1990;16: 167–72

Gedigk P, Bechtelsheimer H, Koch H. Das eosinophile Granulom des Knochens. Med Welt 1964;50:2699–701

Goldman RL. Primary liposarcoma of one. Report of a case. Am J Clin Pathol 1964;42:503–8

Hermichen HG, Wentzensen A. Stabile Osteosynthese nach Beckenschaufelresektion bei intraossärem Ewing-Sarkom. Aktuel Traumatol 1988;18:204–8

Hustu HO, Pinkel D. Lymphoma, Hodgkin's disease and leukemia in bone. Clin Orthop 1967;52:83–93

Ide F, Iwase T, Saito I, Umemura S, Nakajima T. Immunohistochemical and ultrastructural analysis of the proliferating cells in histiocytosis X. Cancer 1984;53: 917–21

Ivins JC, Dahlin DC. Malignant lymphoma (reticulum cell sarcoma) of bone. Proc Mayo Clin 1963;38:375–85

Jaffe HL. Giant-cell reparative granuloma, traumatic bone cyst, and fibrous (fibro-osseous) dysplasia of the jawbones. Oral Surg 1953;6:159–75

Jaffe R, Santamaria M, Yunis EJ, Tannery NH, Agostini RM, Medina J, et al. The neuroectodermal tumour of bone. Am J Surg Pathol 1984;8:885–98

Kadin ME, Bensch KG. On the origin of Ewing's tumor. Cancer 1971;27:257–73

Kauffman SL, Stout AP. Lipoblastic tumors of children. Cancer (Phil) 1959;12:912–25

Kissane JM, Askin FB, Foulkes M, Stratton LB, Shirley SF. Ewing's sarcoma study. Hum Pathol 1983;14:773–9

Kozlowski K, Barylak A, Campbell J, Hoeffel JD, Beluffi G, Masel J, et al. Primary sacral bone tumours in children (report of 16 cases with a short literature review). Austr Radiol 1990;34:142–9

Ladanyi M, Heinemann FS, Huvos AG, Rao PH, Chen QG, Jhanwar SC. Neural differentiation in small round cell tumors of bone and soft tissue with the translocation t (11;22) (q24;q12): an immunohistochemical study of 11 cases. Hum Pathol 1990;21:1245–51

Landing BJ. Lymphohistiocytosis in childhood. Pathologic comparison with fatal Letterer–Siwe disease (disseminated visceral histiocytosis X). Perspect Pediatr Pathol 1987;9:48–74

Lichtenstein L. Histiocytosis X, integration of eosinophilic granuloma of bone, Letterer–Siwe disease and Schüller–Christian disease as related manifestations of a single nosologic entity. Arch Pathol 1953;50:84–102

Lichtenstein L, Jaffe HL. Eosinophilic granuloma of bone with report of case. Am J Pathol 1940;16:595–604

Llombart-Bosch A, Carda C, Peydro-Olaya A, Noguera R, Perez-Bacete M, Pellin A, et al. Soft tissue Ewing's sarcoma. Characterization in established cultures and xenografts with evidence of a neuroectodermic phenotype. Cancer 1990;66:2589–601

Macintosh DJ, Price CHG, Jeffree GM. Malignant lymphoma (reticulosarcoma) in bone. Clin Oncol 1977; 3:287–300

Matejovsky Z, Povysil C. Das Ewing-Sarkom. Neue klinisch-pathologische Aspekte. Zentralbl Allg Pathol 1986;132:11–24

Mickelson MR, Bonfiglio M. Eosinophilic granuloma and its variations. Orthop Clin N Am 1977;8:933–45

Moorefield WG Jr, Urbaniak JR, Gonzalvo AAA. Intramedullary lipoma of the distal femur. South Med J (Bgham Ala) 1976;69:1210–11

Moser RP, Davis MJ, Gilkey FW, Kransdorf MJ, Rosado de Christenson ML, Kumar R, et al. Primary Ewing's sarcoma of rib. Radiographics 1990;10:899–914

Nezelof C. Histiocytosis X: A histological and histogenetic study. In: Rosenberg HS, Bolande RP, eds. Perspectives in pediatric pathology, vol 5. New York: Masson, 1979:153–78

Nezelof C, Barbey S. Histiocytosis. Nosology and pathology. Pediatr Pathol 1985;3:1–41

Nezelof C, Frileux-Herbet F, Cronier-Sachot J. Disseminated histiocytosis X: analysis of prognostic factors based on a retrospective study of 50 cases. Cancer 1979;44:1824–38

Perez-Atayde AR, Grier H, Weinstein H, Delorey M, Leslie N, Vawter G. Neuroectodermal differentiation in bone tumors presenting as Ewing's sarcoma. Proc Int Soc Pediatr Oncol 1985;17:61

Raimer SS, Hollabaugh E. Histiocytic symdromes. Dermatol Clin 1989;7:491–503

Rehak L, Blasko I, Huraj E Jr, Galbavy S. Problems in the diagnosis of Ewing's sarcoma. Acta Chir Orthop Traumatol Cech 1989;56:529–37

Retz LD. Primary liposarcoma of bone. Report of a case and review of the literature. J Bone Jt Surgery 1961;A-43:123–9

Risdall RJ, Dehner LP, Duray P, Kobrinsky N, Robison L, Nesbit ME Jr. Histiocytosis X (Langerhans' cell histiocytosis). Prognostic role of histiopathology. Arch Pathol Lab Med 1983;107:59–63

Ruco LP, Remotti D, Monardo F, Uccini S, Cristiani ML, Modesti A, et al. Letterer–Siwe disease: immunohistochemical evidence for a proliferative disorder involving immature cells of Langerhans' lineage. Virchows Arch A Pathol Anat 1988;413:239–247

Rüschoff J, Rieger CHL, Göbel F-J, Thomas C. Histiocytosis X. Med Welt (Stuttg) 1988;39:886–9

Salzer M, Salzer-Kuntschik M. Zur Frage der sogenannten zentralen Knochenlipome. Beitr Pathol Anat 1965;132:365–75

Scarpa S, D'Orazi G, Modesti M, Modesti A. Ewing's sarcoma lines synthesize laminin and fibronectin. Virchows Arch [A] 1987;410:375–81

Schajowicz F. Eosinophilic granuloma of bone and its relationship to Hand–Schüller–Christian and Letterer–Siwe syndromes. J Bone Jt Surg 1973;B-55:545–65

Schwartz A, Shuster M, Becker SM. Liposarcoma of bone: report of a case and review of the literature. J Bone Jt Surg 1970;A-52:171–7

Short JH. Malignant lymphoma (reticulum cell sarcoma) of bone. Radiography 1977;43:139–43

Smith WE, Fienberg R. Intraosseous lipoma of bone. Cancer (Phil) 1957;10:1151–2

Sneath RS, Carter SR, Grimer RJ. Ewing's sarcoma. Fifteen years of experience. Chir Organi Mov 1990;75:260–1

Spritz RA. The familial histiocytoses. Pediatr Pathol 1985;3:43–57

Telles NC, Rabson AS, Pomeroy TC. Ewing's sarcoma: an autopsy study. Cancer (Phil) 1978;41:2321–9

Toni A, Sudanese A, Ciaroni D, Picci P, Bacci G, Neff JR, et al. The role of surgery in the local treatment of Ewing's sarcoma of the extremities. Chir Organi Mov 1990;75:262–4

Triche TJ. Round cell tumors in childhood: the application of newer techniques to the differential diagnosis. In: Rosenberg HS, Bernstein J, eds. Perspectives in pediatric pathology. New York: Masson, 1982:279–322

Triche TJ, Askin FB. Neuroblastoma and the differential diagnosis of small-, round-blue-cell tumors. Hum Pathol 1983;14:569–595

Triche TJ, Tsokos M, Miser JS, Reynolds CP, Israel MA, Donner L. Peripheral neuroepithelioma. A bone or soft tissue tumor resembling Ewing's sarcoma and distinct from neuroblastoma. Proc Int Soc Pediatr Oncol 1985;17:47

Uehlinger E, Botsztejn C, Schinz HR. Ewingsarkom und Knochenretikulosarkom. Klinik, Diagnose und Differentialdiagnose. Oncologia (Basel) 1948;1:193–245

Willis RA. Metastatic neuroblastoma in bone presenting the Ewing syndrome, with a discussion of "Ewing's sarcoma". Am J Pathol 1940;16:317–31

Tumors of Vascular Origin

BONE HEMANGIOMA
(ICD-O-M-9120/0)

Hemangiomas of bone are infrequent, about 1.2% of all primary bone tumors. In children, they are even more rare, though they do occur. *Bone hemangioma is a benign lesion composed of newly formed blood vessels, capillaries or cavernous blood spaces filled with blood; it leads to a local loss of bone tissue, forming an osteolysis.* In *skeletal hemangiomatosis*, multiple foci are observed throughout the skeleton. This lesion is probably a local hamartoma, rather than a true tumor growth, and therefore should be classified as a dysontogenetic tumor.

Most bone hemangiomas are largely asymptomatic, but local swelling, pain or, occasionally, a pathologic fracture may occur; in the spine, neurologic symptoms may arise.

Radiotherapy is usually successful in vascular bone lesions, but many undergo spontaneous regression with sclerotic reaction.

Sites (*Fig. 2.157*)

The main site of bone hemangiomas is the spine, nearly 60% being found in the vertebral bodies. In 27% of such cases, the cranium (including the jaws) is involved.

Age (*Fig. 2.158*)

Hemangiomas of bone are usually found in adults, mainly in the fifth decade; less than 5% are detected in children or adolescents.

Radiographic Features (*Figs 2.159–2.161*)

An intraosseous hemangioma produces a radiolucent defect, with little bone reaction in its surroundings; this picture is not specific to hemangioma. In the skull, a fairly sharply defined defect is seen (Fig. 2.159); and when expansion is inward as well as outward, a characteristic "sunburst-phenomenon" is often produced by radiating spicules of bone. Vertebral lesions show bony rarefaction of vertebral bodies, with prominent parallel vertical striations or a honeycomb appearance. In the long tubular bones, an osteolytic and ill-defined lesion (Fig. 2.160) or mottled osteolyses are noticed. A hemangioma may also develop in the periosteal region of a bone producing sclerotic broadening of the periosteum with osteolytic foci that reach into the cortex (Fig. 2.161).

Gross Pathologic Features (*Fig. 2.162*)

In section, an ill-defined focus of a dark red, soft and bloody mass is seen in which the bone tissue is completely destroyed. Usually no adjacent bone reaction is visible, but in some cases, especially in the skull, there may be dense, sclerotic trabeculae traversing the involved areas, causing a "soap bubble" appearance.

Histopathologic Features (*Figs 2.163 and 2.164*)

All hemangiomas consist of a conglomerate of newly formed thin-walled vascular channels between which is a fibrous stroma. The tumorous vessels may be blood capillaries (Fig. 2.163); but most lesions show dilated vessels, and so are a cavernous hemangioma (Fig. 2.164).

In *skeletal hemangiomatosis*, multiple osteolytic lesions arise throughout the skeleton, and in some cases a pathologic bone fracture may occur (Fig. 2.165). Radiologic, gross and histologic features are the same as in solitary lesions. A massive osteolysis may occur in the involved bones leading to Gorham–Stout syndrome.

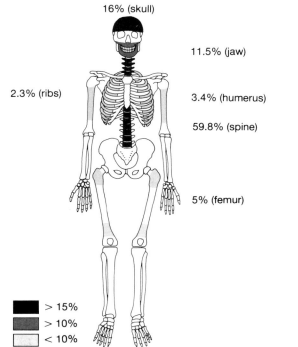

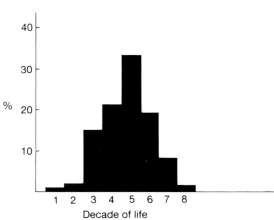

Fig. 2.157. Bone hemangioma: localization. Most of these lesions are found in the spine (60%), skull and jaws. Other sites can be involved, but this is rare.

Fig. 2.158. Bone hemangioma: age distribution. Only 5% of these lesions are found in children or adolescents; most are detected in adults.

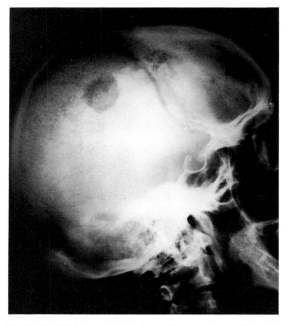

Fig. 2.159. Radiograph of a bone hemangioma of the right side of the skull, showing a sharply defined osteolytic focus including some faint sclerotic densities.

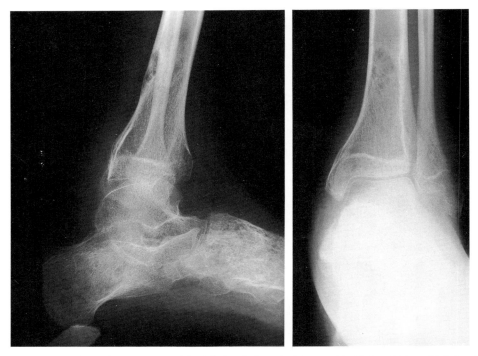

Fig. 2.160. Radiograph of a bone hemangioma of the left distal tibia of a 14-year-old girl, in which an ill-defined lesion with mottled osteolyses is visible. The outer contours of the involved bone are intact; the cortex is not destroyed.

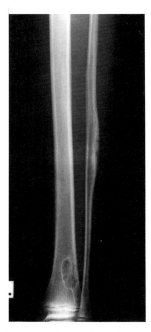

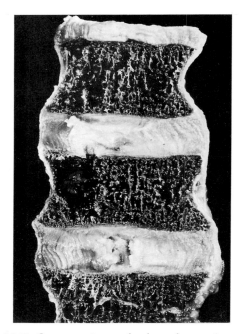

Fig. 2.161. Radiograph of a periosteal bone hemangioma of the left fibular shaft of a 14-year-old girl, showing a broadening of the periosteum, including some osteolytic foci and cortical erosions. (In addition, a non-ossifying bone fibroma of the left distal tibial metaphysis is visible.)

Fig. 2.162. Gross specimen of a bone hemangioma of a vertebral body with an ill-defined osteolysis including a bloody mass in which the bone is destroyed.

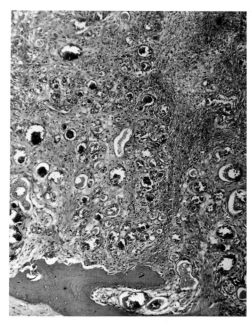

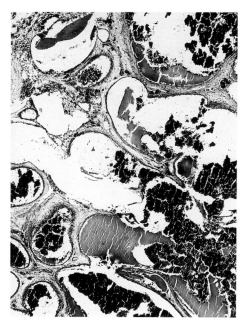

Fig. 2.163. Histologic section of a capillary bone hemangioma with many capillaries in a loose fibrous stroma; there is no new bone formation (H&E, ×32). The adjacent bone trabeculae show deep resorption lacunae.

Fig. 2.164. Histologic section of a cavernous bone hemangioma showing many extremely dilated blood vessels with thin walls and filled with blood (H&E, ×64). No original bone trabeculae are seen within this tumor.

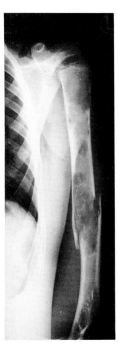

Fig. 2.165. Radiograph of a bone hemangioma of the left humerus of an 11-year-old boy with skeletal hemangiomatosis. There is a large intraosseous osteolysis, expanding the bone and thinning the cortex from the inside, and through this lesion a pathologic fracture is visible.

BONE LYMPHANGIOMA
(ICD-O-M-9176/0)

This very rare, benign vascular bone tumor can best be demonstrated by lymphangiography. *Bone lymphangioma is a benign lesion consisting of newly formed lymph vessels; it destroys the bone, inducing a local osteolysis.* The proliferates of lymphatic vessels arise inside the bone and have radiologic features similar to those of hemangiomas. The tumor may, in rare cases, occur in children; it may cause pathologic bone fracture. Therapy is the same as that for hemangioma.

Sites

Bone lymphangioma is not specific to any part of the skeleton.

Age

There is no predilection for a specific age-group, but children and adolescents can be affected.

Radiographic Features (Fig. 2.166)

A circumscribed local osteolysis or ill-defined, mottled bone destruction indicates pathologic bone destruction, but this is not diagnostic for the lesion. A pathologic bone fracture may occur.

Histopathologic Features (Fig. 2.167)

Between the trabeculae, large lymphatic vessels with very thin walls and filled with lymph fluid are obvious. In the surrounding area, there is edematous fat tissue. In addition, some areas of hemangioma may be present.

In a bone biopsy, it may be extremely difficult to recognize a bone lymphangioma because the lymphatic vessels may be artificially collapsed, so that the underlying lesion is not visible. Lymphangiographies are extremely helpful to confirm the diagnosis.

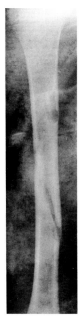

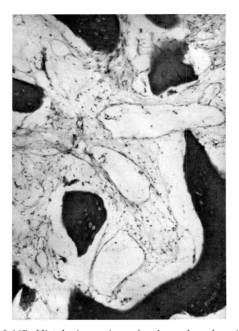

Fig. 2.166. Radiograph of a bone lymphangioma of the right humerus of a 13-year-old boy with a pathologic fracture. Some ill-defined osteolytic foci are seen in the involved shaft.

Fig. 2.167. Histologic section of a bone lymphangioma, showing large lymphatic vessels with thin walls in the medullary cave between the spongy bone trabeculae (H&E, ×50).

MASSIVE OSTEOLYSIS
(Gorham-Stout disease)

This "vanishing" or "phantom" bone disease is associated with angiomas of bone. It is a relatively rare condition, which usually occurs in children and adolescents. *A progressive regional loss of bone with resultant bone instability and deformity is the characteristic symptom of this disease, and no pathognomonic histologic feature is evident.* The process is slowly progressive replacing the bone by fibrous tissue.

There is no satisfactory therapy for this unusual bone disease.

Sites

No predominant sites have been recognized.

Age

The great majority of patients are children or young adults.

Radiographic Features (Fig. 2.168)

The involved bone "vanishes", i.e. no outer contours are visible and there is only a diffuse cloudy shadow representing the former bone. The disease is not limited by the adjacent joints and may expand into the neighboring bone.

Histopathologic Features (*Fig. 2.169*)

A marked increase of intraosseous capillaries can be seen in the lesion; these are blood vessels or lymphatic vessels. The spongy bone trabeculae inbetween are severely reduced. A skeletal angiomatosis is presumed to be the underlying defect. There is no characteristic histologic pattern, and the diagnosis can only be established by also referring to the radiologic image.

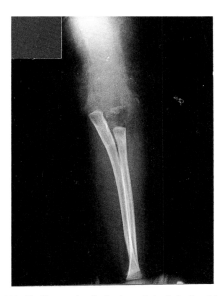

Fig. 2.168. Radiograph of a lesion of the left distal humerus of a 2-year-old child with Gorham–Stout disease, showing complete osteolytic destruction of the bone. The humerus presents merely as a cloudy ("vanished"), undefined shadow.

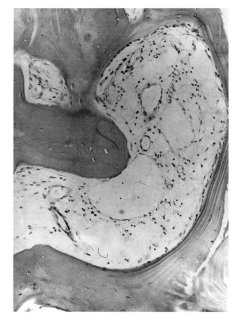

Fig. 2.169. Histologic section of a lesion in Gorham–Stout syndrome, showing many dilated and thin-walled blood vessels in the medullary cavity between the smooth bone trabeculae (H&E, ×82).

HEMANGIOSARCOMA OF BONE
(ICD-O-M-9120/3)

Malignant vascular tumors are extremely rare in bone, comprising, overall, less than 1% of primary malignant bone tumors; they are even more rare in children. *Angiosarcoma (malignant hemangioendothelioma) is a highly malignant growth originating from blood vessels or lymphatic vessels and forming irregular vascular channels, lined by layers of atypical, immature endothelial cells, and accompanied by solid areas of anaplastic cells.*

This tumor has a poor prognosis, and metastases are frequent and occur early on. Radiotherapy and chemotherapy may prolong survival time, but nearly all patients die within 2 years of diagnosis.

Sites and Age

Angiosarcomas may involve multiple bones, and, in a single tumor, the long tubular bones are the most common site. This rare tumor is seen in all age-groups but is scarce in children.

Radiographic Features *(Fig. 2.170)*

In the region of tumor growth, there are multiple osteolytic zones without any reactive bone formation, and, in advanced cases, the bone is completely destroyed. A huge tumor shadow, extending boundaries of bone, may be visible. In all cases, a malignant tumor growth is demonstrated.

Histopathologic Features *(Fig. 2.171)*

An extremely cell-rich tumor tissue is characteristic of this lesion. New blood vessel formations are present, but they may only be faint, the endothelial tumor cells dominating. A severe polymorphism of endothelial cells, including dark nuclei of different sizes, is obvious. Papillary projections of these cells are frequently seen within the tumorous vessels, and atypical mitoses are numerous. The tissue may be extremely undifferentiated, and, in such cases, even immunohistochemical investigations may not indicate a vascular tumor.

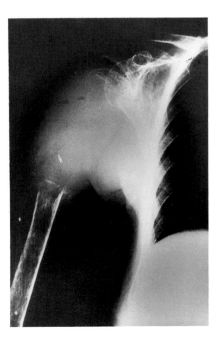

Fig. 2.170. Radiograph of a hemangiosarcoma of bone of the right proximal humerus of a 16-year-old girl; the whole bone is completely destroyed and a huge soft tumor mass is obvious, expanding far into the soft tissues.

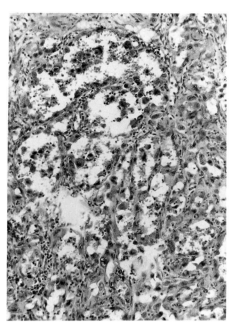

Fig. 2.171. Histologic section of a hemangiosarcoma of bone with atypical blood vessels lined by polymorphous endothelia, possessing polymorphous and hyperchromatic nuclei and many atypical mitoses (H&E, ×82). The endothelial tumor cells are often multilayered, forming papillary projections.

HEMANGIOPERICYTOMA OF BONE
(ICD-O-M-9150/1)

Hemangiopericytoma is an extremely rare primary bone tumor that occurs in every age-group, including children. *The tumor derives from the vascular pericytes and shows an aggressive growth, causing severe local bone destruction in which the histologic aspect does not indicate whether the tumor is benign or malignant.* Those cases that have been observed give no indication of predominant sites or age-groups.

On the radiograph (Fig. 2.172), an osteolytic bone destruction indicating malignancy is seen.

Histologic slides (Fig. 2.173) show a cell-rich tumor tissue with many vascular spaces that are lined by flat endothelial cells and surrounded by a proliferation of round, oval or spindle-shaped cells of rather uniform size, surrounded by reticulin fibrils. Within these tumorous pericytes, cellular and nuclear polymorphy and numerous mitoses may be frequent. However, histologic findings cannot predict the clinical course. Thus, the tumor has to be eliminated completely by operation or radiation.

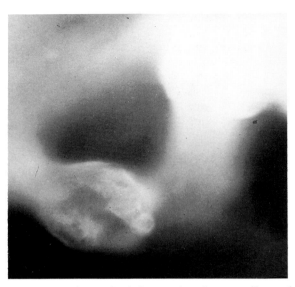

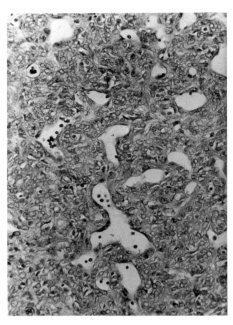

Fig. 2.172. Radiograph of a hemangiopericytoma of bone of the left ischium of a 14-year-old child; there is an expanding lesion, with osteosclerotic and osteolytic areas and no clear margins.

Fig. 2.173. Histologic section of a hemangiopericytoma of bone in which many vascular spaces with small endothelia are seen, surrounded by polymorphous pericytes, including polymorphous and hyperchromatic nuclei with many mitoses, and surrounded by reticulin fibrils (PAS, ×82).

LITERATURE
Tumors of Vascular Origin

Adler CP. Adamantinoma of the tibia mimicking osteofibrous dysplasia (case report). Skeletal Radiol 1990;19:55–8

Adler CP, Klümper A. Röntgenologische und pathologischanatomische Aspekte von Knochentumoren. Radiologe 1977;17:355–92

Adler CP, Träger D. Malignes Hämangioperizytom – ein Weichteil- und Knochentumor. Z Orthop 1989;127:611–5

Agnoli AL, Kirchhoff D, Eggert H. Röntgenologische Befunde beim Hämangiom des Schädels. Radiologe 1978;18:37–41

Angervall L, Kindblom LG, Karlsson K, Stener B. Atypical hemangioendothelioma of venous origin. A clinicopathologic, angiographic, immunohistochemical, and ultrastructural study of two endothelial tumors within the concept of histiocytoid hemangioma. Am J Surg Pathol 1985;9:504–16

Battifora H. Hemangiopericytoma – ultrastructural study of five cases. Cancer 1973;31:1418–32

Boker SM, Cullen GM, Swank M, Just JF. Hemangioma of sternum (case report). Skeletal Radiol 1990;19:77–8

Bullough PG, Goodfellow JW. Solitary lymphangioma of bone. A case report. J Bone Jt Surg 1976;58-A:418–9

Bundens WD Jr, Brighton CT. Malignant hemangioendothelioma of bone. Report of two cases and review of the literature. J Bone Jt Surg 1965;47-A:762–72

Campanacci M, Boriani S, Giunti A. Hemangioendothelioma of bone: a study of 29 cases. Cancer 1980;46:804–14

Cone RO, Hudkins P, Nguyen V, Merriwether WA. Histiocytoid hemangioma of bone: a benign lesion which may mimic angiosarcoma. Report of a case and review of literature. Skeletal Radiol 1983;10:165–9

Dannaker C, Piacquadio D, Willoughby CB, Goltz RW. Histiocytoid hemangioma: a disease spectrum. Report of a case with simultaneous cutaneous and bone involvement limited to one extremity. J Am Acad Dermatol 1989;21:404–9

Davis E, Morgan LR. Hemangioma of bone. Arch Oto-laryngol 1974;99:443–5

De Smet AA, Inscore D, Neff JR. Histiocytoid hemangioma of the distal end of the right humerus (case report). Skeletal Radiol 1989;18:60–5

Dorfman HD, Steiner GC, Jaffe HL. Vascular tumors of bone. Hum Pathol 1971;2:349–76

Dunlop J. Primary hemangiopericytoma of bone: report of two cases. J Bone Jt Surg 1973;55-B:854–7

Eimoto T. Ultrastructure of an infantile hemangipericytoma. Cancer 1977;40:2161–70

Enzinger FM, Smith BH. Hemangiopericytoma – an analysis of 106 cases. Hum Pathol 1976;7:61–82

Fairbank T. Hemangioma of bone. Practioner 1956;177:707–11

Falkner S, Tilling G. Primary lymphangioma of bone. Acta Orthop scand 1956;26:99–110

Garcia-Moral, CA. Malignant hemangioendothelioma of bone: Review of world literature and report of two cases. Clin Orthop 1972;82:70–9

Hartmann WH, Stewart FW. Hemangioendothelioma of bones. Unusual tumor characterized by indolent course. Cancer (Phil) 1962;15:846–54

Kulenkampff H-A, Adler CP. Radiologische und pathologische Befunde beim Gorham–Stout-Syndrom (Massive Osteolyse). Verh Dtsch Ges Pathol 1987;71:574

Kulenkampff H-A, Richter GM, Adler CP, Haase WE. Massive Osteolyse (Gorham–Stout-Syndrom) – Klinik, Diagnostik, Therapie und Prognose. In: Willert H-G, Heuck FHW, eds. Neuere Ergebnisse in der Osteologie. Heidelberg: Springer, 1989:387–97

Kulenkampff H-A, Richter GM, Hasse WE, Adler CP. Massive pelvic osteolysis in the Gorham–Stout syndrome. Int Orthop 1990;14:361–6

Larsson SE, Lorentzon R, Boquist L. Malignant hemangioendothelioma of bone. J Bone Jt Surg 1975;57-A:84–9

Legré G, Payan H, Aubert M. Osseous hemangiopericytoma. Rev Chir Orthop 1966;52:551–4

Marcial-Rojas R. Primary hemangiopericytoma of bone. Review of the literature and report of the first case with metastases. Cancer 1960;13:308–11

Maruyama N, Kumagai Y, Ishida Y. Epitheloid haemangioendothelioma of the bone tissue. Virchows Arch [A] 1985;407:159–65

McMaster M, Soule E, Ivins J. Hemangiopericytoma – a clinico-pathologic study and long-term follow-up of 60 patients. Cancer 1975;36:2232–44

Mirra JM, Kameda N. Myxoid angioblastomatosis of bones. A case report of a rare, multifocal entity with light, ultramicroscopic, and immunopathologic correlation. Am J Surg Pathol 1985;9:450–8

Mirra JG, Chu FC, Fortner JG. The role of radiotherapy in the management of hemangiopericytoma. Report of 11 new cases and review of the literature. Cancer 1977;39:1254–9

Newland RC, Maxwell LE, Constance TJ, Fox RM. Malignant hemangipericytoma: case report and ultrastructural study. Pathology 1978;10:277–83

Nunnery EW, Kahn LB, Reddick RL, Lipper S. Hemangiopericytoma. A light microscopic and ultrastructural study. Cancer 1981;47:906–14

O'Brien P, Brasfield RD. Hemangiopericytoma. Cancer 1965;18:249–52

Ose D, Vollmer R, Shelburne J, McComb R, Harrelson J. Histiocytoid hemangioma of the skin and scapula. Cancer 1983;51:1656–63

Otis J, Hutter RVP, Foote FW Jr, Marcove RC, Stewart FW. Hemangioendothelioma of bone. Surg Gynecol Obstet 1968;127:295–305

Rosenquist CJ, Wolfe DC. Lymphangioma of bone. J Bone Jt Surg 1968;50-A:158–62

Sherman RS, Wilner D. The roentgen diagnosis of hemangioma of bone. Am J Roentgenol 1961;86:1146–59

Tsuneyoshi M, Dorfman HD, Bauer TW. Epithelioid hemangioendothelioma of bone. – A clinicopathologic, ultrastructural, and immunohistochemical study. Am J Surg Pathol 1986;10(11):754–64

Unni KK, Ivins JC, Beabout JW, Dahlin DC. Hemangioma, hemangiopericytoma, and hemangioendothelioma (angiosarcoma) of bone. Cancer 1974;27:1403–14

Warman S, Myssiorek D. Hemangioma of the zygomatic bone. Ann Otol Rhinol Laryngol 1989;98:655–8

Wold LE, Unni KK, Beabout JW, Ivins JC, Bruckman JE, Dahlin DC. Hemangioendothelial sarcoma of bone. Am J Surg Pathol 1982;6:59–70

Yaghmai I. Angiographic manifestations of softtissue and osseous hemangiopericytomas. Radiology 1978;126:653–9

Tumors of Neurogenous Origin

SCHWANNOMA (Neurilemoma, Neurinoma) of Bone
(ICD-O-M-9560/0)

Primary bone tumors of neurogenous origin, benign or malignant, are rare. They do, nevertheless, occur in children. *Schwannoma of bone is a very rare primary bone tumor of nerve sheath origin; it is composed of a nerve-fibre tissue with Schwann cells in twisted rows or palisades (Verocay bodies – Antoni type A pattern) or in a pattern of loosely arranged cells within a wide-meshed, fibrillar stroma (Antoni type B pattern), inducing a local osteolytic lesion.* Such tumors are relatively frequent in soft tissues, where schwannomas may even be malignant; however, the malignant variant is never seen in bone.

Surgical excision is the therapy of choice.

Sites

No specific sites have to be identified for this rare tumor.

Age

Most cases are observed in adults and some in adolescents.

Radiographic Features (*Fig. 2.174*)

Schwannomas produce a cystic-like rarefaction that may be ill-defined or may sometimes have a slightly sclerotic border. The adjacent cortex is thinned and eroded from the inside, but intact in benign lesions. The lesion may occur in any part of a bone, but it is encountered mainly in the shaft or end of a tubular bone.

Histopathologic Features (*Fig. 2.175*)

Spindle-shaped cells of fibrogenic appearance are the basic histologic impression. There are compact bundles and whorls of Schwann cells, with their nuclei aligned in rows or palisades. In cases of Antoni type B pattern, a loose network of myxomatous tissue is visible, together with often irregularly sized nuclei, dark-staining and bizarre, which form Verocay bodies and are reminiscent of a malignant tumor growth. Mitoses are absent, however.

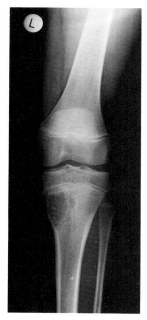

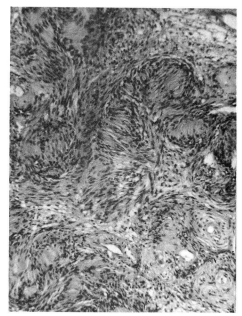

Fig. 2.174. Radiograph of a schwannoma of the left proximal tibial metaphysis of a 15-year-old child, showing a cystic, ill-defined lesion with rarefaction of the cortex from the inside but without destruction of the whole cortex.

Fig. 2.175. Histologic section of a schwannoma of bone; the tissue is fibrous, with compact bundles of Schwann cells and their nuclei aligned in rows or palisades (H&E, ×100). A myxomatous loosening of the tumor tissue may be present. Verocay bodies can be characteristic of this tumor growth.

NEUROFIBROMA AND NEUROFIBROMATOSIS
(Von Recklinghausen's Disease)
(ICD-O-M-9550/1)

Intraosseous neurofibroma is an extremely rare, benign tumor that originates from nerve elements; it consists of a mixture of Schwann cells and loosely arranged connective tissue. Solitary neurofibromas are exceptionally rare; most are associated with neurofibromatosis (von Recklinghausen's disease). Neurofibromatosis is a familial and congenital dysplastic condition, in which there are multiple tumors in the skin (together with café-au-lait patches), soft tissue and nervous system; the skeleton is involved in 39% of cases. Characteristic skeletal changes include growth disorders associated with elephantoid hyperplasia of overlying soft tissue, scoliosis, orbital wall defects, congenital bowing and pseudarthrosis of the lower legs, and erosive defects in bone caused by contiguous neurofibromas of the periosteum and soft tissue. Malignant transformation of neurofibromas may occur.

Sites

The tumors may involve any bone in the skeleton. Most are seen in the mandible, long tubular bones (tibia, femur, humerus) and spine.

Age

Primarily, children are affected, but such tumors may be detected in adult life as well.

Radiographic Features (*Figs 2.176 and 2.177*)

A solitary neurofibroma presents as a well-defined radiolucent defect in the cortical region, together with surrounding sclerosis (Fig. 2.176). Most of the lesions arise in the periosteum and impress the cortex from outside, causing an erosion. In neurofibromatosis, pseudarthrosis of a long bone is a characteristic feature. The tibia is most often affected and may be severely bowed (Fig. 2.177). Some radiolucent foci may be seen in such a bone.

Histopathologic Features (*Fig. 2.178 and 2.179*)

Usually located in the periosteum, a well-delineated tumor tissue, made up of a loose fibrillar matrix with fascicles of collagen fibers and small nerve bundles, is seen surrounded by a fibrous perineurium. The tissue is composed of interlacing bundles of elongated cells with small, haphazardly arranged nuclei. Foci showing myxoid change and lipid-laden histiocytes interspersed with fibrogenic cells are frequent. At the site of a pseudarthrosis, often only fibrous connective tissue is encountered in a biopsy, and neurofibroma cannot identified histologically.

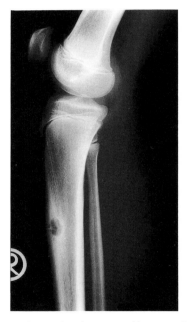

Fig. 2.176. Radiograph of a neurofibroma of the right proximal tibia of a 13-year-old girl, showing a well-defined radiolucent defect surrounded by bony sclerosis in the cortex.

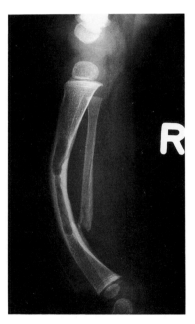

Fig. 2.177. Radiograph of a periosteal neurofibroma of bone: neurofibromatosis of the right tibial shaft of a 10-month-old child is characterized by severe bowing of the tibia and osteolytic intraosseous lesions, including a pathologic fracture. A pseudarthrosis is frequent in such cases.

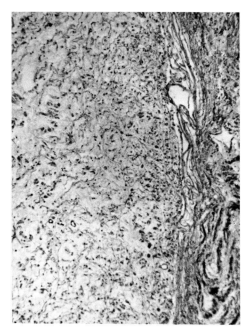

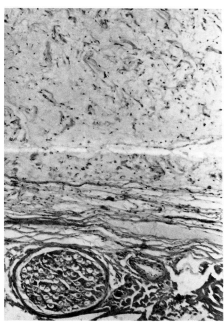

Fig. 2.178. Histologic section of a periosteal neurofibroma, which consists of a loose fibrillar matrix with fascicles of collagen fibers and small nerve bundles, including small, haphazardly arranged nuclei (H&E, ×32).

Fig. 2.179. Histologic section of a periosteal neurofibroma, showing the loose, myxoid tumor tissue and an adjacent nerve (H&E, ×32). No bone tissue is seen in such lesions.

METASTATIC NEUROBLASTOMA
(ICD-O-M-9490/3)

When occurring in bone, neuroblastoma is a secondary tumor metastatic from a primary tumor of the adrenal medulla or the sympathetic chain. *Neuroblastoma itself is a highly malignant tumor in young children, containing extensive undifferentiated round cells; it produces isolated skeletal metastases, mimicking a bone sarcoma.* The metastatic lesion shows a close similarity, radiologically as well as histologically, to other primitive round cell sarcomas of bone, especially Ewing's sarcoma.

Sites

The most common skeletal sites are the skull and metaphyses of the long bones (humerus and femur).

Age

Metastatic neuroblastoma of bone is exclusive to young children. More than 70% of cases are 5 years old or younger.

Radiographic Features (*Fig. 2.180*)

Ill-defined areas of bone destruction that are identical to Ewing's sarcoma are seen. A solitary lesion exhibits a lytic, motheaten or permeating destructive area, interspersed with sclerotic trabeculae. New periosteal bone formation, often parallel to the shaft, may mimic osteomyelitis or Ewing's sarcoma. On the whole, the radiographic features do indicate malignant growth but are not specific for metastatic neuroblastoma.

Histopathologic Features (*Fig. 2.181*)

A completely undifferentiated tumor tissue composed of densely or loosely packed round cells is typical. The small cells simulate lymphocytes containing round and hyperchromatic nuclei, and the cytoplasm is scant. Sometimes, rosette-like structures are visible. In contrast to Ewing's sarcoma, glycogen is absent in most cases, and multinucleated cells may be seen. Nerve fibrils can often be demonstrated with special silver stains, and immunohistological investigations show a positive reaction with neuron-specific enolase (NSE). When such an undifferentiated round-cell tumor tissue is found, Ewing's sarcoma and bone lymphoma should be considered in differential diagnosis; clinical findings (for instance biochemical tests for urinary catecholamine excretion) may secure the final diagnosis.

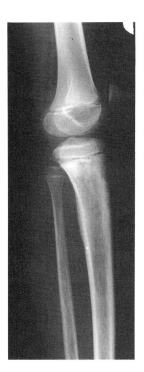

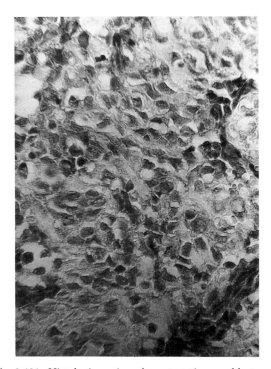

Fig. 2.180. Radiograph of a metastatic neuroblastoma of the head of the left tibia of an 8-year-old girl; an ill-defined area of bone destruction, with mottled lytic and sclerotic changes, is obvious. This poorly defined bone lesion is indicative of a malignant tumor growth.

Fig. 2.181. Histologic section of a metastatic neuroblastoma, showing an undifferentiated cellular tumor tissue that simulates lymphoid cells, with round and hyperchromatic nuclei and scant cytoplasm. The tumor tissue may identified as being of neurogenic origin by immunohistological investigations (neuron-specific enolase, ×450).

LITERATURE
Tumors of Neurogenous Origin

Bachmann-Andersen L, Sorensen SA. Diagnosis of von Recklinghausen neurofibromatosis and the Albright syndrome. Two case reports. Neurofibromatosis 1988;1:120–3

Brodeur GM, Seeger RC, Barrett A, Berthold F, Castleberry RP, D'Angio G, et al. International criteria for diagnosis, staging, and response to treatment in patients with neuroblastoma. J Clin Oncol 1988;6:1874–81

Edeling C-J, Frederiksen PV, Kamper J, Jeppesen P. Diagnosis and treatment of neuroblastoma using metiodo-benzylguanidine. Clin Nucl Med 1987;12:632–7

Gordon EJ. Solitary intrasosseous neurilemmoma of the tibia: Review of intraosseous neurilemmoma and neurofibroma. Clin Orthop 1976;117:271–282

Hall-Craggs MA, Shwa D, Pritchard J, Gordon I. Metastatic neuroblastoma: new abnormalities on bone scintigraphy may not indicate tumour recurrence. Skeletal Radiol 1990;19:33–6

Hunt JC, Pugh DG. Skeletal lesions in neurofibromatosis. Radiology 1961;76:1–20

Huvos AG, Marcove RC. Adamantinoma of long bone – a clinicopathological study of fourteen cases with vascular origin suggested. J Bone Jt Surg 1975;A-57:148–54

Jaffe R, Santamaria M, Yunis EJ, Tannery NH, Agostini RM, Medina J, et al. The neuroectodermal tumour of bone. Am J Surg Pathol 1984;8:885–98

Menendez LR, DiCesare PE, Soto C. Neurofibroma in a patient with von Recklinghausen's disease seen as a malignant schwannoma. A case report. Clin Orthop 1990;254:298–302

Miller G. Die Knochenveränderungen bei der Neurofibromatose Recklinghausen. Fortschr Röntgenstr 1953;78:669–89

Perez-Atayde AR, Grier H, Weinstein H, Delorey M, Leslie N, Vawter G. Neuroectodermal differentiation in bone tumors presenting as Ewing's sarcoma. Proc Int Soc Pediatr Oncol 1985;17:61

Pritchard J, Kiely E, Rogers DW, Spitz L, Shafford EA, Brereton R, et al. Long-term survival after neuroblastoma. N Engl J Med 1987;317:1026–7

Triche TS, Askin FB. Neuroblastoma and the differential diagnosis of small-, round-blue-cell tumors. Hum Pathol 1983;14:569–95

Uhlmann E, Grossman A. Von Recklinghausen's neurofibromatosis with bone manifestations. Ann Intern Med 1940;14:225–41

Weiss SW, Dorfman HD. Adamantinoma of long bone: an analysis of nine new cases with emphasis on metastizing lesions and fibrous dysplasia-like changes. Hum Pathol 1977;8:141–53

3

TUMOR-LIKE BONE LESIONS

True bone tumors are characterized by a continuous and autonomic growth, and another group of local bone lesions may imitate tumor growth, clinically and radiologically. In reality, this group of defects includes only dysplastic or reactive processes without the characteristics of a true benign or even a malignant tumor. All such disturbances are grouped here as "tumor-like bone lesions".

JUVENILE BONE CYST
(ICD-O-M-3340.4)

Cystic bone lesions are relatively common in children and adults, but "bone cyst" is not a true diagnosis. There are many disturbances that may produce a "bone cyst", but only few are real entities. *A juvenile bone cyst (solitary or unicameral cyst) is a benign cystic lesion that develops in children in the center of a metaphysis, expanding the bone; it is smoothly delineated, filled with clear or sanguineous fluid.* It is commonly diagnosed in children or adolescents when it has been causing pain, swelling or stiffness of the adjacent joint. Two-thirds of the patients with such a cyst in a long bone show a pathologic fracture. In some cases, however, this lesion does not show any symptoms and is diagnosed by chance.

A juvenile bone cyst can be treated with curettage and bone grafting, but there is a high recurrence rate in patients less than 10 years of age. Drilling multiple holes into the cyst, optionally with injection of cortisol, can stop the growth of such cysts and can even lead to regression.

Sites

Most juvenile bone cysts are seen in the proximal metaphysis of the humerus or femur, near to the epiphyseal plate. However, they may occur in other long bones (radius, ulna, fibula, tibia, and short tubular bones). During skeletal growth, the cyst may move towards the diaphysis. Usually, there is only one lesion in the skeleton.

Age

Most bone cysts are detected in children or adolescents. However, some are found in adults, when they may present as a "cementoma of long bones" with a solid mass of cementum-like material within the cyst wall.

Radiographic Features *(Figs 3.1 and 3.2)*

The radiograph is essential for the diagnosis of a juvenile bone cyst, and in most cases the diagnosis can be established radiologically. Within the involved metaphysis, a large cystic and centrally located lesion is visible; it is osteolytic, showing no inner features (Fig. 3.1) or some dense and incomplete trabecular densities (Fig. 3.2) that imitate a multicystic appearance. The cyst may abut the ephiseal plate, but in older individuals it is often found in the distal metaphysis, even extending into the diaphysis. Usually, the involved bone area is expanded. The cortex is thinned from the inside and may be eroded, but it is intact unless pathologic fracture has occurred.

Histopathologic Features (Figs 3.3 and 3.4)

Usually, curettage material is available for microscope, and a diagnosis can only be established together with a knowledge of the radiographic features. When larger of pieces tissue

are available, a smooth unicameral cyst without epithelial lining is obvious. The lining membrane consists of a layer of fibrous tissue that may include numerous blood vessels, osteoclastic giant cells, hemosiderin and chronic inflammatory cells. Adjacent to this fibrous wall, a layer of new fibrous bone formation is frequently present (Fig. 3.3). In older lesions, diffuse mineralized masses are deposited, resembling the cementum that is usually seen in cementomas of jaws (Fig. 3.4).

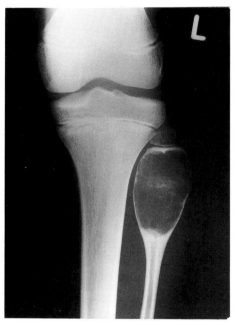

Fig. 3.1. Radiograph of a juvenile bone cyst of the left proximal fibula metaphysis of a 12-year-old boy, showing a central, well-circumscribed cyst expanding the whole metaphysis. The cortex is thinned from the inside, but its outer layer is intact.

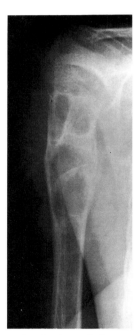

Fig. 3.2. Radiograph of a juvenile bone cyst of the right proximal humerus of a 6-year-old boy. The presence of incomplete bony trabeculae gives the impression of a multicentric cyst. The involved bone is expanded; the cortex is narrowed but intact.

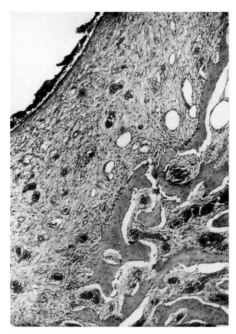

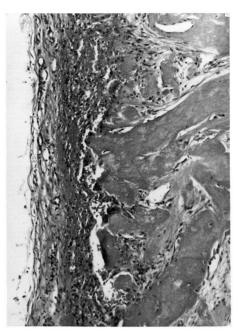

Fig. 3.3. Histologic section of a juvenile bone cyst with a smooth wall of a vascularized granulation tissue and without any epithelial layer (H&E, ×40). In the outer layer of the cyst a network of newly formed bone trabeculae attached by osteoblasts is visible.

Fig. 3.4. Histologic section of a juvenile bone cyst, showing a fibrous cyst wall without any epithelial lining and with deposits inside the wall of a cementum-like material attached by some multinucleated giant cells (H&E, ×80).

ANEURYSMAL BONE CYST
(ICD-O-M-3364.0)

This is a frequent cystic bone lesion that often gives rise to severe diagnostic problems, radiologically as well as histologically. *It is a benign and usually solitary, expansile defect of the vertebrae, the flat bones or the metaphysis of long bones; it consists of a cyst, filled with blood, with an extraosseous part bulging into the soft tissue and producing ill-defined osteolysis.* Many osteoclasts within this lesion provoke an osteolysis of malignant appearance. However, aneurysmal bone cyst should be excluded from neoplastic growths because it regresses after incomplete removal. Features of this lesion are frequently encoun-tered in various true benign and malignant bone tumors. The etiology remains unknown; probably the lesion represents a special type of bone reaction after local damage.

Swelling, pain and tenderness of several months' duration are the most common symptoms; and in about 5% of the cases a pathological bone fracture may occur. Surgical removal of the entire lesion or curettage is the most successful treatment. Embolization has also been performed successfully in some patients. In vertebral bodies, radiation therapy is advocated; but this may provoke postradiation sarcomas.

Sites

Any bone may be involved, but most aneurysmal bone cysts are seen in the vertebrae (27%), long tubular bones (femur, tibia, humerus; 43%), and pelvis (9%). The lesion develops in the metaphyses without penetrating through the epiphyseal plate.

Age

Aneurysmal bone cysts are predominantly found in children and adolescents. Seventy per cent of all patients are younger than 20 years of age; however, the lesion may also occur in adults.

Radiographic Features (Figs 3.5 and 3.6)

In the case of a bone cyst only partly well defined and eccentrically located in the metaphysis of a long tubular bone in a child, an aneurysmal bone cyst is the most favorable diagnosis (Fig. 3.5). It may be circumscribed by a small sclerotic rim, and the osteolytic area often contains septa and ridges, producing a honeycomb pattern. The most characteristic radiological appearance is the "blow-out" character, an osteolytic intraosseous part together with an extraosseous portion bulging into the adjacent soft tissue (Fig. 3.6). In such cases, the cortex is completely destroyed, imitating a malignant growth. The soft-tissue extension is produced by the bulging of periosteum, and new bone formation, recognizable on radiographs indicating the periphery of an aneurysmal bone cyst, usually occurs.

Histopathologic Features (Figs 3.7 and 3.8)

The tissue is made up of large and small, smoothly demarcated cystic spaces without any epithelial lining (Fig. 3.7). Within the cavities, coagulated blood may be present. The cavities are outlined by a loose fibrous wall that contains an inner layer of cell-rich granulation tissue with many multinuclear giant cells of osteoclastic origin (Fig. 3.8). The outer layer of the cystic wall is composed of a dense fibrous tissue in which osteoid deposits and even new-formed woven bone trabeculae may be seen. Solid portions may be predominantly fibrous, including a lacework of osteoid or newly formed bone trabeculae or, in a "solid aneurysmal bone cyst", a cell-rich granulation tissue including multiple osteoclastic giant cells. In cases with solid portions, it may become difficult to make the differential diagnosis of aneurysmal bone cyst, resorptive giant cell granuloma in hyperparathyroidism, reparative giant cell granuloma of jaws, giant cell granuloma of short tubular bones, osteoblastoma, osteoclastoma, or even a malignant tumor growth such as telangiectatic osteosarcoma. Careful clinical, radiologic and histological investigations have to be performed in order to find the correct diagnosis.

In conclusion, an aneurysmal bone cyst is not a real bone tumor but rather a tumor-like bone reaction caused by local bone damaging. It may arise spontaneously or following a local trauma or in conjunction with a real benign or even a malignant bone tumor.

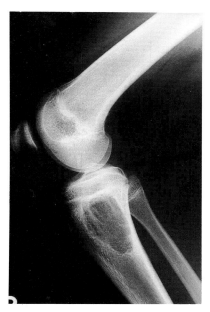

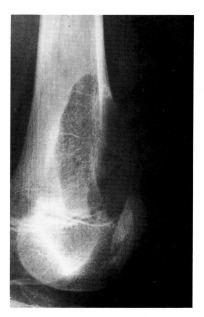

Fig. 3.5. Radiograph of an aneurysmal bone cyst of the right proximal tibial metaphysis of a 16-year-old girl; the cyst is well-defined, with some sclerotic densities in it. An incomplete marginal sclerosis is visible.

Fig. 3.6. Radiograph of an aneurysmal bone cyst of the right distal femoral metaphysis of a 9-year-old girl. The cyst has an eccentric position within the bone and shows a clear extraosseous portion bulging into the soft tissue. The cortex of this area is completely destroyed; however, this is not a sign of malignancy. The inside of the cyst is sharply delineated.

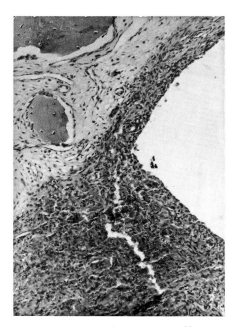

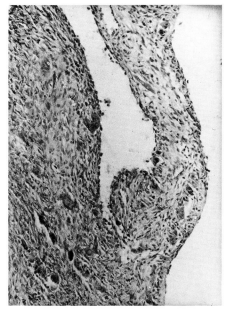

Fig. 3.7. Histologic section of an aneurysmal bone cyst. The cyst wall is smooth, with cell-rich granulation tissue including many multinuclear osteoclastic giant cells (H&E, ×50). No epithelial layer is seen. The cyst may be filled with blood.

Fig. 3.8. Histologic section of an aneurysmal bone cyst walled by a loose fibrous and granulation tissue, including many multinuclear giant cells (PAS, ×50). Inside, the cyst is smooth without any epithelial layer. Usually, the whole lesion consists of many such cavities of different sizes.

LOCALIZED MYOSITIS OSSIFICANS

A tumor-like lesion that gives the impression of a parosteal tumor growth may develop in the soft tissue near to a bone. Usually, it is preceded by local trauma. *This localized myositis ossificans is a non-neoplastic condition associated with a local trauma, occurring on the external surface of a bone or in soft tissue; it is characterized by proliferation of fibrous tissue together with severe osseous and often cartilaginous metaplasia.* The lesion is extraosseous, periosteal or parosteal and develops within 14 weeks after the precipitating trauma. Some months later, mineralized bone visible on radiographs, occurs within the lesion. Often, a rapid proliferation together with tremendous increase in size may give the impression of a malignant growth. In reality, however, it is merely a reactive heterotopic ossification. A localized painful swelling is the most common symptom. Such a lesion can usually be identified radiologically and, when in its proliferating stage, should not be treated by any surgical operation. Otherwise, a high recurrence rate is registered.

Post-traumatic localized myositis ossificans should be distinguished from "myositis ossificans progressiva" which is a congenital, hereditary and fatal disease.

In most cases localized myositis ossificans can be recognized radiologically. Following conservative therapy, this absolutely benign lesion undergoes almost total regression. Any remaining hard bony mass that bothers the patient can be excised later.

Sites

A post-traumatic parosteal lesion may develop in any bone region, but most cases occur in the region of the femur or humerus.

Age

Most cases are children or young adults; the lesion often is associated with sports injuries.

Radiographic Features (Figs 3.9 and 3.10)

Heterotopic ossification may develop near a bone as a roundish, well-delimited, dense nodule that is separated from the underlying cortex or periosteal region by a radiolucent zone (Fig. 3.9). It has an ovoid or rounded shape. The center of this focus has a radiolucent core surrounded by a densely calcified zone of bony appearance. Sometimes, and especially in the proliferating stage, the lesion is ill-defined, having a speckled appearance without any zoning, and seems to emerge from the periosteum (Fig. 3.10).

Histopathologic Features (Figs 3.11 and 3.12)

Under the microscope, an active fibroblastic proliferation is the dominant feature. In the early proliferation stage, within the vascular connective tissue polymorphous spindle cells with hyperchromatic nuclei and numerous mitotic figures are visible, giving the impression of a soft-tissue sarcoma. In the surrounding area, dead and dying or regenerating muscle fibers are present. In addition, strands of new osteoid tissue and well-formed osseous trabeculae, sometimes together with cartilage, are formed, and from these features a periosteal osteosarcoma might be diagnosed histologically. However, an excised lesion demonstrates three different zones: (a) the central area shows a cell-rich granulation tissue, often with polymorphous spindle cells and occasionally with atypical mitotic figures; (b) in the middle zone, this granulation tissue becomes more organized, and uncalcified osteoid deposits are seen (Fig. 3.11); (c) the outermost margins of the lesion consist of well-formed woven bone that is more or less calcified (Fig. 3.12). Usually, the lesion is sharply demarcated by a fibrous pseudocapsule. In most cases it can be recognized radiologically.

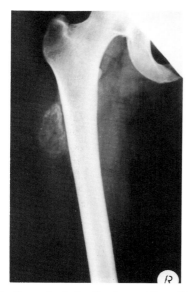

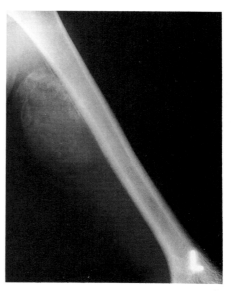

Fig. 3.9. Radiograph of a localized myositis ossificans in the right proximal thigh in a 15-year-old girl. There is a large, roundish focus of mottled density in the parosteal soft tissue, clearly separated from the bone by a radiolucent zone. A denser bony zone is seen in the periphery of the lesion, with a radiolucent center. The femur is intact.

Fig. 3.10. Radiograph of a localized myositis ossificans in the left upper arm of a 16-year-old boy, showing an ill-defined, roundish and speckled shadow adjacent to the long tubular bone, which is intact. There is a bony density in the periphery of this parosteal lesion.

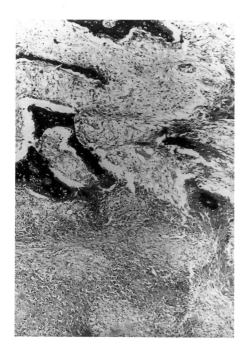

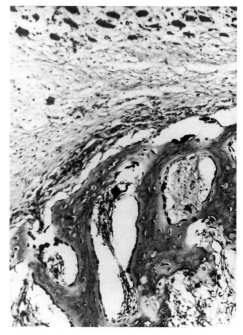

Fig. 3.11. Histologic section of a localized myositis ossificans, showing a loose fibrous tissue rich in proliferating fibroblasts, in which the more central zone has osteoid deposits and the outer zone newly formed bone trabeculae (H&E, ×64). Mitoses are numerous in the proliferating stage.

Fig. 3.12. Histologic section of a localized myositis ossificans, showing the periphery of the lesion where the outer zone of newly formed bone trabeculae is lined by osteoblasts and, adjacent, the muscle is penetrated by scars (H&E, ×82).

MELORHEOSTOSIS

This very rare osteosclerotic bone lesion, first described by Léri in 1928, may induce the impression of a bone tumor. *Melorheostosis is a nonhereditary, painful and progressive hyperostosis of unknown etiology that involves one or more long bones of the extremities; it commences in childhood.* Some cases may be symptomless, but in most cases the bone appositions on the bone surface induce clinical symptoms.

In melorheostosis we are dealing with a congenital bone dysplasia and not with a real tumorous growth. This disease shows a good prognosis with cessation of proliferation in later life. If the appositional bone masses provoke symptoms, they can be eliminated operatively.

Sites

Most lesions occur in the lower extremities.

Age

Beginning in childhood, surface bone proliferation of this kind may proliferate rapidly, but in adult life proliferation decreases and painful articular contracture may develop.

Radiographic Features *(Fig. 3.13)*

A bulging bone mass is apparent; it covers the involved bone, giving an impression of wax flowing down a candle. The new-formed bone material may be extremely dense, so that the whole bone seems to be enlarged by a bony mass.

Gross Pathological Features *(Fig. 3.14)*

In a macerated specimen, a bony mass covers the surface of the bone and bulges into the surrounding tissue.

Histopathological Features *(Fig. 3.15)*

Histologically, the only feature is irregularly arranged and heavily calcified bone; this alone is not diagnostic. Thus, melorheostosis can only be diagnosed by its radiologic appearance.

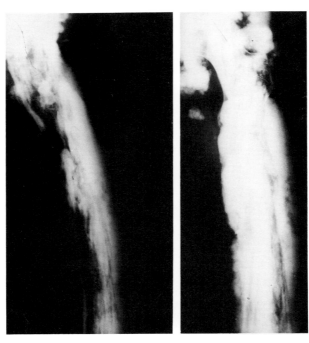

Fig. 3.13. Radiograph of a melorheostosis of the left femur of a 12-year-old child. The bone is deformed and covered by extensive bone masses that overly the shaft; the impression is of a candle, down which wax is flowing.

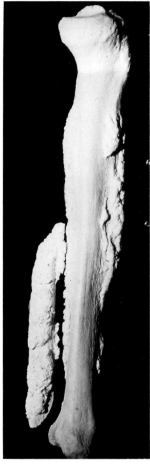

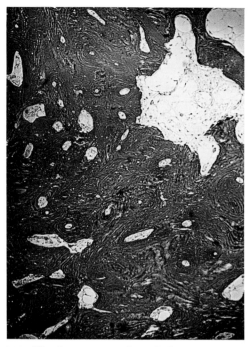

Fig. 3.15. Histologic section of a melorheostosis, showing a dense sclerotic bone tissue with Havers' osteons but without any osteoblasts (H&E, ×50). Between these parosteal bone masses, fat tissue is visible.

Fig. 3.14. Gross specimen of a melorheostosis of the tibia. On this maceration specimen it becomes obvious that the pathologic bone masses are laid down on the outside of the long tubular bone, projecting far into the soft tissue.

GIANT CELL REACTION OF SHORT TUBULAR BONES
(ICD-O-M-4411/0)

In the short tubular bones of the feet and hands, a destructive lesion may occur that gives the impression of a malignant tumor growth. *Here we are dealing with a benign, non-tumorous and reactive granulation tissue, including many osteoclastic giant cells, that destroys the bone; the lesion is caused by a traumatic bone damage.* This lesion is, radiologically and histologically, very similar to an aneurysmal bone cyst.

Simple curettage of the lesion, and replacement by bone chips, should be the treatment of choice, and no more invasive management is necessary. The damaged bone recovers afterwards.

Sites

The short tubular bones of feet, and occasionally the hands, are exclusively involved.

Age

This lesion may develop at any age, but occurs most often in children and adolescents.

Radiographic Features (Fig. 3.16)

The involved part of the short tubular bone is expanded, with a cystic brightening and opaque center. The cortex is partly thinned and partly thickened but usually intact. The lesion is not clearly demarcated and may give the impression of malignant tumor growth.

Histopathologic Features (Figs 3.17 and 3.18)

The interior of the lesion includes a cell-rich granulation tissue, with many blood vessels, composed of multiple osteoclastic giant cells (Fig. 3.17). The most characteristic feature is a prominent proliferation of atypical osteoid (Fig. 3.18), very similar to an osteosarcomatous tissue. In reality, however, we are dealing merely with a reaction lesion similar to an aneurysmal bone cyst that should not be confused with a malignant tumor growth.

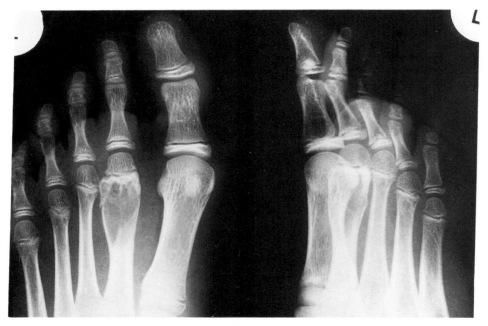

Fig. 3.16. Radiograph of a giant cell reaction of the second left metatarsal bone of an 11-year-old girl; the bone is expanded and includes an ill-defined cystic osteolysis with an opaque center. The cortex is thinned from the inside, but is mostly intact.

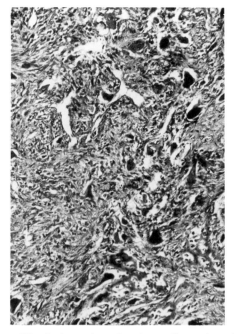

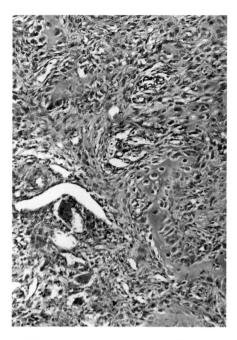

Fig. 3.17. Histologic section of a giant cell reaction of the short tubular bone, demonstrating a cell-rich granulation tissue with many blood vessels and multiple osteoclastic giant cells (Goldner, ×64). The original spongiosa is completely destroyed.

Fig. 3.18. Histologic section of a giant cell reaction of the short tubular bone, showing a vascularized granulation tissue in which there is heavy deposition of atypical osteoid (H&E, ×64). This granulation tissue is a characteristic feature of this lesion.

REPARATIVE GIANT CELL GRANULOMA OF THE JAW BONES
(ICD-O-M-4413/0)

Reparative giant cell granuloma of the jaw bones is another reactive lesion seen in children and adolescents; it may appear to be a "bone cyst" or may have a destructive area that gives the impression of being a malignant growth. *It is a nontumorous lesion, occurring in the jaw bones, that consists of a granulation tissue rich in osteoclastic giant cells and is a reactive organization tissue following traumatic bone damage.* An osteoclastoma or "brown tumor" in hyperparathyroidism must be excluded in diagnosis, but most giant cell lesions in the jaws are reparative giant cell granulomas. A simple curettage is the adequate therapy, and complete healing can be expected.

Sites

The mandible is the preferred localization of this disease.

Age

Most patients are between 10 and 25 years of age.

Radiographic Features *(Fig. 3.19)*

On the radiograph, the lesion appears as a roundish or oval area of radiolucency, including some faint trabeculae; usually, it is defined by a thin marginal sclerosis. The involved jaw bone is expanded and the cortex is thinned from the inside but is not perforated. In general, a definitive preoperative diagnosis cannot be established from the rather nondescript radiographic appearance, and a biopsy is required for diagnosis.

Histopathologic Features *(Fig. 3.20)*

The cystic bone lesion is filled with a cell-rich granulation tissue, with a fairly loose, vascular stroma composed of small spindle-shaped cells, including hemorrhagic extravasation. The proliferating fibroblasts contain isomorphic, roundish or elongated nuclei, and some of them may appear hyperchromatic, but mitoses are rare. Multinuclear giant cells are sparse, small and unevenly distributed, and sometimes delicate trabeculae of newly formed osteoid and bone are seen.

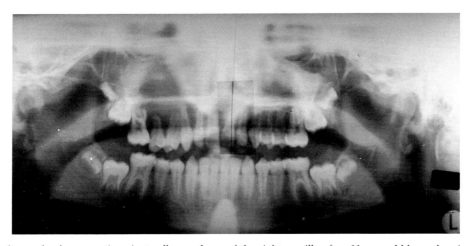

Fig. 3.19. Radiograph of a reparative giant cell granuloma of the right maxilla of an 11-year-old boy, showing a roundish radiolucent focus defined by a thin marginal sclerosis.

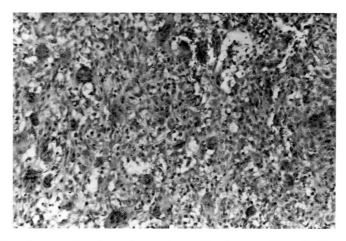

Fig. 3.20. Histologic section of a reparative giant cell granuloma of jaw bones, with a cell-rich granulation tissue, including proliferating fibroblasts and small multinucleated giant cells in an uneven distribution (H&E, ×64). Osteoid deposits and new woven bone trabeculae may occur in such lesions.

LITERATURE

Adler CP. Knochenzysten. Beitr Pathol Anat 1973;150: 103–31

Adler CP. Teleangiectatic osteosarcoma of the femur with features of an aggressive aneurysmal bone cyst. Skeletal Radiol 1980;5:56–60

Adler CP. Klassifikation der Knochentumoren und Pathologie der gutartigen und semimalignen Knochentumoren. Klinisch-radiologisches Seminar, Bd X. Stuttgart: Thieme, 1980

Adler CP. Granulomatöse Erkrankungen im Knochen. Verh Dtsch Ges Pathol 1980; 64:359–65

Adler CP, Härle F. Zur Differentialdiagnose osteofibröser Kiefererkrankungen. Verh Dtsch Ges Pathol 1974;58: 308–14

Adler CP. Recidivierende cortikale diaphysäre aneurysmatische Knochenzyste der Tibia. Verh Dtsch Ges Pathol 1974;58:256–8

Adler CP, Schmidt A. Aneurysmale Knochenzyste des Femurs mit malignem Verlauf. Verh Dtsch Ges Pathol 1978;62:487

Adler CP, Uehlinger E. Grenzfälle bei Knochentumoren. Präneoplastische Veränderungen und Geschwülste fraglicher Dignität. Verh Dtsch Ges Pathol 1979;63:352–8

Austin LT Jr, Dahlin DC, Royer EQ. Giant-cell reparative granuloma and related conditions affecting the jawbones. Oral Surg 1959;12:1285–95

Baker DM. Benign unicameral bone cyst: a study of forty-five cases with long-term follow-up. Clin Orthop 1970;71: 140–51

Biesecker JL, Marcove RC, Huvos AG, Mike V. Aneurysmal bone cysts: a clinicopathologic study of 66 cases. Cancer (Phil) 1970;26:615–25

Bonk U. Zur Problematik der Riesenzelltumoren und Riesenzellgranulome im Kieferknochen. In: Schuchardt K, Pfeifer G. Grundlagen, Entwicklung und Fortschritte der Mund-, Kiefer- und Gesichtschirurgie, Bd. XXI. Stuttgart: Thieme, 1976:161–4

Boseker EH, Bickel WH, Dahlin DC. A clinicopathologic study of simple unicameral bone cysts: Surg Gynecol Obstet 1968;127:550–60

Campbell CJ, Papademetrious T, Bonfiglio M. Melorheostosis: a report of the clinical, roentgenographic and pathological findings in fourteen cases. J Bone Jt Surg 1968;A-50:1281–304

Clough JR, Price CHG. Aneurysmal bone cysts. J Bone Jt Surg 1968;B-50:116–27

Cohen J. Simple bone cysts. Studies of cyst fluid in six cases with a theory of pathogenesis. J Bone Jt Surg 1960; A-42:609–16

Connolly J, Secor M. Cortisone treatment of pathologic fracture through a bone cyst. Nebr Med J 1982;67:286–7

Crane AR, Scarano JJ. Synovial cysts (ganglia) of bone. Report of two cases. J Bone Jt Surg 1967;A-49:355–61

Dabska M, Buraczewski J. Aneurysmal bone cyst: pathology, clinical course and radiologic appearance. Cancer (Phil) 1969;23:371–89

Fahey J, O'Brien E. Subtotal resection and grafting in selected cases of solitary unicameral bone cysts. J Bone Jt Surg 1973;A-55:59–68

Gold RH, Mirra JM. Melorheostosis. Skeletal Radiol 1977; 2:57–8

Green A, Ellswood WH, Collins JR. Melorheostosis and osteopoikilosis – with a review of the literature. Am J Roentgenol 1962;87:1096–111

Hove E, Sury B. Melorheostosis: Report on five cases with follow-up. Acta Orthop Scand 1971;42:315–19

Hughston JC, Whatley GS, Stone MM. Myositis ossificans traumatica (myo-osteosis). Sth Med J (Bgham, Ala) 1962; 55:1167–70

Jaffe HL. Giant-cell reparative granuloma, traumatic bone cyst, and fibrous (fibro-osseous) dysplasia of the jawbones. Oral Surg 1953;6:159–75

Lagier R, Cox JN. Pseudomalignant myositis ossificans. A pathological study of eight cases. Hum Pathol 1975;6: 653–65

Lodwick GS. Juvenile unicameral bone cyst. A roentgen reappraisal. Am J Roentgenol 1958;80:495–504

Martin SJ, Schiller JE. Unicameral bone cyst of the second metatarsal with pathologic fracture. J Am Pediatr Med Assoc 1987;77:143–7

Neer CS, Francis KC, Marcove RC, Terz J, Carbonara PN. Treatment of unicameral bone cyst. A follow-up study of one hundred seventy-five cases. J Bone Jt Surg 1966; A-48:731–45

Norman A, Schiffman M. Simple bone cyst: factors of age dependency. Radiology 1977;124:779–82

Oppenheim WL, Galleno H. Operative treatment versus steroid injection in the management of unicameral bone cysts. J Pediatr Orthop 1984;4:1–7

Reynolds J. The "fallen fragment sign" in the diagnosis of unicameral bone cysts. Radiology 1969;92:949–53

Robins PR, Peterson HA. Management of pathologic fractures through unicameral bone cysts. JAMA 1972;222: 80–1

Sanerkin NG, Mott MG, Roylance J. An unusual intraosseous lesion with fibroblastic, osteoclastic, osteoblastic, aneurysmal and fibromyxoid elements. "Solid" variant of aneurysmal bone cyst. Cancer 1983;51:2278–86

Savastana AA. The treatment of bone cysts with intracyst injection of steroids. Rhode Island Med J 1979;62:93–5

Schulz A, Märker R, Delling G. Central giant cell granuloma. Histochemical and ultrastructural study on giant cell function. Virchows Arch [A] 1976;371:161–70

Skajaa T. Myositis ossificans. Acta Chir Scand 1958;116: 68–72

Spence KF, Bright RW, Fitzgerald SP. Solitary unicameral bone cysts: Treatment with freeze-dried crushed cortical bone allograft. J Bone Jt Surg 1976;A-58:636–41

Tillmann B, Dahlin DC, Lipscomb PR, Stewart JR. Aneurysmal bone cyst – an analysis of ninety-five cases. Mayo Clin Proc 1968;43:478–95

4

RADIOGRAPHIC APPROACH TO THE DIAGNOSIS OF PRIMARY BONE TUMORS

INTRODUCTION

The early diagnosis of primary bone tumors – particularly malignant ones – is very difficult in childhood. Unfortunately, the malignant bone tumors are all too often obvious by the time of presentation, and hence at an advanced stage.

One of the main reasons for diagnostic problems is the rarity of primary bone malignancy in childhood (0.48/100 000/year) and therefore a lack of experience among medical practitioners. The second source of problems is the impossibility of recognizing the growth in the asymptomatic phase. We do not know how long the asymptomatic phase lasts and it may be that metastases become symptomatic before the primary focus is detected. Finally, the early symptomatic phase of primary bone tumors has unusual characteristics, which make correct diagnosis difficult:

Unusual clinical history – age, signs and symptoms

Unusual radiographic and/or histologic appearances

Unusual clinical course

The most common symptom of primary malignant bone tumor is protracted skeletal, joint or muscular pain, often poorly localized, away from the affected area. As skeletal and muscle pain is common in healthy, growing individuals, possibly due to strain, "obscure skeletal pains" are often recognized. Often a diagnosis of rheumatic disease is erroneously made in children with primary bone malignancy. As trauma is a daily occurrence in childhood, so preliminary diagnosis of accidental or stress injury is not unusual. Knee pain is often the main symptom in hip pathology, whereas primary pelvic tumors, particularly those of iliac bone, present as hip, buttock and/or knee pain. This sclerodermal pain pattern makes it difficult to localize the affected area. A tumor may mimic irritable hip or Perthes' disease. Waisting of the limb in a case of femoral tumor, subsequent to decreased mobility because of pain, may raise suspicion of a spinal cord lesion and result in unnecessary myelography and computed tomography (CT) or magnetic resonance imaging (MR) of the spine. Painful spinal scoliosis is a common primary sign in vertebral tumors.

Even when the tumor becomes radiologically evident, diagnosis in the very early stages is extremely difficult (Table 4.1). The small, localized lesion may mimic a normal anatomical variant, trauma or an inflammatory lesion. Accidental or stress injury may be diagnosed, particularly when a cortical tumor is accompanied by periosteal reaction. In cases of osteolytic, circumscribed lesions, osteomyelitis in its acute or chronic form (especially Brodie's abscess) is a common misdiagnoses. Detailed clinical history and clinical examination usually allows one to separate bone tumor from inflammatory bone disease (Table 4.2). The latter presents with localized swelling, limitation of passive and active movements, pain on pressure, often history of past fever incident, increased erythrocyte sedimentation rate (ESR) and white blood cell count (WBC), findings rarely found in malignant bone tumors, with exception of Ewing's sarcoma. Pathological frac-

Table 4.1. Differential diagnoses of primary bone tumors

Ossification variants
Trauma – stress fracture
Infection – acute osteomyelitis, primary chronic
        osteomyelitis (Brodie's abscess, Garré's
        osteomyelitis, plasma cellular osteomyelitis,
        etc.)
Eosinophilic granuloma (histiocytosis X)
Soft tissue tumors
Metastases
Benign versus malignant bone tumor
Residua of orthopedic procedures

Table 4.2. Clinicial and family history and laboratory evaluation in the diagnosis of bone tumors

	Benign tumor	Malignant tumor
Clinical history		
Swelling	Nonsymptomatic	Painfull, warm
Tumor growth	Very slow	Rapid
Other signs and symptoms	Usually none; rarely, localized pain	Protracted, difficult-to-localize pain; loss of weight; anemia
Family history	Tumor or tumorous condition in the family (neurofibromatosis, cherubism, etc.)	
Laboratory evaluation	White blood count, sedimentation rate, enzymatic investigations	

ture occurs as the first manifestation in about 10% of patients with primary bone tumors. It is characteristic of unicameral bone cysts, fibrous dysplasia and neurofibromatosis.

Biochemical tests may occasionally be useful. Catecholamines may be positive in obscure metastases which are due to neuroblastoma. A monostotic lesion in a healthy child with eosinophilia is a strong indicator for eosinophilic granuloma. Primary lymphoma of bone may be accompanied by abnormal white cells. Markedly increased ESR is a strong indication of osteomyelitis in a child who is not emaciated. Moderately increased ESR is not uncommon in Ewing's sarcoma and primary bone lymphoma.

Radiography is one of the keys to diagnosis. The important features are outlined in Figure 4.1.

Plain radiography is the first diagnostic test to make if a primary bone tumor is suspected. However the advent of bone scintigraphy, CT and MR made the diagnosis of bone tumor much easier.

Bone scintigraphy is a test of very high sensitivity and very low specificity. It is the best and/or simplest test for evaluation of obscure skeletal pain. By imaging the local physiology of bone it achieves greater sensitivity than standard radiographic procedures in detailing trauma, inflammation and neoplastic processes. It shows extension of malignant (and some benign) tumors and detects bony metastases. Extraosseous accumulation of the isotope may detect a variety of unsuspected soft tissue pathologies – benign and malignant lesions, trauma, congenital abnormalities or ectopic calcifications.

Computed tomography has dramatically changed the diagnostic approach to pediatric bone oncology. Because of its improved contrast and resolution, intraosseous and extraosseous tumor extension and marrow involvement is well demonstrated. By displaying cross-sectional anatomy it makes the anatomically complex regions – vertebral column, pelvis, shoulder – much easier to evaluate. It is a very sensitive method for early detection of calcification. All of this information is of utmost importance in planning the management of the patient – chemotherapy, surgery, radiation. Follow-up therapy can be well monitored, as early soft-tissue changes (recurrence) are demonstrated early on. Contrast enhancement gives additional CT information, particularly in relation to the vessels. Finally, fat-containing tumors can be diagnosed by CT.

Magnetic resonance imaging prompted further advances in the diagnosis of primary bone tumors. It is inferior to CT for the evaluation of calcification, ossification, cortical destruction and endoperiosteal reaction, as it produces a poor signal from bone and contributes little in the direct evaluation of bone structures. However, the different signal intensities produced by fat, muscle, hyaline cartilage, ligament, tendon and fibrocartilage give excellent soft tissue contrast. Therefore, MR is the best noninvasive method for delineating intra- and extraosseous extension of the tumor. It is the best noninvasive method for detecting bone marrow changes, as it identifies excellently edema and hemorrage. This may be helpful in differentiation between tumor, trauma and infection. The involvement of a neurovascular bundle can usually be demonstrated well. Tumor characteristics can be identified by MR in several conditions – lipomas, angiolipomas, angiomas, aneurismal bone cysts. Multidirectional MR makes the interpretation of images much easier and more acceptable. MR has further advantages in that it has no known biochemical hazards, does not produce ionizing radiation and does not give rise to streak artefacts. The development of contrast agents will have further impact development of MR for diagnosis.

Angiography for the diagnosis of primary bone tumors has decreased dramatically with the advent of CT and, particularly, MR. Its most common applications are (a) to delineate anatomy when a vascularized graft is used in limb salvage procedures, and (b) in planning embolization procedures.

It is clear that no single technique will provide an accurate diagnosis of bone tumor. A combination of three approaches must be used:

1. Clinical diagnosis (history, signs, symptoms)
2. Radiologic diagnosis
3. Histologic diagnosis

Only then can diagnosis be made with any certainty.

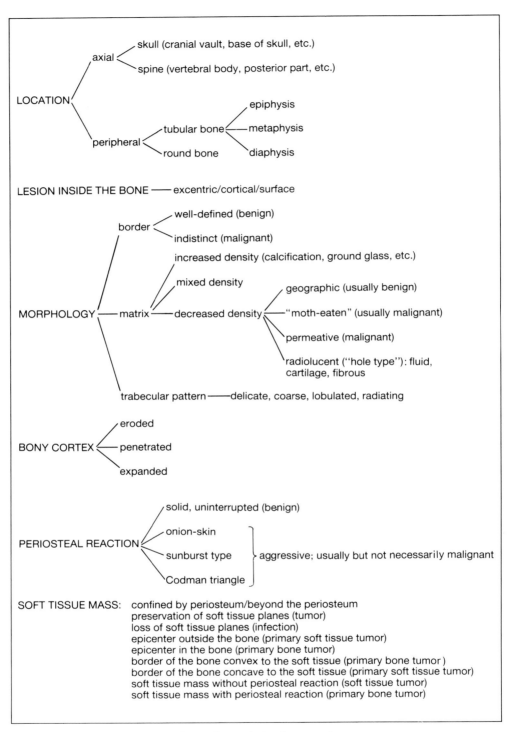

Fig. 4.1. Radiographic analysis of primary bone tumors.

LITERATURE
Introduction

Berger PE, Kuhn JP. Computed tomography of tumours of the musco-skeletal system in children. Radiology 1978; 127:171–5

Bernard C, Galloy MA, Hoeffel JC, et al. IRM en Pediatrie Med Infant 1988;95:727–42

Cohen MD, Klatte EC, Baehner R, et al. Magnetic resonance imaging of bone marrow disease in children. Radiology 1984;151:715–18

Dumontier C, Rigault P, Padovani JP, Touzet PH, Finidori G, Mallet JF. Tumeurs cartilagineuses de l'enfant. Chir Pediatr 1989;30:91–7

Edeiken J. A systematic approach to the diagnosis of primary tumours of Bone. Radiologic and other biophysical methods in tumor diagnosis. Mosby Year Book, St Louis 1975:125–37

Frank JA, Ling A, Patronas NJ, et al. Detection of malignant bone tumours: MR imaging vs scintigraphy. AJR 1990;155:1043–8

Harvie JN. Radiographic principles of bone tumors and tumor-like lesions. CRC Crit Rev Diagn Radiol 1978; 11:21–36

Helvig H. Frühdiagnose maligner Knochentumoren im Kindesalter. Pädiat Prax 1980;23:79–85

Kanal E, Burk L, Brunberg JA, et al. Pediatric musculoskeletal magnetic resonance imaging. Radiol Clin N Am 1988;26:211–39

Kransdorf MJ, Jelinek JS, Moser RP Jr, et al. Soft-tissue masses: diagnostic using MR imaging. AJR 1989;153:541–7

Kricun ME. Radiographic evaluation of solitary bone lesions. Orthop Clin N Am 1983;14:39–63

Meulenter DC, Majd M. Bone scintigraphy in the evaluation of children with obscure skeletal pain. Pediatrics 1987;79:587–92

Murray IPC. Bone scanning in the child and young adult.

Part I. Skeletal Radiol 1980;5:1–14

Murray IPC. Bone scanning in the child and young adult. Part II Skeletal Radiol 1980;5:65–76

Pettersson H, Gillespy T, Hamlin DJ, et al. Primary musculoskeletal tumors: examination with MR imaging compared with conventional modalities. Radiology 1987;164:237–41

Riddlesberger MM. Computed tomography of the musculoskeletal system. Radiol Clin N Am 1981;19:463–77

Rösli AJ. Zur Röntgendiagnostik von Knochentumoren. Orthopäde 1976;5:129–36

Sundaram M, McGurie MH. Computed tomography of magnetic resonance for evaluating the solitary tumour or tumour-like lesion of bone. Skeletal Radiol 1988;17:393–401

Sundaram M, McLeod RA. MR imaging of tumor and tumorlike lesions of bone and soft tissue. AJR 1990;155:817–24

Tehranzadeh J, Mnaymneh W, Ghavam C, et al. Comparison of CT and MR imaging in musculoskeletal neoplasms. J Comp Assist Tomogr 1989;13:466–72

Tschäppeler H. Die Computertomographie bei primären Knochentumoren im Kindesalter. Radiologe 1984;24:217–21

Unger E, Moldofsky PH, Gatenby R, et al. Diagnosis of osteomyelitis by MR imaging. AJR 1988;150:605–10

Vanel D, Di Paola R, Contesso G. Magnetic resonance imaging in musculoskeletal primary malignant tumours. In: Kressel HY (ed) Magnetic resonance annual. New York: Raven Press, 1987:237–61

Vanel D. Analyse radiologique d'une tumeur osseuse. Radiologie 1989;9:15–20

Vanel D. Strategie d'exploration radiologique d'une tumeur osseuse primitive. Rev Immunol Med 1990;2:213–9

Vogler JB, Murphy WA. Bone marrow imaging. Radiology 1988;168:679–93

SKULL TUMORS

Primary tumors and tumorous conditions of the cranial vault, with the exception of eosinophilic granuloma and epidermoid/dermoid cyst, are rare in childhood. The chordoma is an important although very rare primary tumor of the base of the skull.

Cranial eosinophilic granuloma is the most common form of skeletal involvement. Although single cranial lesions are not rare, multifocal forms of the disease are more common. Cranial involvement presents as a radiolucent, circumscribed, "washed-out" defect with beveled edges involving the diploë at both outer and inner tables (Fig. 4.2). In a stage of repair it may be surrounded by a sclerotic margin. When advanced and widespread, it may present as "geographic skull" (Fig. 4.2e).

Epidermoid/dermoid cyst presents as a round, sharply circumscribed, small translucency in one of the bones of the cranial vault (Fig. 4.3). It has tendency to regress. If growth is rapid, it causes expansion of both inner and outer tables. Dermoid cysts are localized more in the midline, whereas epidermoid cysts are more likely to be positioned laterally. Radiologically they cannot be differentiated. The differential diagnosis of

Table 4.3. Primary cranial vault tumors and primary tumors of the base of the skull

Common	Rare		Common metastases
	Benign	Malignant	
Eosinophilic granuloma	Fibro-osseous tumours	Ewing's sarcoma	Leukemia
Epidermoid/dermoid cyst	Osteoma	Osteosarcoma	Neuroblastoma
Fibrous dysplasia (polyostotic)	Hemangioma	Lymphoma	Ewing's sarcoma
	Fibrous dysplasia (monostotic)		Lymphoma
	Osteoid osteoma		Osteosarcoma
	Osteoblastoma		
	Progonoma		
	Aneurysmal bone cyst		

Table 4.4. Primary tumors of the base of the skull

"Common"	Rare
Chordoma	Eosinophilic granuloma
	Chondrosarcoma
	Metastases

Table 4.5. Differential diagnosis of the primary tumors of the skull; clinical history and physical examination allows easy recognition of most of the conditions

Osteomyelitis (tuberculosis)
Metastases
Myelomeningocoele (usually midsagittal plane)
Dermal sinus (usually midsagittal plane)
Surgical holes
Thinning of the occipital squama
Foramina parietalia per magna
Neurofibromatosis (defects along the lambdoid suture and sphenoid bone)
Aplasia cutis congenita (defects in the posterior part of the parietal bone)
Meningeal tumors
Sarcoidosis
Idiopathic "doughnut lesions"

epidermoid/dermoid cyst is with fibrous lesions (Fig. 4.4).

All other primary tumors of the cranium are rare in childhood and seldom show characteristic radiographic features, with the exceptions of hemangioma, aneurysmal bone cyst, osteoma and progonoma. The multifocal, generalized form of fibrous dysplasia is common in the skull and has diagnostic features in more advanced stages (see Fig. 4.166a). It is very rare as a localized, monostotic lesion of the cranial vault in children.

The cranium and vertebrae are the most common sites of osseous hemangioma (Fig. 4.5). In the early stages, hemangiomas are sometimes discovered on radiographs performed for other reasons. In the newborn, a soft-tissue hemangioma may extend into the bone. At later stages,

cranial hemangioma expands the bone, causing pain. Widening of the bone, with exaggerated vertical striations – sun ray skull – or a coarse honeycomb pattern, are the typical radiographic appearances of bony hemangioma. On CT there is increased contrast enhancement of the lesion, and on MR it is characterized by a low signal on T1-weighted images and a very high signal on T2-weighted images.

Aneurysmal bone cyst is a very rare lesion of the cranial vault, only single cases being reported in childhood. The lesion expands both extra- and intracranially (Fig. 4.6). The cerebral symptoms are a common complication. The characteristic CT and MR findings include a multiloculated cystic appearance with gravity-dependent fluid levels, irregular contrast enhancement and preservation of the periosteum. The nuclear scan shows characteristic appearances – a large, localized expansile hot lesion (Fig. 4.6, inset).

Osteoma is a common cranial lesion, the paranasal sinuses and cranial vault being the most common location (Fig. 4.7). The tumor presents as a localized sclerotic lesion. The differential diagnosis includes reactive (post-traumatic and postinflammatory) lesions, long-standing osteochondromas, "bony islands", osteoid osteoma/ osteoblastoma complex and fibro-osseous lesions with extensive ossification. Reactive hyperostosis from meningioma is extremely rare in childhood.

Osteochondroma occurs in any bone with enchondral ossification. Osteochondroma of the cranial vault is a very unusual lesion indeed (Fig. 4.8).

Progonoma (melanotic neuroectodermal tumor of infancy) is a tumor of the first year of life, located in the maxilla in about two-thirds of cases, and in the skull, mandible and brain in about a third. Approximately 150 cases have been reported in the literature. This is a well-documented tumor with characteristic radiographic and histologic appearances; catecholamines may be elevated. Any primary tumor with rapid growth in the first year of life is progonoma until proved otherwise. The radiographic appearances are that of a malignant tumor. CT and MR present much better the details of the lesion and show some features which may be helpful in the diagnosis (Fig. 4.9). Complete cure follows surgical resection, and metastases are very rare.

Monostotic fibrous lesions usually show radiographic features of a benign lesion – lytic defect with or without sclerotic border – but without specific characteristics (Fig. 4.4). The histologic diagnosis is also often difficult, as there is a variable percentage of fibroplastic tissue and osseous and vascular components; the lesions therefore defy strict classification. In a longstanding lesion, myxomatous degeneration increases the diagnostic difficulties (Figs 4.10 and 4.11).

Chondromyxoid fibroma (Fig. 4.11), osteoid osteoma/osteoblastoma complex (Fig. 4.12) and other benign tumors have been sporadically reported. They do not show obvious radiographic characteristics, and a rational diagnosis of the lesions is unlikely.

The primary malignant tumors of the cranial vault are very rare in children. Their incidence in childhood is not known as there are only a few, usually single, case reports, and cases are sometimes reported as part of adult series. Osteosarcoma, Ewing's sarcoma and lymphoma (Figs 4.13 and 4.14) do not have characteristic appearances in their early stages; the differential diagnosis between benign lesions and osteomyelitis is difficult if not impossible. The later features of a malignant lesion are apparent in osteosarcoma, which usually presents as an osteosclerotic, and in Ewing's sarcoma and lymphoma as an osteolytic, lesion. Post-radiation osteosarcomas are becoming more and more common. In our experience, every destructive bone lesion in the field of previous radiotherapy is osteosarcoma until proved otherwise.

Primary osteomyelitis of the skull is very rare. Usually it follows sepsis, sinusitis or direct injury (accidental or post-surgical).

Monostotic metastatic cranial bone lesions (Fig. 4.15), secondary to an unrecognized primary tumor are extremely rare in childhood. This clinical presentation is most common with neuroblastoma (Fig. 4.16). The radiographic appearances are that of a destructive, malignant bone lesion. Usually there are clinical signs and symptoms suggesting a systemic disease. However, the primary lesion may be occult. A plain abdominal radiograph may reveal suprarenal calcifications. If the latter is normal and intravenous pyelography (IVP) and/or ultrasound and the plain chest radiograph are normal, then biochemical investigation will show increased catecholamine levels in serum and urine. Rarely, CT or MR may be necessary to localize the lesion.

The only important – although rare – tumor of the base of the skull in childhood is chordoma (Fig. 4.17). About 40% of the patients present with the tumor localized at the cranial end of the spinal column. About 40 cases of cranial chordoma were reported in children up to 1990. The clinical history is long, with variable neurologic symptoms and signs. Although plain X-ray of the skull shows destruction of the sphenoid, the exact location of the lesion as well as its relation to the surrounding tissues can be seen only if CT, and preferably MR, are performed. Occasionally, sphenoid bone destruction can be seen in eosinophilic granuloma, but pituitary involvement is almost always present (Fig. 4.2e). Clivus meningioma and metastases are important differential diagnoses in adults.

The results of surgical interventions and normal anatomical variants should hardly ever cause confusion with primary tumors of the skull (Figs 4.18–4.20).

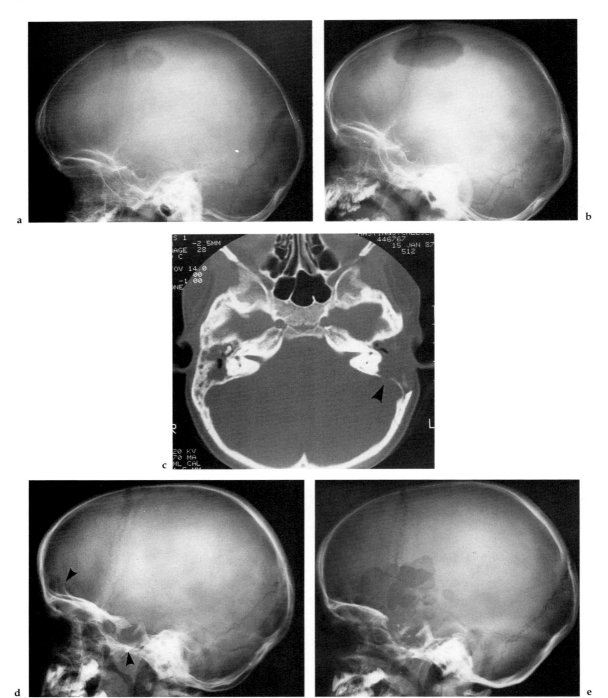

Fig. 4.2. Eosinophilic granuloma (histiocytosis X). **a** A radiolucent lesion in the anterior part of the right parietal bone; **b** 10 months later the lesion has enlarged and extended through the coronal suture into the frontal bone (18-month-old boy). **c** Extensive destructive changes in the left temporal bone and the middle ear (*arrow*) (7-year-old girl). **d,e** Eosinophilic granuloma in a 4-year-old boy with diabetes insipidus: **d** destructive changes in the body of the sphenoid, including the floor of the pituitary fossa, together with similar minor changes in the frontal bone (*arrows*); **e** 11 months later, progressive destruction gives a "geographic pattern" to the lytic cranial vault defects.

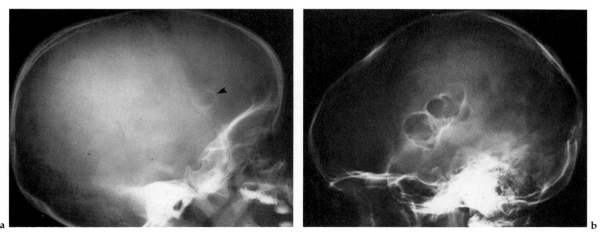

a   b

Fig. 4.3. Epidermoid cyst. **a** A small, round lesion with sclerotic rim in the posterior part of the frontal bone (*arrow*) (3-year-old girl). **b** An unusually large epidermoid cyst images as a multilocular osteolytic lesion with sclerotic margin (12.5-year-old girl).

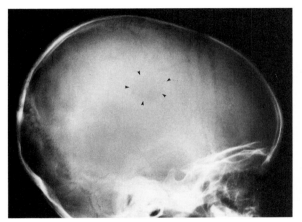

Fig. 4.4. Fibrous dysplasia. A round, radiolucent defect in the left parietal bone (20-month-old girl). The clinical diagnosis was eosinophilic granuloma; a biopsy indicated blood clot and the skeletal survey revealed discrete, polyostotic changes which progressed with time to the characteristic changes of fibrous dysplasia.

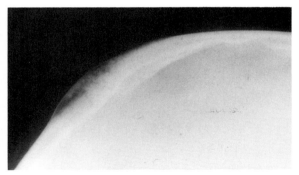

Fig. 4.5. Hemangioma. This 7-year-old girl had a 6-month history of right posterior parietal mass. Plain radiography demonstrates a lytic lesion (2 × 2 × 1.5 cm) with multiple irregular striations within the mass. (From Dr W McAlister, Mallinckrodt Institute of Radiology, St Louis, USA, with permission.)

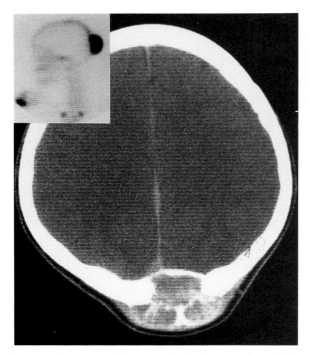

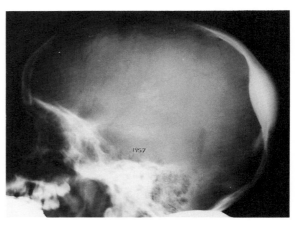

Fig. 4.7. Osteoma. This 6.5-year-old girl had a hard painless mass in the posterior parietal region, progressively enlarging for 6 months. A large area of dense compact bone can be seen in the posterior parietal region. (From Kozlowski et al. 1991, with permission.)

Fig. 4.6. Aneurysmal bone cyst. This 13-year-old girl had a 4-month history of swelling in the occipital area. There is an expansile lesion within the preserved periosteum, and there is irregular contrast enhancement. *Inset*: intensive uptake on bone scan. (From Kozlowski et al. 1991, with permission.)

Fig. 4.8. Osteochondroma. A lump in the right temporoparietal area was noted 3 months before this 15-year-old boy admission. There is a large osteosclerotic, exostosis-like lesion in the right temporoparietal region. (From Kozlowski et al. 1991, with permission.)
▼

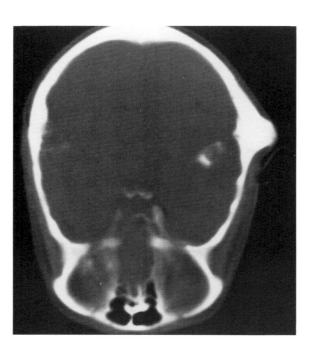

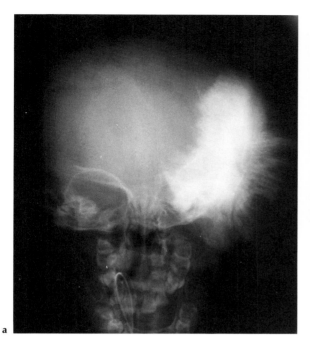

a

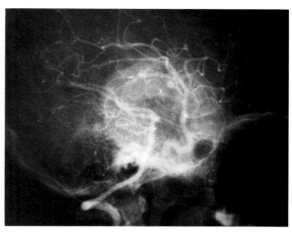

Fig. 4.10. Benign fibro-osseous tumor. Mass involving the right temporal region was noted 1 year prior to admission of this 9-year-old boy. The mass is vascular and sharply delineated by intravenous contrast medium. (From Kozlowski et al. 1991, with permission.)

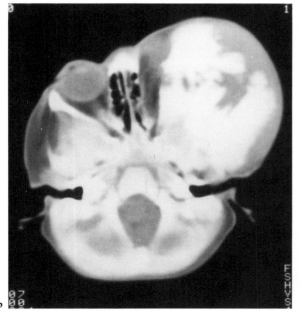

b

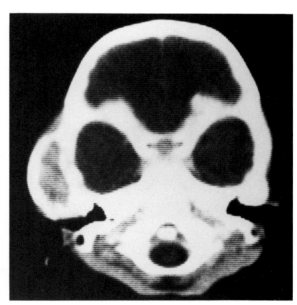

Fig. 4.9. Progonoma. This 9-month-old girl had presented with swelling involving the left forehead at the age of 2 weeks; it increased in size. **a** At 9 months of age the radiograph shows a large, sclerotic mass with spiculation along the lateral and medial border of the left temporal and left frontal bone, with invasion of the orbit, **b** CT demonstrates an irregularly sclerotic mass in the left temporal region, extending along the lateral wall of the orbit. (From Kozlowski et al. 1991, with permission.)

Fig. 4.11. Chondromyxoid fibroma or fibromyxoma (diagnosis uncertain). At the age of 14 months a hard lump was detected at the upper end of this girl's right ear. The CT, at 17 months, shows a soft tissue mass adjacent to the right temporal bone, surrounded by a thick, calcified shell at the periphery. (From Kozlowski et al. 1991, with permission.)

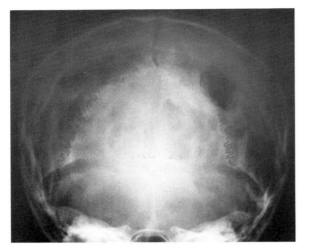

Fig. 4.12. Osteoblastoma. A lump in the left occipital region slowly in creasing in size was noted several months before admission of this 9-year-old girl. An osteolytic defect with beveled edges is seen in the occipital squama on the left. (From Kozlowski et al. 1991, with permission.)

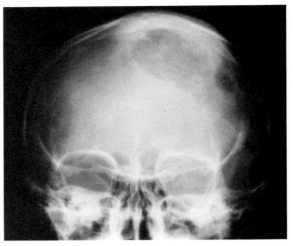

Fig. 4.13. Ewing's sarcoma. A left parietal mass increasing in size was noted about 3 months before admission of this 6.5-year-old boy. There is a lytic lesion in the left parietal region. (From Kozlowski et al. 1991, with permission.)

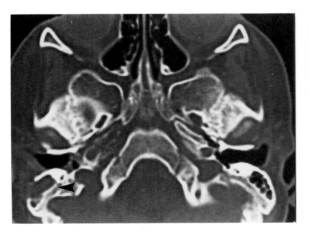

Fig. 4.14. Lymphoma. This 3-year-old boy had a 6-week history of otitis media with right facial paralysis resistant to treatment. There is a destructive lesion in the right petrous apex (*arrow*). (From Kozlowski et al. 1991, with permission.)

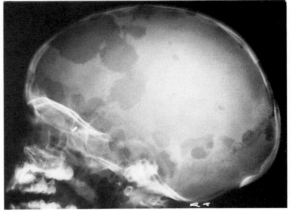

Fig. 4.15. Ependymoma – metastases 3.5-year-old girl operated at the age of 1 year 8 months for a fourth ventricular ependymoma.

Fig. 4.17. Chordoma. **a** Ophthalmoplegia was noted in this 3.5-year-old girl 5 months prior to admission with progression of symptoms and signs; blastic and lytic changes can be seen in the sphenoid and basioccipital bones (from Dr W McAlister Mallinckrodt, Institute of Radiology, St Louis, USA, with permission). **b** Progressive dysphagia and dysphonia were observed in this 6-year-old girl over several weeks; increasing retropharyngeal soft tissue swelling can be seen, together with osteolytic changes in the clivus (*arrow*) (from Dr A Taccone, Instituto G. Gaslini, Genoa, Italy, with permission). **c** This 13-year-old girl had progressive rhinodyspnea for 2 years; the MR shows beautifully the large clivus tumor extending both anteriorly and in the nasopharynx and posteriorly into the spinal canal and base of the skull (*diamond*); note the displacement of the lower pontine and medullary cisterns (from Kozlowski et al. 1991, with permission).

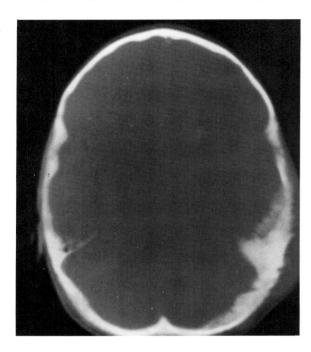

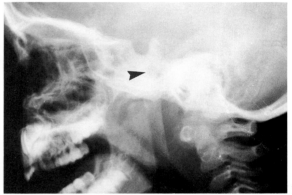

Fig. 4.16. Neuroblastoma metastasis from an occult adrenal lesion. This 4-year-old boy presented with a left temporooccipital mass 3 weeks before admission; he was entirely well and otherwise asymptomatic. The CT shows a large infiltrative lesion in the left temporooccipital region. Vanillyl-mandelic acid was elevated. (From Kozlowski et al. 1991, with permission.)

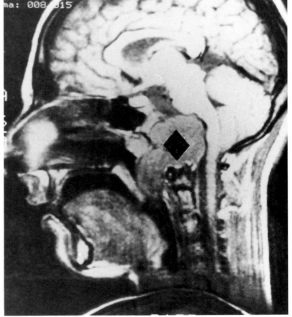

b

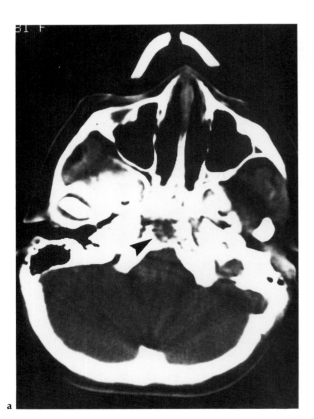

a

c

Fig. 4.17

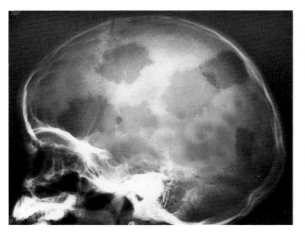

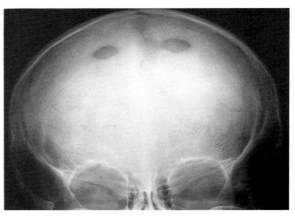

Fig. 4.18. Burr holes: diagnosis is easy when the history is known (10-year-old girl).

Fig. 4.19. Foramina parietalia, a developmental variant (7-year-old girl).

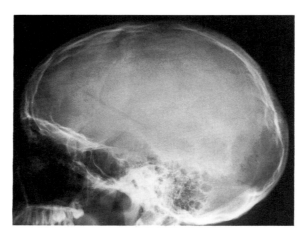

Fig. 4.20. Thinning of the occipital squama, a developmental variant (9-year-old boy).

LITERATURE
Skull Tumors

Arthur RJ, Brunelle F. Computerised tomography in the evaluation of expansile lesions arising from the skull vault in children – a report of 5 cases. Pediatr Radiol 1988;18: 294–301

Atkinson Jr GO, Davis PC, Patrick LE, Winn KJ, Ball TI, Wyly JB. Melanotic neuroectodermal tumour of infancy. MR findings and a review of the literature. Pediatr Radiol 1989;20:20–2

Baker RS, Goldstein SJ. Radiological case of the month. Am J Dis Child 1988;142:979–80

Benson JE, Goske M, Han JS, Brodkey JS, Yoon YS. Primary osteogenic sarcoma of the calvaria. Am J Neuroradiol 1984;5:810–13

Bertoni F, Unni KK, Beabout JW, Harner SG, Dahlin DC. Chondroblastoma of the skull and facial bones. Am J Clin Pathol 1987;88:1–9

Bourjat P, Flament J, Forest M. Kyste anevrysmal de l'orbite. J Radiol 1979;60:643–5

Braendli AF, Bulfamante GP. Unusual osteoblastoma of the skull. Helv Paediatr Acta 1986;41:505–8

Crone-Münzebrock, Heller M, Jend HH. Computertomographische Diagnostik bei Patienten mit Histiocytosis X. Röntgenblatter 1984;37:381–4

Dehner LP, Sibley RK, Sauk JJ, Vickers RA, Nesbit ME, Leonard AS, et al. Malignant melanotic neuroectodermal tumour of infancy. A clinical, pathologic, ultrastructural and tissue culture study. Cancer 1979;43:1389–410

DeMarino DP, Dutcher PO Jr, Parkins ChW, Hengerer AS. Histiocytosis X: otologic presentations. Int J Pediatr Otorhinol 1985;10:91–100

Di Rocco C, Jannelli A, Fileni A, Moschini M. Solitary osteolytic lesions of the skull vault in children. Neurochir 1982;25:57–61

Enzinger FM, Smith BH. Hemangiopericytoma. An analysis of 106 cases. Hum Pathol 1976;7:61–82

Gutjahr P, Meyer WW, Spranger J. Case Report 28. Skeletal Radiol 1977;1:253–5

Hoeffel JC, Galloy MA, Mainard L, Bretagne MC. Les lacunes de la voûte du crane chez l'enfant. Aspects radiologiques. Med Infant 1992;99:7–22

Huvos AG, Sundaresan N, Bretsky SS, Butler A. Osteogenic sarcoma of the skull: a clinicopathologic study of 19 patients. Cancer 1985;1214–21

Kopperman M, Antoine JE. Primary lymphangioma of the calvarium. AJR 1974;121:118–20

Kornreich L, Grunebaum M, Ziv N, Cohen Y. Osteogenic sarcoma of the calvarium in children: CT manifestations. Neuroradiology 1988;30:439–41

Kozlowski K. Case Report 614. Skeletal Radiol 1990;19: 305–7

Kozlowski K, Campbell J, McAlister W. Primary, rare cranial and base of the skull tumours in children. Radiol Med, 1991;81:213–24

Larson SE, Boquist L, Bergdahl L. Ewing's sarcoma. A consecutive series of 64 cases diagnosed in Sweden 1958–1967. Clin Orthop Rel Res 1973;95:263–72

Lichtenstein L, Sawyer WR. Benign osteoblastoma – further observation and report of twenty additional cases. J Bone Jt Surgery 1964;46:755–65

Lodge T. Developmental defects in the cranial vault. Br J Radiol 1975;48:421–34

Martinez-Madrigal F, Vanel D, Luboinski B, Terrier Ph. . Case report 670. Skeletal Radiol 1991;20:299–301

Mathias K, Weigel K. Ungewöhnliche Komplikation eines eosinophilen Granuloms des Schädels. Fortschr Röntgenstr 1978;128:767–9

Matsumo J, Towbin RB, Ball WS Jr. Cranial chordomas in infancy and childhood. A report of two cases and review of the literature. Pediatr Radiol 1989;20:28–32

Meyers PA. Malignant bone tumours in children: Ewing's sarcoma. Hematol/Oncol Clin N Am 1987;1:667–73

Mohan V, Gupta RP, Arora MM. Tuberculosis of the calvaria mimicking eosinophilic granuloma. Aust Radiol 1988;32:147–8

Mohdan V, Gupta SK, Mohanty S. Chronic pyogenic osteomyelitis of the calvarial bones. Aust Radiol 1987;31:389–90

Pochaczewski R, Yen YM, Sherman RS. The roentgen appearance of benign osteoblastoma. Radiology 1960;75: 429–37

Rafinski R. Przypadek kostniaka luski kosci skroniowej. Otolaryng Polska 1968;22:593–4

Rustiadji, Chunadi E, Koosnadi S, Kozlowski K. Posttraumatic aneurismal bone cyst in the temporal bone. La Radiologia Medica 1989;78:386–7

Saha MM, Agarwal KN, Bhardwaj OP. Calvarial bone defects in neurofibromatosis. A case report. AJR 1969;105: 319–21

Scott JA, Augustyn GT, Gilmor RJ, Mealey J Jr, Olson EW. Magnetic resonance imaging of a venous angioma. Am J Neuroradiol 1985;6:284–6

Tehranzadeh J, Jenkins JJ, Horton JA. Case Report 249. Skeletal Radiol 1983;10:276–80

Thiebot J, Clavier E, Challine B, Henry J. Localisation tumoralé sphénoidalé isolée chez enfant révélatrice d'une histiocytose X. J Radiol 1987;68:309–11

Williams RN, Boop WC. Benign osteoblastoma of the skull. Case report. J Neurosurg 1984;41:769–72

Yannopoulos K, Born AF, Griffiths C. Osteosarcoma arising in fibrous dysplasia of the facial bones. Am J Surg 1964; 107:556–64

JAW   TUMORS

Jaw tumors are rarely seen in children even in large children's hospitals. Their variety surpasses that of tumors of the rest of the skeletal system. The jaws share with the rest of the skeleton the nonodontogenic and metastatic tumors but are almost unique sites of odontogenic cysts and tumors. Additionally, many soft tissue tumors (perimandibular, oral, pharyngeal and neck tumors) extend into jaws.

Few jaw tumors show characteristic radiographic findings. The anatomical structure of the jaws is such that many of the characteristic features of nonodontogenic tumors are poorly defined or absent. The most common presentation of both nonodontogenic and odontogenic tumors or tumor-like conditions is a lytic or cyst-like lesion.

Some jaw tumors show interesting features with respect to the clinical course, location and radiographic findings. The new modalities – CT, MR, US and nuclear scan – are often very helpful not only in defining the exact anatomical location and extent of the tumor but also in showing diagnostic features not shown on plain radiography.

The clinical history may be a very important source of information; for example, familial fibrous dysplasia localized to the jaws occurs in cherubism (Fig. 4.21), and odontogenic cysts (Fig. 4.22) occur in nevoid basal cell carcinoma syndrome. In any infant with a rapidly growing jaw tumor melanotic progonoma, a tumor of the first year of life, is the most likely diagnosis (Fig. 4.23). In a patient with a malignant tumor after radiotherapy, postradiation osteosarcoma has to be excluded (Fig. 4.24). The diagnostic "floating teeth" pattern can be the presentation of histiocytosis X, with mandibular involvement

being more common than maxillary (Fig. 4.25). In most instances, skeletal survey will detect polyostotic involvement in histiocytosis X. In a patient with a bleeding disorder, an intraosseous or subperiosteal hematoma may present as a cystic lesion. At later, reparative stages it may resemble a malignant bone tumor.

Aneurysmal bone cyst presents as unilocular or multilocular, sometimes expansile, lesion (Fig. 4.26). The appearances are less characteristic than in the long bones.

Metastases (neuroblastoma, lymphoma) are easy to diagnose because the site of the primary lesion is usually already known.

The relatively common postinflammatory tumor-like lesion, giant cell reparative granuloma, presents as a radiolucent, expansile lesion (Fig. 4.27).

Few of the odontogenic tumors have diagnostic features. The most common in children is odontoma (Fig. 4.28). This lesion is usually symptomless and discovered accidentally following an unerupted, maldeveloped or maligned primary or secondary tooth. It presents at all stages from an unorganized, more or less calcified mass of dental tissue to the formation of a complete tooth. Usually small, odontomas may become large in rare instances. Multiple odontomas, familial cases and associations with various syndromes have been reported. A cementoma is localized in the proximity of the tooth root (Fig. 4.29). In its immature (noncalcified) stage it presents as a cyst-like lesion. In the mature (calcified) stage it often has characteristic features, being a well-circumscribed, calcified mass with a peripheral, radiolucent halo and attachment to the root of an erupted permanent molar tooth. Ameloblastoma, a rare

Table 4.6. Jaw tumors

| Common | Rare | | Differential diagnosis |
	Benign	Malignant	

Giant cell reparative granuloma
Histiocytosis (eosinophilic
  granuloma)
Odontoma
Cementoma
Aneurysmal bone cyst
	All other benign odontogenic
	  and nonodontogenic
	  tumors
		Osteosarcoma
		Ewing's sarcoma
		Fibrosarcoma
		Lymphoma
			Soft tissue tumors
			Osteomyelitis
			Metastases (neuroblastoma, leukemia,
			  lymphoma)
			Syndrome associations (cherubism,
			  Nevoid basal cell carcinoma, etc.)
			Caffey's disease

tumor in childhood, presents as a multiloculated or unilocular radiolucency (Fig. 4.30). The relatively common fibroma, like other odontogenic tumors, does not have characteristic radiographic features (Fig. 4.31).

Microscopic diagnosis is indispensable in the exact diagnosis of odontogenic tumors.

The perimaxillary and perimandibular tumors are demonstrated very well by CT and MR. The varying imaging characteristics of the tumors may give a clue to the underlying histology. It is better, in cases of perimandibular and perimaxillary soft tissue tumors, for the radiologist to describe the anatomical details and leave the diagnosis for the pathologist (Fig. 4.32).

Primary jaw osteomyelitis (Fig. 4.33) is rare in childhood. Usually it is secondary to tooth or sinus infection or direct trauma.

Actinomycosis presents as an obscure inflammatory process or neoplastic lesion (Fig. 4.34). Microscopic and laboratory examinations are of critical significance.

Caffey's disease, in which one of the first clinical signs may be jaw swelling, usually has diagnostic radiographic features (Fig. 4.35). There is massive, symmetrical cortical thickening with bone widening. During the healing phase there might be thin cortex with a widened, enlarged mandible.

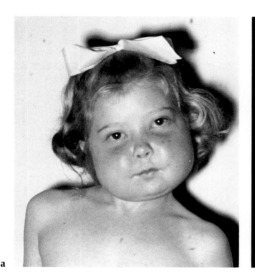
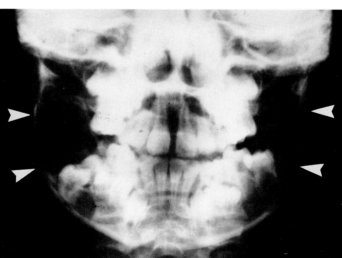

a   b

Fig. 4.21. Cherubism. **a** Marked swelling of the cheeks; both the upper and the lower jaw are affected (7-year-old girl). **b** Extensive radiolucent lesions in the rami of the mandible (*arrows*). (From Kozlowski et al. 1981, with permission.)

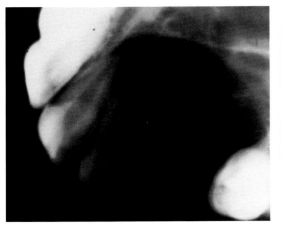

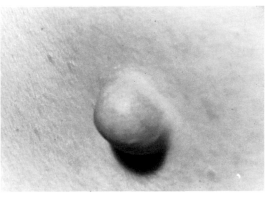

Fig. 4.22. Multiple nevoid basal cell carcinoma syndrome. **a** Large jaw cyst in a 13-year-old. **b** Skin cyst in a 32-year-old. (From Kozlowski et al. 1974, with permission.)

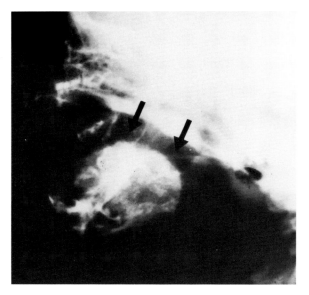

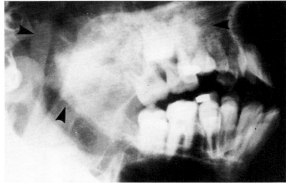

Fig. 4.23. Melanotic progonoma (pigmented neuro-ectodermal tumor of infancy). A partly calcified tumor is eroding and expanding the right side of the body of the mandible (6-week-old boy). (From Kozlowski et al. 1981, with permission.)

Fig. 4.24. Postradiation osteosarcoma. A soft tissue lump was removed from this 12-year-old boy's left lower lip at the age of 6 years. A large irregularly sclerotic lesion, with a spiculated pattern of new subperiosteal bone formation, is present (*arrows*).

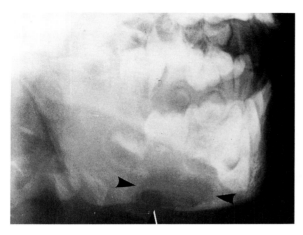

Fig. 4.25. Histiocytosis X (monostotic eosinophilic granuloma). There had been increasing swelling of the left side of the jaw for several months. There is a large osteolytic defect with cortical destruction (*arrows*). (From Kozlowski et al. 1981, with permission.)

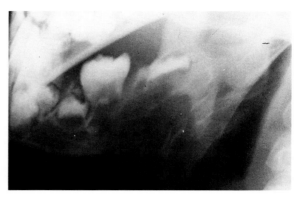

Fig. 4.27. Giant cell reparative granuloma. The 5-year-old girl had swelling of the right mandibular angle for several weeks. An infected second molar had been extracted 3 weeks earlier. (From Kozlowski et al. 1970, with permission.)

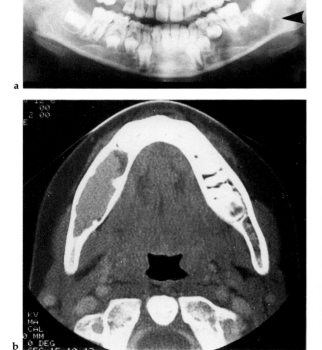

Fig. 4.26. Aneurysmal bone cyst. Large cyst with a slightly irregular border in the left mandible (8.5-year-old girl).

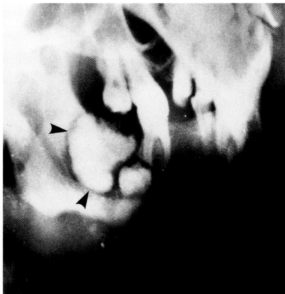

Fig. 4.28. Complex odontoma. Large, uniformly dense mass in the posterior left mandibular region, surrounded by a radiolucent halo (17-year-old boy). (From Piekarczyk et al. 1986, with permission.)

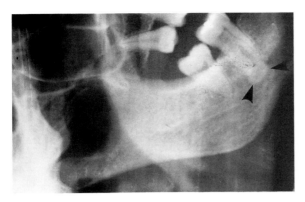

Fig. 4.29. Cementoma. A small, oval radio-opaque mass with sharp borders located at the root of L7 (17-year-old girl). (From Kryst et al. 1985, with permission.)

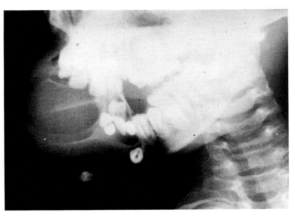

Fig. 4.30. Ameloblastoma. A huge tumor involves the central and right lateral side of the mandible (10-year-old boy). (From Pramulio et al. 1985, with permission.)

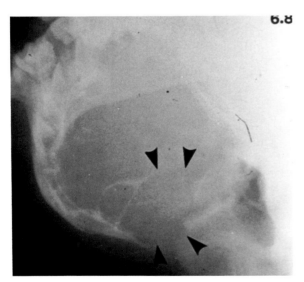

Fig. 4.31. Odontogenic fibroma. This 2-year-old boy had swelling of the right mandibular angle from the age of 9 months. A large destructive lesion is seen in the right side of the mandible. (From Kees et al. 1985, with permission.)

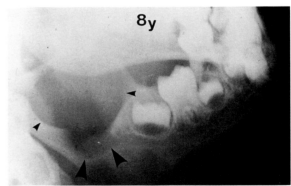

Fig. 4.32. Embryonal rhabdomyosarcoma. There had been increasing swelling of the left cheek of this 8-year-old girl for several weeks. The intercondylar notch is enlarged (*small arrows*) and a destructive bone lesion is present (*large arrows*). (From Kozlowski et al. 1981, with permission.)

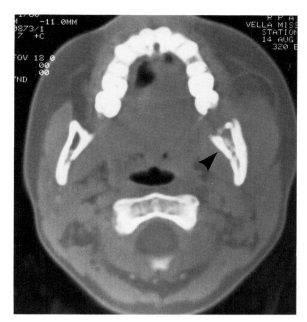

Fig. 4.33. Primary mandibular osteomyelitis. This 11.5-year-old girl presented with swelling and pain in the right side of the mandible.

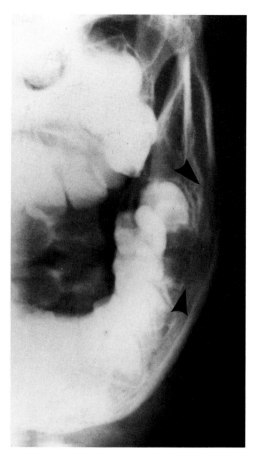

Fig. 4.34. Actinomycosis (*arrows*). This 9-year-old girl presented with slightly swollen and painful area in right side of the mandible.

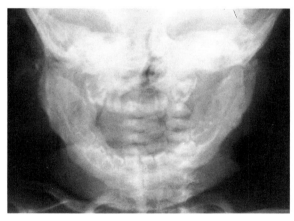

Fig. 4.35. Caffey's disease: mandibular hyperostosis (9-month-old boy).

LITERATURE
Jaw Tumors

Baker CHG, Tishler JM. Review article. Malignant disease in the jaws. J Can Assoc Radiol 1977;28:129–41

Blank E, Runckel DN. Case report 119. Skeletal Radiol 1980;5:179–82

Düker J. Röntgenologische Differentialdiagnose der Kiefer-zysten. Radiologe 1984;24:537–46

Finkelstein JB. Osteosarcoma of the jaw bones. Radiol Clin N Am 1970;8:425–43

Horner K, Forman GH, Smith NJD. Atypical simple bone cysts of the jaws. I Recurrent lesions. Clin Radiol 1988;39:53–7

Howe GL. Haemorrhagic cysts of the mandible. Br J Oral Surg 1965;3:55–76

Kees A, Vandervord JG, Thompson Ph, Godfrey E, Kozlow-ski K. Odontogenes fibrom der Mandibula bei einem 2 Jahre alten Kind Chir Praxis 1985;34:315–21

Kozlowski K, Baker P, Glasson M. Multiple nevoid basal cell carcinoma syndrome. Pediatr Radiol 1974;2:185–90

Kozlowski K, Gorska M, Depowski M, Sikorska B. Tumeures osséuses rares, primitives ou secondaires de l'enfant. A propos de neuf observations. Ann Radiol 1970;13:219–28

Kozlowski K, Masel J, Sprague P, Tamaela A, Kan A, Middleton R. Mandibular and para-mandibular tumours in children. Report of 16 cases. Pediatr Radiol 1981;11:183–92

Kozlowski K, Turner G. Stickler syndrome. Report of the second Australian family. Pediatr Radiol 1975;3:230–4

Kryst L, Piekarczyk J, Kozlowski K. Cementoma. Aust Radiol 1985;29:275–8

Ord RA. Osteomyelitis of the mandible in children – clinical presentations and review of management. Brit J Oral Maxillofac Surg 1987;25:204–17

Piekarczyk J, Mlosek K, Kozlowski K. Odontoma. Report of 8 cases. Aust Radiol 1986;30:213–16

Pramulio THS, Said HM, Kozlowski K. Huge ameloblas-toma of the jaw. Report of three cases. Aust Radiol 1985;29:308–10

Revel MP, Vanel D, Mamelle G, Piekarski JD, Franc J, Meunier M. MRI of neoplasms of the facial region. Study of 97 examinations. Diagn Intervent Radiol 1990;2:53–59

Sartoris DJ, Arkoff RS, Parker BR. Aggressive fibromatosis of the mandible in childhood. Skeletal Radiol 1983;10:154–6

Som PM, Lawson W, Cohen BA. Giant-cell lesions of the facial bones. Radiology 1983;147:129–34

Taconis WK, van Rijssel ThG. Fibrosarcoma of the jaws. Skeletal Radiol 1986;15:10–13

Waldron ChA, Shafer WG. The central giant cell reparative granuloma of the jaws. Am J Clin Pathol 1966;45:437–47

Waldron ChA. Nonodontogenic neoplasms, cysts and allied conditions of the jaws. Semin Roentgenol 1971;6:414–425

Wass SH. Melanotic adamantinoma of the mandible of a child aged 5 months. Proc R Soc Med 1968;41:281–3

VERTEBRAL TUMORS

Primary tumors of the spine tend to be discovered late in spite of the introduction of new imaging modalities – nuclear scan, CT and MR. Preoperative radiographic diagnosis has improved, but in many instances the exact character of a tumor remains a matter of conjecture because neither early specific clinical nor radiographic criteria are present.

The most important clinical signs of primary vertebral tumors are protracted back pain and abnormal spine alignment, usually scoliosis. The duration of symptoms in patients with undiagnosed vertebral tumors varies between a few days to several years. Spinal alignment is normal in midsacral and posterior spinal process lesions. Spinal curves disappear after successful therapy.

In a review of 22 cases of osteoid osteoma and osteoblastoma, patients were found to have had protracted back pain for 6–36 weeks' duration at the time of diagnosis (Azouz et al. 1986). Another review of 13 patients, all aged below 21 years, with osteoid osteoma and osteoblastoma of the sacral bone, showed that the avarage duration of the symptoms was 33 months (Capanna et al. 1986).

It is our experience that children with protracted back pain with or without scoliosis and stiffness of the back and normal radiography findings should undergo an isotope scan. A negative scan excludes malignant bone lesions and most of the benign bone lesions. It also directs the CT and MR examination to the appropriate level. In cases of paraspinal and intraspinal lesions, MR and/or myelography are preferable.

Osteoid osteoma and osteoblastoma are the most common primary vertebral tumors in children (Figs 4.36–4.39). Typical osteoid osteoma presents as a painful lesion smaller than 1.5–2.0 cm with a small nidus surrounded by sclerosis. Osteoblastomas are larger than 1.5–2.0 cm, with mixed osteosclerotic and/or osteolytic features and progressive growth. The vertebral column is a preferred location of osteoid osteoma and more specifically of osteoblastoma. Up to 10% of osteoid osteomas and 40% of osteoblastomas are localized in the spine. About 70% of osteoid osteomas and 60% of osteoblastomas occur in the first two decades of life, predominantly in teenagers. Osteoid osteoma is more painful, and analgesics of the

Table 4.7. Primary malignant vertebral tumors

Common		Rare		Differential diagnosis
Benign	Malignant	Benign	Malignant	

Eosinophilic granuloma
Osteoid osteoma
Osteoblastoma
Aneurysmal bone cyst
	Ewing's sarcoma	Exchondroma
		Enchondroma
			Osteosarcoma
			Lymphoma
			Malignant vascular tumors
			Chordoma
				Trauma (fracture, anterior and
				    posterior intervertebral disk
				    herniation)
				Osteomyelitis (including
				    tuberculosis and discitis)
				VERTEBRA PLANA:
				    eosinophilic granuloma,
				    Ewing's sarcoma, trauma,
				    osteomyelitis
				ANISOSPONDYLY: all
				    diseases causing
				    osteoporosis (osteogenesis
				    imperfecta, steroid therapy,
				    leukemia), metastatic bone
				    disorders (leukemia/
				    lymphoma,
				    neuroblastoma), trauma,
				    bone dysplasia
				PLATYSPONDYLY: bone
				    dysplasia

salicylate group are more effective in relieving pain in osteoid osteoma than in osteoblastoma.

All patients with osteoid osteoma show a typical positive "hot spot" which makes spot films, tomograms and myelography unnecessary. Plain films and tomograms may show the nidus, but CT depicts the location and extent of the lesion much better.

Both osteoid osteoma and osteoblastoma are predominantly lesions of the posterior part of the vertebra (pedicles and neural arch). A primary lesion in the vertebral body is rare, but extension of osteoblastoma of the pedicle into the vertebral body is common. The radiographic appearances of osteoblastoma are much more versatile and therefore its diagnosis is much more difficult than that of osteoid osteoma. Whereas the differential diagnosis of osteoid osteoma is primarily with unifocal metastases – a rare occurrence in childhood – osteoblastoma must be differentiated from aneurysmal bone cyst, osteomyelitis, Ewing's sarcoma, other rare primary benign and malignant vertebral tumors, and intra- and paraspinal tumors.

In eosinophilic granuloma (histiocytosis X), the spine is the most commonly affected area of the skeleton after the calvarium (Fig. 4.40a–d). The radiographic diagnosis is easy if there are multifocal lesions or if the classical manifestation of vertebra plana is present. In early stages and when the location is the posterior part of the vertebrae, the diagnosis might be very difficult. Two further confusing findings in the usually asymptomatic patients are neural defects (accompanied by hip and limb pain, muscle wasting, walking difficulties) and paravertebral mass.

The radiographic appearances of uncharacteristic eosinophilic granuloma are sometimes that of a lytic, aggressive process. As the vertebral body collapses it becomes more sclerotic. The appearances are similar to that of Ewing's sarcoma. In the case of a small, localized lesion in the vertebral body, osteomyelitis should be considered. If the lesion is localized in the posterior part of the vertebrae, the differential diagnosis is even more complicated and includes osteoblastoma, aneurysmal bone cyst, inflammatory processes and congenital malformations (specifically the absent pedicle syndrome). Tuberculosis should be considered in patients who have lung changes, have a positive tuberculin test or come from countries where tuberculosis is common.

The spine is a common location of aneurysmal bone cyst (Fig. 4.41). According to Hay et al. (1978) 78 cases of spinal aneurysmal bone cyst were reported in the English literature up to 1978, and they added 14 cases of their own, nine of which were in children under 17 years of age. Out of 160 cases of aneurysmal cysts, Schajowicz (1981) records that 21 were vertebral.

Aneurysmal bone cyst shows a predilection for the lumbar spine, and the posterior parts of the vertebrae are more often affected. It presents as an osteolytic, expansile lesion with a tendency to compress the spinal cord and/or spinal roots. CT demonstrates very well the cortical rim with a sharp interface between the extraosseous mass and adjacent tissue planes. Fluid levels have also been demonstrated. MR is even more specific than CT.

The differential diagnosis of the early stages of aneurysmal bone cyst is very difficult and includes both malignant (Ewing's sarcoma, osteosarcoma) and benign (osteochondroma, osteoblastoma) tumors, eosinophilic granuloma, inflammatory processes and congenital malformations. Later, when the tumor enlarges, the predominant differential diagnosis is osteoblastoma. Secondary aneurysmal bone cyst developing on primary lesion should always be remembered.

Osteochondroma of the spine (Figs 4.42 and 4.43) is rare in childhood. As it is usually a part of exchondromatosis (diaphyseal aclasia) there is little difficulty in recognizing the tumor. Diagnostic difficulties do arise when the tumor is single, small and in an unusual location, for example in the coccyx (as we have observed in one of our patients). There are only few reports of spinal osteochondroma in children. The disease becomes more common with advancing age. The presentation is usually that of an asymptomatic, painless, hard mass, but several cases with spinal cord compression have been reported. In one of our patients with exchondromatosis, a cervical spine exostosis caused swallowing difficulties. CT and MR exactly delineate the tumor and its relationship to the spinal canal and neural foramina.

Ewing's sarcoma (Fig. 4.44) is the most common malignant spinal tumor in children, with a wide spectrum of clinical presentation. The history is usually that of back pain for several weeks, but this can be months or days. Intra- and perispinal soft tissue masses are common features of Ewing's sarcoma. Neurologic signs are a frequent occurrence. Sudden progressive spinal cord symptoms – paresthesias, sensory loss, weakness of muscles, paraplegia, bladder dysfunction – have all been reported. Ewing's sarcoma is often accompanied by constitutional symptoms (fever, leukocytosis, anemia, weight loss).

The most common radiographic feature is permeating destruction of the vertebral body with compression fracture. Mixed or sclerotic appearances of the vertebral body are not rare in our experience. The tumor occasionally extends into the pedicles and the primary lesion is rarely in the posterior part of the vertebra. Calcification of the paraspinal mass may mimic the radiographic appearances of neuroblastoma.

The main differential diagnoses of vertebral Ewing's sarcoma are inflammatory lesions and eosinophilic granuloma. In cases with a large soft tissue mass a perivertebral or an intervertebral tumor, usually neuroblastoma, should be considered. All the reports stress the difficulties in correct and early recognition of Ewing's sarcoma.

Other primary malignant vertebral tumors – osteosarcoma, lymphoma, chondrosarcoma – are very rare in childhood. Vertebral osteosarcoma in children is almost always secondary to irradiation. Lymphoma is usually one of the presentations of a multifocal condition.

Chordoma, a slow-growing tumor, rarely occurs in childhood. It accounts for about 1% of primary bone tumors, and is encountered in twice as many males as females. Chordoma arises from ectopic notochord remnants in the vertebral bodies and sacrum. More than half of the lesions occur in the sacrum, more than a third at the base of the skull and the rest in the spine. In the rare child cases the tumor is limited to the skull and the cervical spine. The clinical symptoms and signs are most often neurologic complaints – pain, leg numbness, bowel and bladder incontinence, and sacral mass. The symptoms may last for years before the diagnosis is made. Radiographic examination shows destructive changes in the dorsum sellae, posterior clinoid processes and a soft tissue mass in the nasopharynx (see Fig. 4.17). A caudal location, with destructive changes in the sacrum and an adjacent soft tissue mass, is extremely rare in childhood (see Fig. 4.88).

Vertebral metastases in childhood are common in neuroblastoma and leukemia (Fig. 4.45). Usually the diagnosis is already known by the time that the vertebral changes become apparent.

The differential diagnoses of primary vertebral tumors are osteomyelitis (Figs 4.46 and 4.47) and trauma (Figs 4.48 and 4.49). Congenital anomalies and normal anatomical variants should seldom cause confusion (Fig. 4.50).

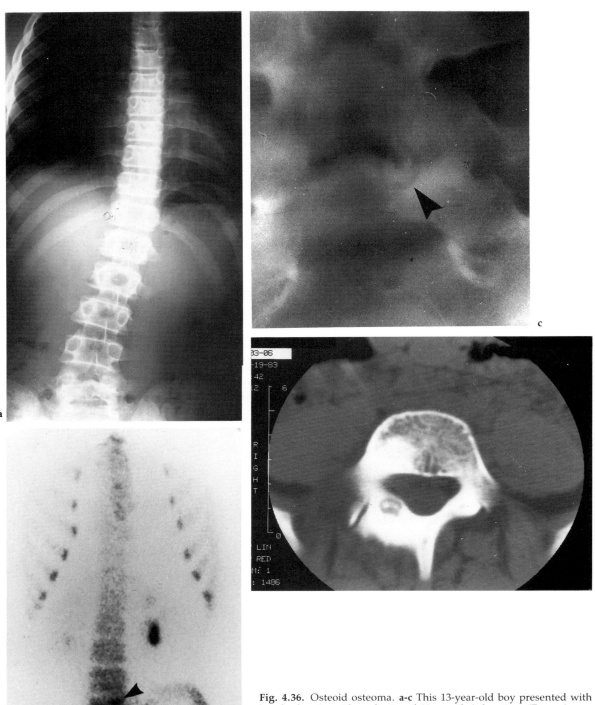

Fig. 4.36. Osteoid osteoma. **a-c** This 13-year-old boy presented with low back pain with scoliosis, of 18 months' duration. (From Azouz et al. 1986, with permission.) **a** Lumbar scoliosis convex to the left is seen on the radiograph of an apparently normal spine. **b** Increased isotope uptake in L5 (*arrow*). **c** The tomogram shows clearly a nidus in the lamina of L5 (*arrow*). **d** This 15-year-old girl presented with back pain, revealed by aspirin, over a period of 9 months. There was sclerosis of the left pedicle and vertebral body. The CT shows clearly a nidus protruding into the spinal canal.

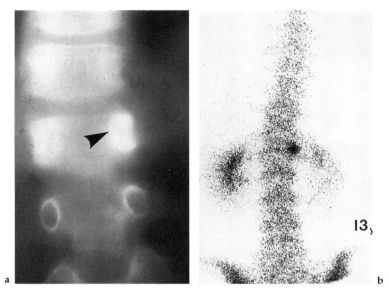

Fig. 4.37. Osteoblastoma. This 13-year-old girl had back pain for several months and scoliosis to the right. **a** Sclerosis of the left pedicle of L1 (*arrow*). **b** Intensive concentration of the isotope in the L1. (From Kozlowski et al. 1984, with permission.)

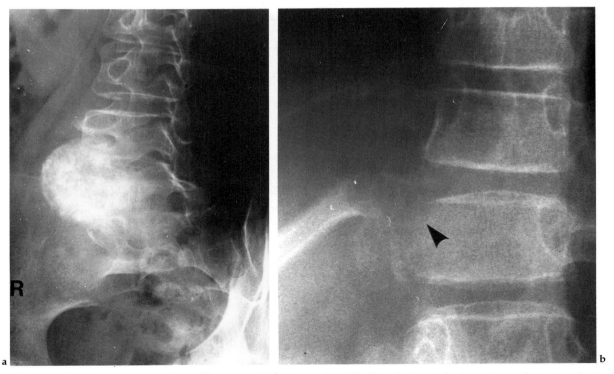

Fig. 4.38. Variable appearances of osteoblastoma. **a** This 13-year-old girl had low back pain for 9 months; scoliosis is evident and there is a large, osteosclerotic expansile lesion in the right pedicle of L5. **b** This 12-year-old girl had back pain for 10 months and had scoliosis; there is a large expansile osteolytic and osteosclerotic lesion in the lamina, pedicle and transverse process of T6 (*arrow*). (*continued overleaf*)

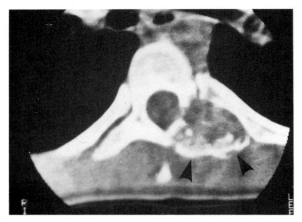

Fig. 4.38. (*continued*) Variable appearances of osteoblastoma. **c** This 13-year-old boy presented with sudden onset of pain in the right thoracic region, worse at night; there is a large osteolytic lesion involving right posterior elements and body of T11 (*arrows*). (From Azouz et al. 1986, with permission.)

Fig. 4.40. Eosinophilic granuloma (histiocytosis X). **a,b** Monofocal eosinophilic granuloma in a 2.5-year-old boy who presented with increasing back pain over several weeks. (From Kozlowski et al. 1984, with permission.) **a** Extensive destructive changes in L2 vertebral body. **b** Radiography performed 1 month later showed typical appearances of vertebral histiocytosis X – vertebra plana. Such quick progress of the changes would be unlikely in Ewing's sarcoma. **c** Monofocal eosinophilic granuloma in a 6-year-old girl who had had back pain for several months; there is verbebra plana (*arrow*). **d** Multifocal eosinophilic granuloma; an expasile lesion is seen in the left pedicle of L4, with an area of bone loss within this pedicle (*arrow*); the plain radiograph showed an ill-defined lytic lesion in the widened pedicle (11-year-old girl).

$\longrightarrow$

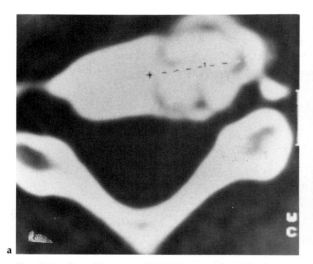

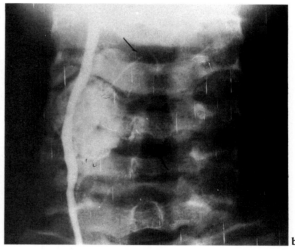

Fig. 4.39. Osteoblastoma. This 10-year-old girl had progressive cervical pain for 2 years and torticollis. **a** Osteosclerotic lesion of a diameter up to 1 cm in the body of C5, a very rare location for osteoblastoma. **b** Arteriography shows a highly vascularized tumor with feeding branches from several vessels. (From Azouz et al. 1986, with permission.)

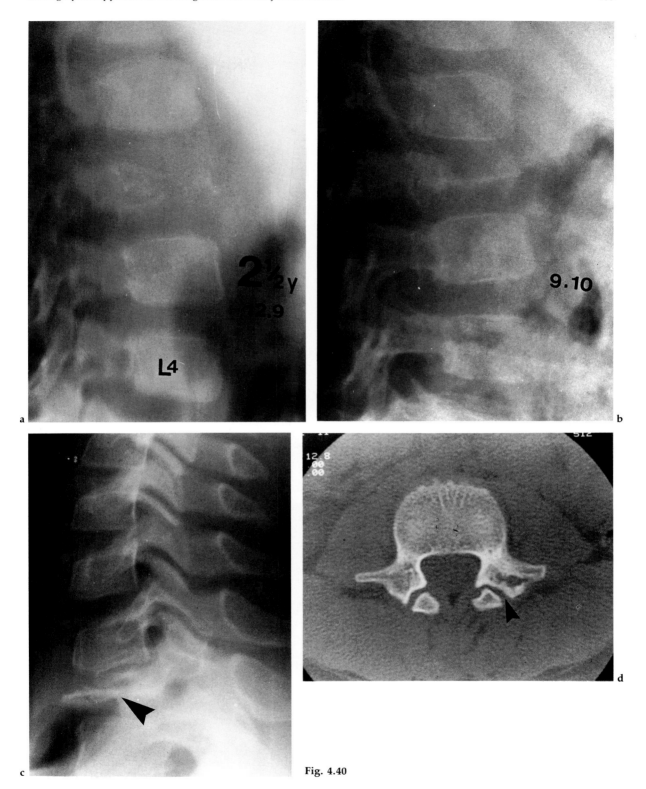

Fig. 4.40

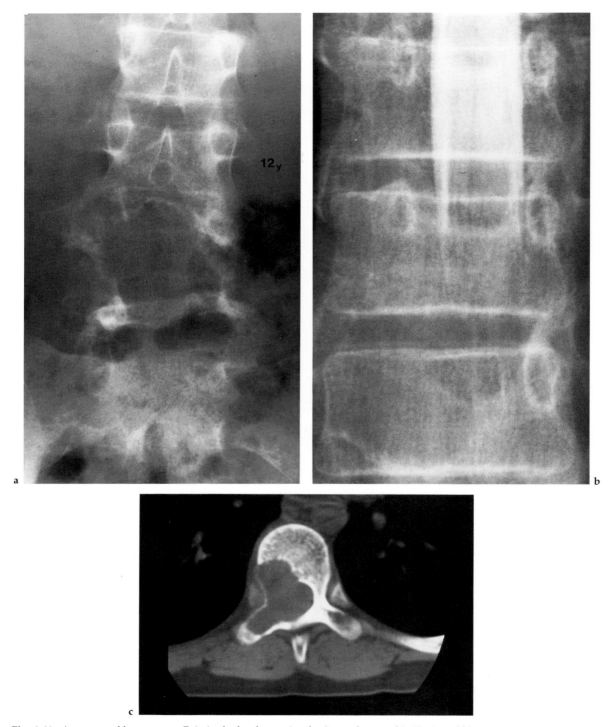

Fig. 4.41. Aneurysmal bone cyst. **a** Pain in the lumbar region for 8 months was this 12-year-old boy's presenting symptom: lytic, expansile lesion in the pedicle of L4 extending into the vertebral body and surrounded by a thin shell of bone. (From Kozlowski et al. 1984, with permission.) **b,c** This 13-year-old boy had a history of neuroblastoma and presented with back pain over a period of 6 weeks: **b** myelography demonstrates that the right pedicle of T8 is absent, and a total block at the level of T7; **c** a large, lytic, expansile lesion in the right posterior elements of T8 extending into the spinal canal and vertebral body.

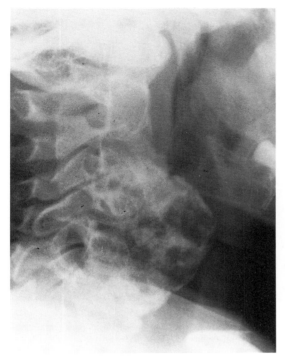

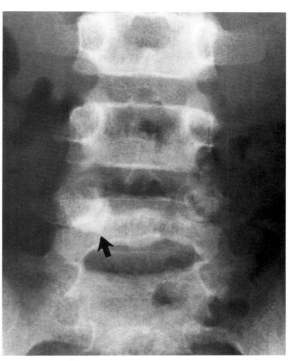

Fig. 4.42. Exchondroma. An 8-year-old boy with exchondromatosis presented with difficulty in swallowing and a lump in the neck. There are several clusters of calcification at the level of C7 and T1. (From Kozlowski et al. 1984, with permission.)

Fig. 4.43. Ostechondroma in a 7-year-old boy with rhabdomyosarcoma. A bone scan made earlier showed focal tracer accumulation in the region of the right side of the L5 vertebral body. There is a sclerotic lesion in the right pedicle of L5 (*arrow*). (From Kozlowski et al. 1987, with permission.)

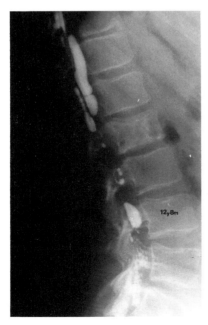

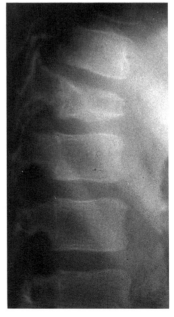

Fig. 4.44. Ewing's sarcoma. This 12-year-old girl experienced back pain for several months. Extensive osteolytic and osteosclerotic changes are seen in the body of L2.

Fig. 4.45. Leukemia. Flattening with anterior wedging of T12 vertebral body in a 9-year-old girl who developed sudden back pain.

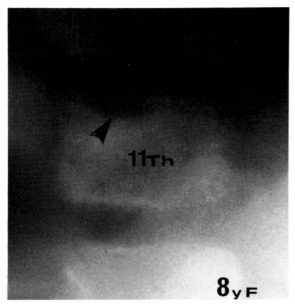

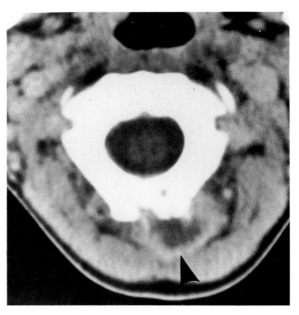

Fig. 4.46. Multifocal, chronic osteomyelitis of unknown etiology. Defect in the posterior, superior aspect of T11 vertebral body (*arrow*) (8-year-old girl). (From Kozlowski et al. 1985, with permission.)

Fig. 4.47. Osteomyelitis. This 5.5-year-old boy had neck pain for 3 weeks after circumcision; the plain radiographs were normal. A periosteal soft tissue abscess (*arrow*) is seen.

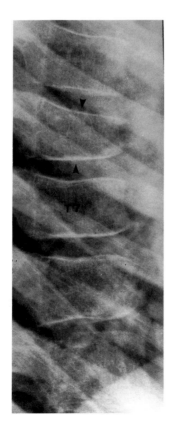

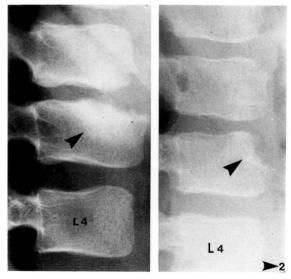

Fig. 4.49. Anterior intervertebral disk herniation (*arrows*). This type of spinal injury is common in boys active in contact sports. Often it is misdiagnosed as osteomyelitis, sometimes as eosinophilic granuloma. (From Kozlowski 1977, with permission.)

◄ **Fig. 4.48.** Trauma. Flattening with anterior wedging of T8 vertebral body (*arrows*), resulting from a fall (9-year-old boy).

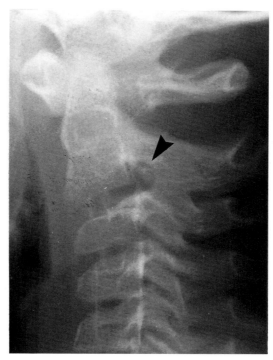

Fig. 4.50. Pseudo-osteoid osteoma – foramen transversarium, a congenital abnormality. The central density is a portion of the spinal process projected through the lucency of the foramen (*arrow*).

LITERATURE
Vertebral Tumors

Allen BL, Jinkins WJ. Vertebral osteonecrosis associated with pancreatitis in a child. J Bone Joint Surg 1978;60-A: 985–7

Ameri MR, Zurbriggen S, Wagner HP. Das solitäre eosinophile Granulom der Wirbelsaüle. Radiol Clin Biol 1974;43: 318–27

Azouz EM, Kozlowski K, Marton D, et al. Osteoid osteoma and osteoblastoma of the spine in children. Pediatr Radiol 1986;16:25–31

Barea FL, Peralto JLR, Lopez JG, Grueso FSP. Case report 694. Skeletal Radiol 1991;20:539–42

Beltran J, Simon DC, Levy M, et al. Aneurysmal bone cysts: MR imaging at 1.5 T[1]. Radiology 1986;158:689–90

Blery M, Le Roux B. Osteome osteoide vertebral. A propos de six cas. Ann Radiol 1978;21:59–63

Bonakdarpour A, Mayer DP, Clancy M, Steel H, Petersen

RO. Case report 208. Skeletal Radiol 1982;8:319–21

Bruïne FT, Kroon HM. Spinal chordoma: radiographic features in 14 cases. AJR 1988;150:861–3

Capanna R, Albisinni U, Picci P, et al. Aneurysmal bone cyst of the spine. J Bone J Surg 1985;67-A:527–31

Capanna R, Ayala A, Bertoni F, et al. Sacral osteoid osteoma and osteoblastoma: a report of 13 cases. Arch Orthop Trauma Surg 1986;105:205–10

Cory DA, Fritsch SA, Cohen MD, et al. Aneurysmal bone cysts: imaging findings and embolotherapy. AJR 1989;153: 369–73

Daffner RH, Linetsky L, Zabkar JH. Case report 433. Skeletal Radiol 1987;16:428–32

Eftekhari F, Wallce S, Chuang VP, et al. Intra-arterial management of giant-cell tumors of the spine in children. Pediatr Radiol 1982;12:289–93

Faure C, Boccon-Gibod L, Herve J, Pernin P. Case report 154. Skeletal Radiol 1981;6:229–31

Gamba JL, Martinez S, Apple J, Harrelson JM, Nunley JA. Computed tomography of axial skeletal osteoid osteomas. AJR 1984;142:769–72

Greinacher L, Gutjahr P. Tumorbedingte Veränderungen im Röntgenbild der kindlichen Wirbelsäule. Monatsschr Kinderheilkol 1976;124:519–26

Greinacher I, Gutjahr P. Histiocytosis X. Röntgenbefunde an der Wirbelsäule des Kindes. Radiologe 1978;18:228–32

Hay MC, Paterson D, Taylor TKF. Aneurysmal bone cyst of the spine. J Bone J Surg 1978;60-B:406–11

Hoeffel JC, Brasse F, Schmitt M. About one case of vertebral chondroblastoma. Pediatr Radiol 1987;17:392–6

Howe JW, Baumgard S, Yochum TR, Sladich MA. Case report 449. Skeletal Radiol 1988;17:52–5

Immenkamp M. Das eosinophile Granulom der Wirbelsäule. Z Orthop 1985;123:227–34

Janin Y, Epstein JA, Carras R, Khan A. Osteoid osteomas and osteoblastomas of the spine. Neurosurgery 1981;8: 31–8

Kaernbach A, Strecker EP, Schäfer JH. Aggressive aneurysmale Knochencyste der Wirbelsäule im Kindesalter. Radiologe 1978;18:279–83

Kirwan EO'G, Hutton PAN, Pozo JL, Ransford AO. Osteoid osteoma and benign osteoblastoma of the spine. Clinical presentation and treatment. J Bone J Surg 1984;66-B:21–6

Klaassen MA, Hoffman G. Ewing's sarcoma presenting as spondylolisthesis. Report of a case. J Bone J Surg 1987;69-A:1089–92

Kozlowski K. Anterior intervertebral disc herniation in children. Pediatr Radiol 1977;6:32–5

Kozlowski K, Beluffi G, Masel J, et al. Primary vertebral tumours in children. Report of 20 cases with brief literature review. Pediatr Radiol 1984;14:129–39

Kozlowski K, Beluffi G, Feltham C, James M, Nespoli L, Tamaela L. Multifocal, chronic osteomyelitis of unknown etiology. A further report. Fortschr Röntgenstr 1985;142: 440–6

Kozlowski K, Scougall J, Stevens M. Solitary osteochondroma of the spine. Report of two unusual cases in children. Fortschr Röntgenstr 1987;146:462–4

Kraeft H, Holschneider AM, Gratzl O, Meister P, Hecker WCh. Aneurysmatische Knochenzyste der Brustwirbelsäule mit Rippen- und Lungenbeteiligung. Z Kinderchir 1980;29:262–7

Lanzieri ChL, Solodnik P, Sacher M, Herman G. Computed tomography of solitary spinal osteochondromas. J Comput Assist Tomogr 1985;9:1042–4

Lundeen MA, Herring JA. Osteoid osteoma of the spine: sclerosis in two levels. A case report. J Bone J Surg 1980;62-A:476–8

Malghem J, Maldague B, Esselinckx W, Noel H, DeNayer P, Vincent A. Spontaneous healing of aneurysmal bone cysts. A report of three cases. J Bone Joint Surg 1989;71-B: 645–50

Mau H. Das osteoid-osteom der Wirbelsäle. Z Orthop 1982; 120:761–6

Mnaymneh W, Brown M, Tejada F, Morrison G. Primary osteogenic sarcoma of the second cervical vertebra. Case report. J Bone J Surg 1979;61-A:460–3

Mohan V, Arora MM, Gupta RP, Issat F. Aneurysmal bone cyst of the dorsal spine. Arch Orthop Trauma Surg 1989; 108:390–3

Pettine KA, Klassen RA. Osteoid osteoma and osteoblastoma of the spine. J Bone J Surg 1986;68-A:353–61

Schajowicz F. Tumors and tumorlike lesions of bones and joints. New York: Springer-Verlag, 1981

Schwimer SR, Bassett LW, Mancuso AA, Mirra JM, Dawson EG. Giant cell tumor of the cervicothoracic spine. AJR 1981;136:63–7

Shives TC, Dahlin DC, Sim FH, Pritchard DJ, Earle JD. Osteosarcoma of the spine. J Bone J Surg 1986;68-A:660–8

Twersky J, Kassner EG, Tenner MS, Camera A. Vertebral and costal osteochondromas causing spinal cord compression. AJR 1975;124:124–9

Urso S, Alessi G, Risi D, Migliorini A, Pacciani E. Osteoma osteoide ed osteoblastoma a localizzazione vertebrale. Radiol Med 1987;73:13–20

Weinstein JB, Siegel MJ, Griffith RC. Spinal Ewing's sarcoma: misleading appearances. Skeletal Radiol 1984;11: 262–5

Wooten WB, Summer TE, Crowe JE, Ayala A. Case report 64. Skeletal Radiol 1978;3:65–7

CLAVICULAR TUMORS

Clavicular tumors are rare, comprising about 1% of all bone neoplasms. Often the clavicle is one of the locations of the multifocal diseases eosinophilic granuloma, leukemia or fibrous dysplasia.

Review of the literature on clavicular tumors shows that primary malignant lesions are more common than benign ones. In childhood, both are very rare. Eosinophilic granuloma (histiocytosis X) is the most common benign lesion (Fig. 4.51), and Ewing's sarcoma and osteosarcoma the most common malignant lesions (Fig. 4.52). All the other primary bone tumors or tumorous conditions do occur occasionally:

aneurysmal bone cyst, simple bone cyst, osteoid osteoma.

The most important lesion in the differential diagnosis is the common clavicular osteomyelitis (Figs 4.53–4.55). Usually the clinical history, signs, symptoms and blood tests allow correct diagnosis. Condensing clavicular osteomyelitis may sometimes cause confusion, especially if the lesion is unifocal and not part of a multifocal

chronic osteomyelitis or pustulosis plantopalmaris. Sternoclavicular hyperostosis is a condition of adults. The clavicle is affected in the majority of patients with Caffey's disease.

Other medical disorders involving clavicular changes should cause no diagnostic problems. Post-traumatic and congenital anomalies are usually easy to differentiate from clavicular tumors.

Table 4.8. Clavicular tumors

Benign	Malignant	Differential diagnosis
Eosinophilic granuloma Rarely other benign tumors, as unifocal disease	Ewing's sarcoma Osteosarcoma	Osteomyelitis Caffey's disease Trauma Congenital abnormalities

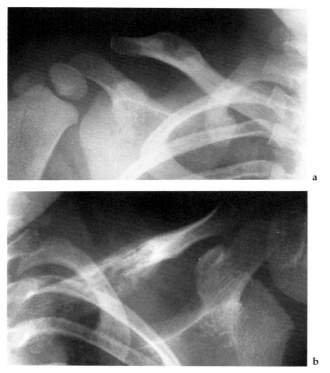

Fig. 4.51. Eosinophilic granuloma (histiocytosis X). **a** This 5-year-old girl had had a painful right shoulder for several weeks; there is a radiolucent expansile lesion with cortical invasion at the outer end of the right clavicle. **b** This 4-year-old girl fell on her left shoulder 7 weeks previously and was in pain; on examination, no abnormality was detected. 10 days before radiography, a lump over the left clavicle and tenderness were noticed. The lesion is expansile, destructive and with extensive periosteal reaction.

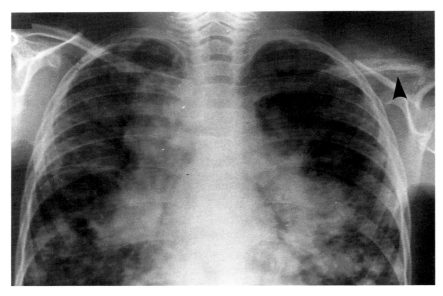

Fig. 4.52. Undifferentiated, non-epithelial malignant tumor – possibly Ewing's sarcoma. This 7-year-old boy had increasing swelling of the left clavicle over a period of 4 months, and cough, dyspnea and loss of weight for 2 months. Extensive clavicular destruction with periosteal thickening (*arrow*), and massive pulmonary metastases are seen. (From Kozlowski et al. 1970; with permission.)

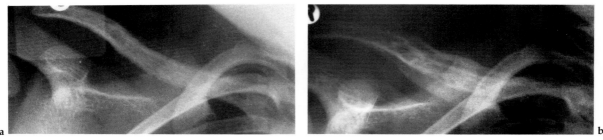

Fig. 4.53. Staphyloccoccal osteomyelitis. The radiographs were taken 2 (**a**) and 4 weeks (**b**) after the diagnosis. Note similarity between **b** and Fig. 4.51b.

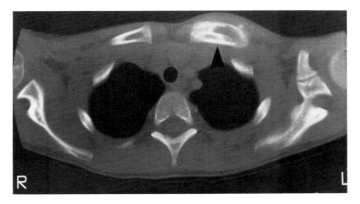

Fig. 4.54. Staphylococcal osteomyelitis. This 10-year-old boy had fractured his left clavicle at the ages of 3 and 7 years. He presented with clavicular pain over a period of a month. Extensive clavicular destruction with periosteal thickening may be seen (*arrow*).

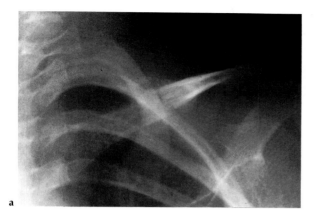

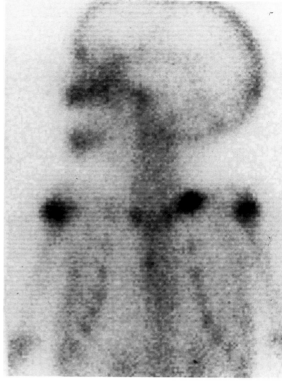

Fig. 4.55. Staphylococcal osteomyelitis. **a** Osteoporosis of the medial part of the left clavicle; there is indefinite fracture line in the midpart with soft tissue mass or callus formation. **e** Highly positive but nonspecific nuclear scan. (1.5-year-old boy.)

LITERATURE
Tumors of the Clavicle

Alman BA, Goldberg MJ. Solitary osteochondroma of the clavicle. J Ped Orthop 1991;11:181–3

Franklin JL, Parker JC, King HA. Nontraumatic clavicle lesions in children. J Pediatr Orthop 1987;7:575–8

Gardiner GA. Clavicular nonosteogenic fibroma. Am J Dis Child 1974;127:737–5

Gerscovich EO, Greenspan A, Szabo RM. Benign clavicular lesions that may mimic malignancy. Skeletal Radiol 1991; 20:173–80

Glay A. Destructive lesions of the clavicle. J Assoc Can Radiol 1961;12:117–125

Healey JH, Land JM, Erlandson RA, et al. Solid leukemic tumor. An uncommon presentation of a common disease. Clin Orthop 1985;194:248–51

Herring JA. Lesion of the clavicle. J Pediatr Orthop 1986;6: 236–8

Jurik AG, Moller BN. Inflammatory hyperostosis and sclerosis of the clavicle. Skeletal Radiol 1986;15:284–90

Klein MJ, Lusskin R, Becker MH, et al. Osteoid osteoma of the clavicle. Clin Orthop 1979;143:162–4

Kozlowski K, Gorska M, Depowski M, Sikorska B. Tumeurs osséuses rare primitives ou secondaires de l'enfant. A propos de neuf observation. Ann Radiol 1970;13:219–28

Mackay RMI, Gandhi RK. Eosinophilic granuloma of the clavicle. Br J Surg 1963;50:552–4

Smith J, Yuppa F, Watson RC. Primary tumors and tumor-like lesions of the clavicle. Skeletal Radiol 1988;17:235–47

SCAPULAR TUMORS

Scapular tumors are rare in childhood, with the exception of exchondromata which are found often in children affected by exchondromatosis. The scapula may be affected in enchondromatosis and multifocal fibrous dysplasia.

Eosinophilic granuloma (histiocytosis X) is a relatively common condition which should be considered in any monostotic destructive process (Fig. 4.56). Aneurysmal bone cyst may occasionally be encountered. All the other benign scapular bone tumors are rare.

The most common malignant tumors of scapula are Ewing's sarcoma (Fig. 4.57), osteosarcoma (Fig. 4.58), lymphoma (Fig. 4.59) and chondrosarcoma (Fig. 4.60). Malignant vascular tumors such as haemangioendothelioma occur sporadically.

The most important lesions in the differential diagnosis are Caffey's disease (infantile cortical hyperostosis) in infancy (Fig. 4.61) and osteomyelitis later in life (Fig. 4.62). Soft tissue tumors which impinge on the scapula may mimic primary scapular tumors.

The examinations of choice for the demonstration of the anatomical details are CT and MR. The diagnosis and differential diagnosis of primary scapular bone tumors is much easier when these new modalities are used.

Table 4.9. Scapular tumors

Benign	Malignant		Differential diagnosis
	Common	Rare	
Osteochondroma (exchondromatosis)	Ewing's sarcoma Osteosarcoma	Lymphoma Chondrosarcoma Malignant vascular tumors	Osteomyelitis Caffey's disease Soft tissue tumors Trauma Osteolysis
Eosinophilic granuloma (histiocytosis X)			
Aneurysmal bone cyst			
Fibrous dysplasia (multifocal)			
All other primary benign scapular bone tumors are rare			

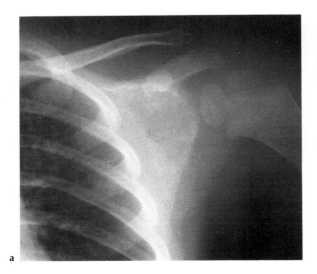

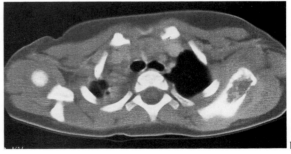

Fig. 4.56. Eosinophilic granuloma (histiocytosis X). This 18-month-old girl fell on her left shoulder 2 weeks before presentation and had a tender mass over the right scapula. **a** Poorly-defined radiolucent defect with some irregular calcification extending into the glenoid. **b** CT scan showing that, in spite of some cortical invasion, there is little if any soft tissue mass. (*continued*)

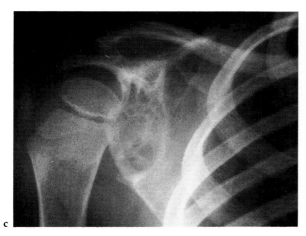

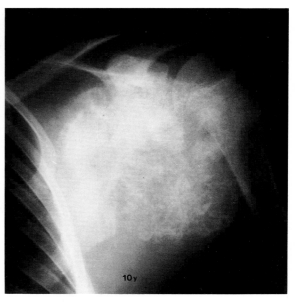

c

Fig. 4.56 (*continued*) **c** A 2-year-old girl presented with pain in the right shoulder over several weeks. A large, polycystic destructive lesion is seen in the glenoid region of the right scapula.

Fig. 4.58. Osteosarcoma. A 10-year-old girl presented with a 2-week histroy of pain in the left arm radiating into the wrist. There is a large tumor in the region of the left scapula, with extensive osteosclerotic and osteolytic changes in the scapula. The girl died 16 months after the initial diagnosis. (From Kozlowski 1980, with permission.)

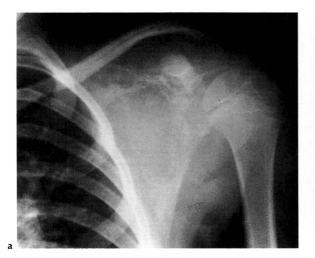

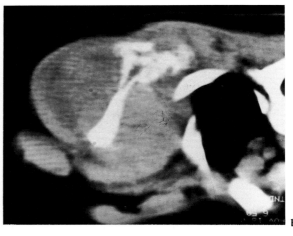

a b

Fig. 4.57. Ewing's sarcoma. Increasing pain in the right shoulder for several months was this 5-year-old girl's presentation. **a** Extensive destructive process in the upper part of the right scapula. **b** CT clearly shows the large soft tissue mass.

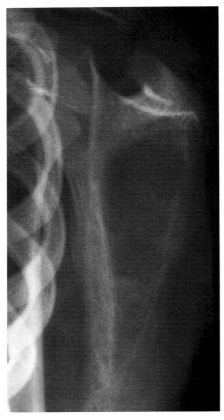

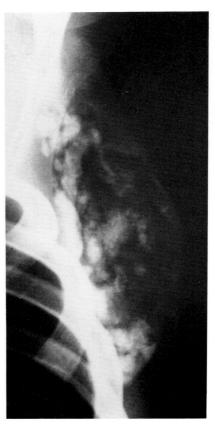

Fig. 4.59. Lymphoma. This 7-year-old boy experienced pain in the left shoulder for several months. A large, destructive lesion with abundant periosteal reaction is seen in the left scapula.

Fig. 4.60. Chondrosarcoma. This 11-year-old boy had a progressively painful left shoulder after a fall some weeks previously and was experiencing limitation of arm movements. A large, expansile lesion, with multiple irregular calcifications, is present in the left scapula.

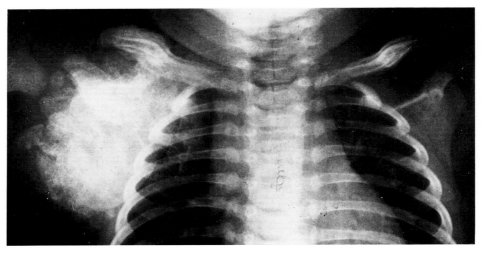

Fig. 4.61. Caffey's disease (infantile cortical hyperostosis). Extensive hyperostosis of the right scapula; both clavicles are also affected (8-month-old boy).

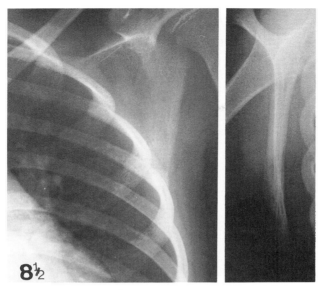

Fig. 4.62. Osteomyelitis. This 8.5-year old girl had fever and shoulder pain for 3 weeks. Lamellar, periosteal thickening is well-demonstrated in the axial view.

LITERATURE
Scapular Tumors

Abdul-Karim FW, Pathria MN, Heller JG, Sorensen RU. Case report 664. Skeletal Radiol 1991;20:227–9

Gold RH, Mirra JM. Case Report 234. Skeletal Radiol 1983;10:57–60

Freedman S, Taber P, Alter A. Benign osteoblastic lesion in the scapula of a child. Am J Dis Child 1972;123:236–7

Hope JW, Gould RJ. Scapular lesions in childhood. AJR 1962;88:496–502

Kozlowski K. Osteiod sarcoma with unusual clinical and/or radiographic appearances. Pediatr Radiol 1980;9:167–70

Pratt GF, Dahlin DC, Ghormley RK. Tumours of scapula and clavicle. Surg Gynecol Obstet 1958;106:536–44

Samilson RL, Morris JM, Thompson RW. Tumours of the scapula. A review of the literature and an analysis of 31 cases. Clin Orthop 1968;58:105–15

Smith J, McLachlan DL, Huvos AG, et al. Primary tumours of the clavicle and scapula. AJR 1975;124:113–23

STERNAL TUMORS

In a child with a primary destructive sternal lesion the diagnosis is osteomyelitis until proved otherwise (Fig. 4.63). We have not seen any child with primary sternal bone tumor, though one of our patients with polyostotic eosinophilic granuloma showed positive sternal nuclear scan

Both the benign and malignant primary sternal tumors are extremely rare in childhood

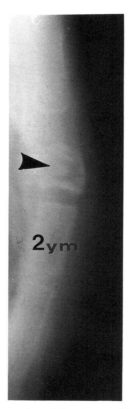

Fig. 4.63. Osteomyelitis. This 3-year-old boy presented with swelling over the sternum painful on palpation. There is a destructive lesion in the proximal ossification center of the body of the sternum. A sequester is present inside the abscess (*arrow*).

RIB TUMORS

The symptoms and signs of the primary rib tumors are fairly uniform: thoracic, sometimes shoulder or pleuritic, rarely abdominal, pain and localized swelling. A history of preceding trauma, supposedly causing the disease, is frequently ascertained. This probably causes subclinical, pathologic fractures or local hemorrhages which are not demonstrated on radiographs. Horner syndrome, superior vena cava syndrome, pseudoabdominal tumor in cases of lower rib involvement and systemic manifestations suggesting rib infection have all been sporadically reported. Benign tumors usually cause less disability. Often they are an incidental finding on a routine chest radiograph or a radiograph taken because of prolonged chest pain – due to a pathologic fracture – after a minor trauma.

Most of the primary rib tumors in children are benign. Osteochondromas and enchondromas are found in conjunction with exchondromatosis and enchondromatosis (Fig. 4.64). Similarly, multifocal fibrous dysplasia (Fig. 4.65) and multifocal eosinophilic granuloma with rib involvement are easily recognizable. If osteolytic, multifocal lesions are demonstrated, polyostotic angiomatosis should be considered.

All the single, benign primary bone tumors and tumorous conditions are rare, aneurysmal bone cyst and eosinophilic granuloma being most common. Aneurysmal bone cyst presents as a localized destructive process and in the early stages may mimic malignant bone tumors, particularly Ewing's sarcoma and eosinophilic granuloma. Later, the lesion "balloons" out, but it does not extend through the cortex and there is little permeative destruction at its periphery (Fig. 4.66). The soft tissue mass is absent or small in comparison to the primary lesion. MR may show blood inside the lesion. In eosinophilic granuloma (histiocytosis X), a rare monofocal rib lesion (Fig. 4.67), the permeative destruction is more localized than in Ewing's sarcoma and the transition zone is limited to a short segment. There is usually some cortical destruction, with little periosteal reaction. The soft tissue mass, if present, is much smaller than would be expected in Ewing's sarcoma. The illness is usually not systemic. Eosinophilia is a strong indication for eosinophilic granuloma.

Other benign rib tumors – osteoid osteoma (Fig. 4.68), simple bone cyst, chondroblastoma – have been reported occasionally. The characteristic radiographic features of those lesions so spectacularly demonstrated in the long bones are virtually absent in the ribs.

Of the malignant tumors of the ribs, Ewing's sarcoma is the most common. It accounts for about 10–22% of all Ewing sarcoma cases (children and adults). In our series of 20 cases, the youngest patient was 18 months old and the symptoms lasted between 3 days and 1 year. The most important radiographic signs are rib destruction and soft tissue mass, often with

Table 4.10. Rib tumors

Common		Rare		Differential diagnosis
Benign	Malignant	Benign	Malignant	
Osteochondroma Enchondroma Fibrous dysplasia (polyostotic) Eosinophilic granuloma (polyostotic)	Ewing's sarcoma	Eosinophilic granuloma (monostotic) Fibrous dysplasia (monostotic) Aneurysmal bone cyst Osteoid osteoma Benign vascular tumors Osteoma Intraosseous neuroblastoma/ ganglioneuroma	Osteosarcoma Lymphoma Chondrosarcoma Malignant vascular tumors	Osteomyelitis (including tuberculosis and actinomycosis) Neurogenic tumors – neuroblastoma and ganglioneuroma Soft tissue tumors – intra- and extrathoracic Metastases Other rare conditions as tuberous sclerosis and intraosseous rheumatic nodule

extrathoracic extension and pleural effusion. Three major radiographic patterns can be observed in Ewing's sarcoma:

1. A lytic, permeative process with a wide zone of transition, relatively little cortical destruction, and some bone expansion and periosteal reaction (Fig. 4.69a,b).
2. Complete lysis of a portion of the rib – "disappearing rib" (Fig. 4.69c).
3. A mixed, osteolytic and osteosclerotic lesion with some rib expansion, the rarest pattern (Fig. 4.69d).

A large, adjacent soft tissue mass is always present in Ewing's sarcoma. Only in the initial stages is the lesion localized to the bone only.

Although the plain chest radiograph is the easiest and cheapest examination for rib destruction and soft tissue mass, the anatomical characteristics of the tumor, its relation to the thoracic cage, mediastinum and diaphragm, and accompanying pleural effusion cannot be well demonstrated until CT or MR are performed. Nuclear scan may show involvement in more than one rib, which probably reflects early bone metastases or infiltration of the adjacent ribs by the tumor.

Other primary malignant bone tumors of the ribs are very rare in children. Lymphoma does not show any characteristic bone changes that allow it to be differentiated from Ewing's sarcoma. Osteosarcoma, chondrosarcoma and fibrosarcoma are occasionally seen; chondrosarcoma should be considered as the most likely malignant tumor in patients with rib enchondroma or enchondromatosis.

The differential diagnosis of rib tumors has been much easier since the advent of nuclear scan, CT and MR. The anatomic details of the tumor and surrounding tissues, as well some tumor characteristics, can be beautifully displayed. Rib metastases, in which the primary tumor had not been diagnosed, are extremely rare in children. Rib metastases are common in neuroblastoma and leukemia as an expression of polyostotic involvement. Similarly, there is usually little difficulty in recognizing rib osteomyelitis. If the symptomatology of rib osteomyelitis mimics that of tumor (Fig. 4.70), then some rare bacterium or tuberculosis is likely to be the cause. Aspergillosis invades the ribs from a pre-existing soft tissue lesion. Rib trauma should not cause confusion: there is usually a history of injury, excessive sport activity, soft tissue involvement and pain on palpation. Respiratory and stress fractures resulting from physiotherapy are easily recognized if the clinical history is not neglected. In child abuse cases, even if trauma is denied there are other clinical and radiographic signs supporting the diagnosis of non-accidental injury.

Most important in the differential diagnosis of primary rib tumors are soft tissue tumors of the thorax, lungs, pleura (fibrous, muscular, vascular and neural tissue tumors) (Fig. 4.71). The soft tissue mass of an intrathoracic tumor often occupies a large part of the hemithorax and a pleural effusion may be present. If the soft tissue mass spreads to the ribs, then more than one rib is affected. The neurogenic tumors, particularly by extrinsic pressure, erode the ribs, widen the intercostal spaces and often spread into the spinal canal. In such cases, deformity of the ribs is greater than the destruction; the opposite is true in the primary rib tumors.

There are only few conditions which present with diagnostic radiographic changes. These include chest mesenchymoma (see Fig. 4.158), a characteristic tumor of infancy, and tuberous sclerosis.

With proper history, basic biochemical tests, plain chest radiographs, nuclear studies and/or skeletal survey, the diagnosis of rib tumors can be established in most cases. This high percentage can be even elevated if CT and MR are performed. There will remain a small number of cases in which the clinicoradiographic diagnosis will fail because of unusual or rare pathology, as in the case of rheumatic nodule within the rib, as reported by Brantley et al. (1987). There will also remain some cases in which the histologic diagnosis remain uncertain.

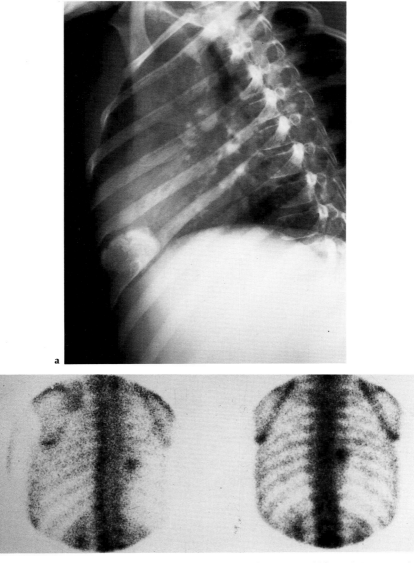

Fig. 4.64. Osteochondroma. **a** Lump in the anterior part of the 7th left rib (12-year-old boy). **b** Lump in the posterior part of the 8th right rib. Positive nuclear scan. (Courtesy of Dr L Morris, Adelaide Children's Hospital.)

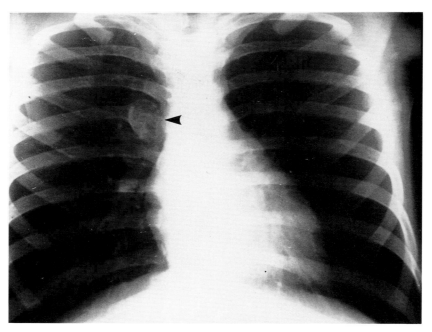

Fig. 4.65. Fibrous dysplasia. Unusual deformity of the posterior end of the 5th right rib (10-year-old girl) (*arrow*). Other bone changes typical of fibrous dysplasia were also present. (From Kozlowski et al. 1989, with permission.)

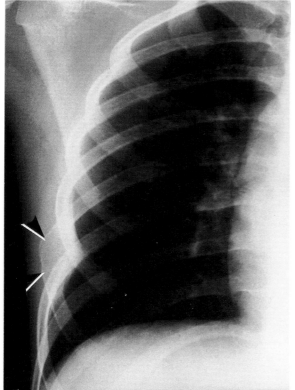

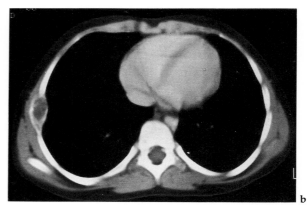

Fig. 4.66. Aneurysmal bone cyst. This 9-year-old girl presented with localized right-sided chest pain and a palpable lump at the level of 6th rib. **a** Destructive, slightly expansile lesion at the 6th right rib in the midaxillary line (*arrow*). **b** CT shows localized lytic lesion without soft tissue mass. (From Kozlowski et al. 1989, with permission.)

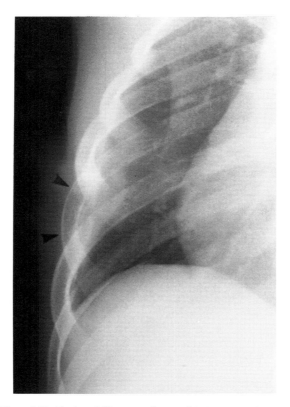

Fig. 4.67. Eosinophilic granuloma (histiocytosis X). A painless mass was present in the right chest wall of this 6.5-year-old boy for 2 months. Destructive changes are seen in the 6th right rib (*arrows*). (From Kozlowski et al. with 1989, with permission.)

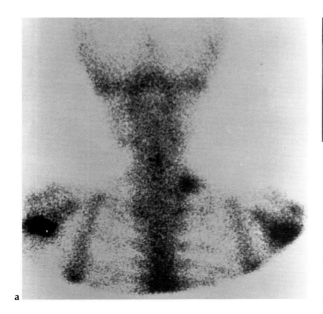

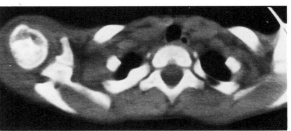

Fig. 4.68. Osteoid osteoma. This 6.5-year-old boy presented with a 2-month history of night pain in the lower neck responding to aspirin. **a** Positive nuclear scan. **b** Osteolytic defect in the posterior part of the 1st rib. (From Kozlowski et al. 1989, with permission.)

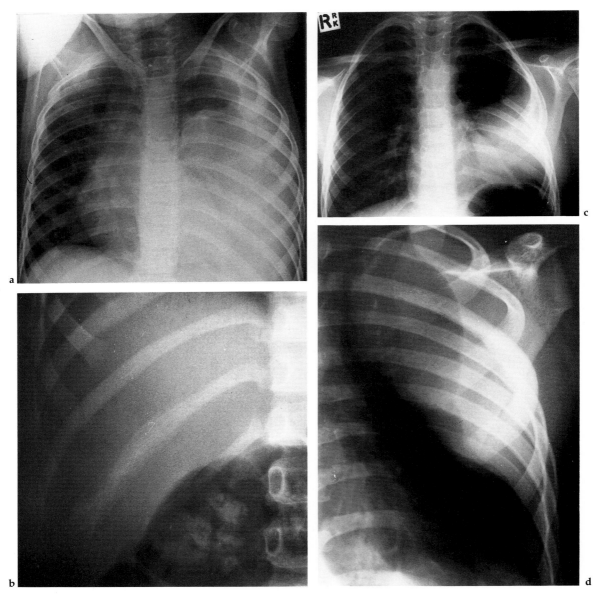

Fig. 4.69. Ewing's sarcoma. **a** This 8-year-old girl had a history of pain in the left chest for 6 months, anorexia and weight loss. There are opacification of the left chest with pleural effusion and osteolytic changes in the 6th left rib. **b** This 7-year-old boy had enlargement of the 11th right rib after a kick. The diagnosis was subperiosteal hematoma; 10 months later he presented with "swollen" 11th rib. There is permeative destruction of the 11th rib with some periosteal reaction. **c** Chest discomfort, weight loss and cough for 2 months were this 7-year-old boy's symptoms. He had a "disappearing rib". Lytic destruction of the anteromedial part of the 6th left rib was seen. CT showed a large soft tissue mass with extrathoracic extension. **d** Presenting with increasing shoulder pain for 6 weeks, general malaise, loss of weight and weakness, this 10-year-old boy had osteosclerosis of the 4th left rib, with a large soft tissue mass. Routine radiography 10 months earlier which showed minimal changes was reported as normal. (**a, c, d** From Kozlowski et al. 1989, **b** from Kozlowski et al. 1976, with permission.)

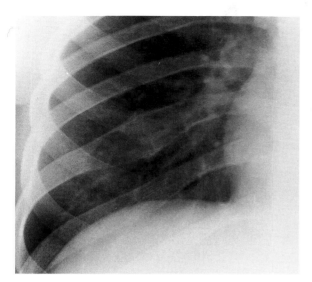

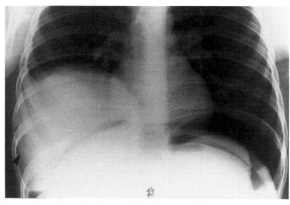

Fig. 4.71. Mesothelioma. This 7-year-old boy had dyspnea and cachexia. He was followed up for 1 year because of the abnormal appearance of his left lung. Destructive changes in the 9th right rib are seen.

Fig. 4.70. Granulomatous osteomyelitis. This 7-year-old boy presented with lump attached posteriorly to the 9th right rib. An earlier radiograph showed fracture. One month later, a lytic lesion is seen. (From Kozlowski et al. 1989, with permission.)

LITERATURE
Rib Tumors

Abadou H, Bernard C, Bretagne MC, Marchal AM, Derelle J, Hoeffel JC. L'imagerie dans les tumeurs costales primitives chez l'enfant et l'adolescent. À propos de 10 cas. Med Infant 1988;95:855–64

Berard J, de Beaujeu MJ, Valla JS. Les tumeurs primitives se côtes chez l'enfant et l'adolescent. A propos de 15 cas. Chir Pediatr 1982;23:387–92

Brantley SD, Schksinger AE, Orzel JA, McQuaid KJ. Intraosseous rheumatoid nodule. Pediatr Radiol 1987;17:432–4

Derbekyan V, Azouz M. Radiological case of the month. Am J Dis Child 1984;138:885–6

Dutton RV, Singleton EB. Tuberous sclerosis: a case report with aortic aneurysm and unusual rib changes. Pediatr Radiol 1975;3:184–6

Joseph WL, Fonkalsrud EW. Primary rib tumours in children. Am Surg 1972;38:338–42

Kaiser G, Locher GW. Ungewöhnliche Rippentumoren beim Kind: Ein Beitrag zur klinischen und patologisch-anatomischen Besonderheit atypisch lokalisierter Riesenzelltumoren und aneurismatischer Knochenzysten. Z Kinderchir 1975;16:234–46

Klein GM. Chondromyxoid fibroma. An unusual location. Clin Orthop Rel Res 1982;164:249–51

Kozlowski K, Bale P, Reye RDK. Difficulté du diagnostic radiographique des tumeurs primitive. Ann Radiol 1976;19:781–90

Kozlowski K, Campbell J, Morris L, Sprague P, Taccone A, Beluffi Marcinski A, Porta F, Stevens M. Primary rib tumors in children. (Report of 27 cases with short literature review.) Austr Radiol 1989;33:210–22

Leb I, Denes J, Schläffer E. Riesenzelltumor der Rippe im Mindesalter. Z Kinderchir 1976;19:413–16

Levine E, Levine C. Ewing's tumour of rib. Radiologic

findings and computed tomography – contribution. Skeletal Radiol 1983;9:227–33

Locher GW, Kaiser G. Giant-cell tumours and aneurysmal bone cysts of ribs in childhood. J Pediatr Surg 1975;10: 103–8

Marchal AL, Hoeffel JC, Bocquillon H, Brasse F, Olive D. Atteintes pleurales par contiguïté ou métastases dans les tumeurs osséuses malignes primitives de l'enfant. J Radiol 1986;67:303–7

McCarthy EF, Dorfman HD. Vascular and cartilaginous hamartoma of the ribs in infancy with secondary aneurysmal bone cyst formation. Am J Surg Pathol 1980;4: 247–53

Mitchell ChD. Rib sarcoma with multiple bone metastases. Med Pediatr Oncol 1985;13:298

Oakley RH, Carty H, Cudmore RE. Multiple benign

mesenchymomata of the chest wall. Pediatr Radiol 1985; 15:58–60

Shulman HS, Wilson SR, Harvie JN, Cruickshank B. Unicameral bone cyst in a rib in a child. AJR 1977;128: 1058–60

Strom FK, Eilber FR, Mirra J, Morton DL. Neurofibrosarcoma. Cancer 1980;45:126–9

Sundaram M, McGuire MH, Naunheim K, Schajowicz F. Case report 467. Skeletal Radiol 1988;17:136–40

Tulloh HP, Harry D. Osteoblastoma in a rib in childhood. Clin Radiol 1969;20:337–8

Ushigome S, Takakuwa T, Takagi M, Sato Y. Case report 263. Skeletal Radiol 1984;11:151–4

Weigel W. Ewing-Sarcome der Rippen bei Kindern. Z Kiderchir 1979;28:28–38

PELVIC TUMORS

The most common malignant bone tumor of the pelvis is Ewing's sarcoma. In children and adults the frequency of iliac involvement is approximately 11%, pubic 3% and ischial 2%.

The delay in diagnosis is usually several months, partly due to the misleading history of trauma. Pain, limping and a mass are the most important symptoms and signs. The pain is variable and poorly localized in different areas. Described as hip, groin, thigh, buttock, knee and rarely abdominal or back pain, it diverts attention from the affected area. At the time of diagnosis an abdominal mass is present in about 50% of patients.

Although the plain radiograph is the best single method in assessment of the tumor and in predicting the histologic diagnosis, CT and MR give much better information regarding the exact extension of the tumor and associated soft

tissue mass. The nuclear scan is the method of choice for detection of early metastases.

The radiographic appearances of Ewing's sarcoma are variable. Diffuse osteosclerosis, diffuse osteoporosis, permeative osteolysis and mixed forms have been reported (Figs 4.72 and 4.73).

Other primary malignant pelvic bone tumors are very rare and there are few characteristic radiographic features useful in differential diagnosis. Osteosarcoma of the pelvis is very rare in childhood. No characteristic features are present in the early stages of the disease. Primary bone lymphoma shows appearances similar to the permeative type of Ewing's sarcoma (Fig. 4.74). Chondrosarcoma, a common primary tumor in adults, has been observed in children only very rarely in the first decade of life. It presents as a lesion with mottled calcifications

(Fig. 4.75). Multiple enchondromas if present are important supportive evidence.

Chondroblastoma of the triradiate cartilage is a locally agressive lesion causing extensive lytic bony destruction and presenting with an intrapelvic soft tissue mass.

Two most important entities in the differential diagnosis of Ewing's sarcoma are eosinophilic granuloma (histiocytosis X) and osteomyelitis. Eosinophilic granuloma is often multifocal. Monostotic eosinophilic granuloma usually presents as an osteolytic, well-circumscribed lesion similar to the osteolytic form of Ewing's sarcoma. However, the soft tissue mass is small or absent in the former (Fig. 4.76). In the ischial and pubic bones, eosinophilic granuloma may present as a lytic, circumscribed lesion simulating simple bone cyst or aneurysmal bone cyst, or as a permeative lesion with periosteal reaction simulating Ewing's sarcoma or osteomyelitis.

The monostotic benign primary bone tumors, apart from eosinophilic granuloma, are rare in childhood. This rarity is increased by the fact that lesions which are often discovered accidentally on radiographs performed for other reasons and do not show radiographic signs of malignancy are not biopsied. So the true nature of the lesions remains uncertain.

Aneurysmal bone cyst usually presents with typical radiographic findings: expansile, washed out lesion with a thin shell of cortical bone showing total abscence or only minimal periosteal reaction (Fig. 4.77).

Other benign pelvic tumors have occasionally been reported. These include osteoid osteoma/ osteoblastoma complex, hemangioma and osteoma, as well as other rare primary bone tumors (Figs 4.78 and 4.79). Monostotic pelvic fibrous dysplasia occurs very rarely in childhood (Fig. 4.80). The lesion should be followed up for malignant degeneration. With new modalities the specific diagnosis of some of these rare tumors – aneurismal bone cyst, osteoid osteoma – is possible.

Osteomyelitis of the pelvis has usually a short history. Laboratory findings are in keeping with an inflammatory disease (Fig. 4.81a–c). In rare instances, low-grade osteomyelitis may cause diagnostic difficulties (Fig. 4.81d).

Traumatized apophysis – stress apophysis and traumatic apophysis – should cause no confusion. They have a characteristic history, occur in a specific age-group (teenagers and young adults) and show diagnostic radiographic appearances (Fig. 4.82). The ischial tuberosity, anterior inferior iliac spine and anterior superior iliac spine are affected in decreasing frequency. These traumatic lesions are sometimes misdiagnosed as osteosarcoma or osteomyelitis. Healed fractures of pelvic bones may sometimes present confusing appearances unless the history is known to the radiologist.

Table 4.11. Primary tumors of the pelvis

Common		Rare		Differential diagnosis
Benign	Malignant	Benign	Malignant	
Eosinophilic granuloma	Ewing's sarcoma	Exchondroma (monostotic)	Lymphoma	Osteomyelitis
Aneurysmal bone cyst		Enchondroma (monostotic)	Chondrosarcoma	Trauma
Osteochondroma (polyostotic)		Fibrous dysplasia	Osteosarcoma	(apophyseolysis,
Enchondroma (polyostatic)		(monostotic)	Malignant vascular	stress
Fibrous dysplasia (polyostotic)		Osteoid osteoma/	tumors	apophysis)
Osteoma		osteoblastoma		Anatomical
		Simple bone cyst		variants
		Chondroblastoma		Soft tissue tumors
		Giant cell tumors		Osteochondritis
				ischiopubica

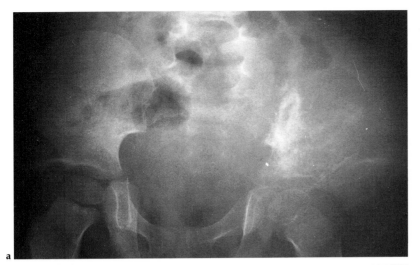

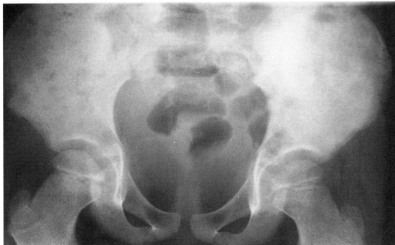

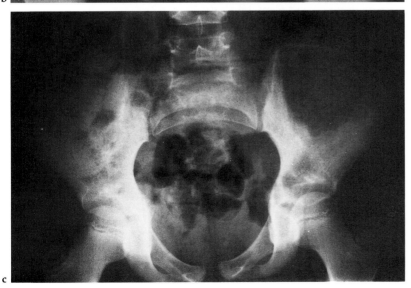

Fig. 4.72. Ewing's sarcoma. **a** Left iliac fossa swelling extending into the left buttock, and extensive destructive changes in the left iliac bone with some osteosclerosis at the medial aspect (2.5-year-old boy). **b** Three-year old boy with a history of 8 month of pain in the left knee and a limp for 2 months. There is a mass in the left iliac fossa and osteosclerosis and slight overgrowth of the left ilium with minimal periosteal thickening at the lateral aspect of the body of the left ilium. **c,d** This 6.5-year-old girl presented with a history of 8 weeks of pain and swelling in the left inguinal region. **c** Large osteolytic defect in the left ilium; minimal osteosclerotic reaction at the medial aspect (from Dr J Campbell, Orlando, USA). (*continued*)

Fig. 4.72 (*continued*) Ewing's sarcoma. **d** Extensive destruction of the left ilium, and a large soft tissue mass.

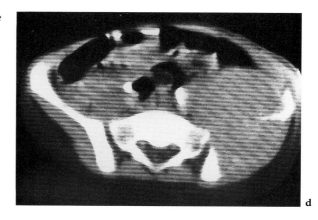

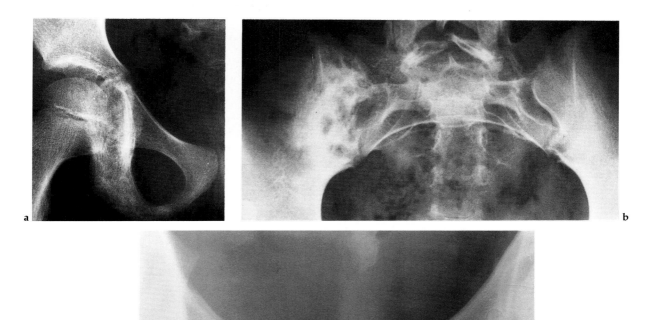

Fig. 4.73. Ewing's sarcoma. **a** This 6.5-year-old girl presented with pain and swelling of the right buttock and perineum for 4 weeks. There are mixed osteolytic and osteosclerotic destruction of the right ischium and a large soft tissue mass. **b** This 12-year-old girl presented with pain in the right sacroiliac region for 1 year; osteomyelitis was seriously considered in the differential diagnosis. **c** This 14-year-old girl presented with progressive pain in the right groin. An enlarged, osteosclerotic right superior pubic ramus with mature periosteal apposition is seen. (**a** From Dr J Campbell, Orlando, USA, **f,g** from Kozlowski et al. 1989, with permission.)

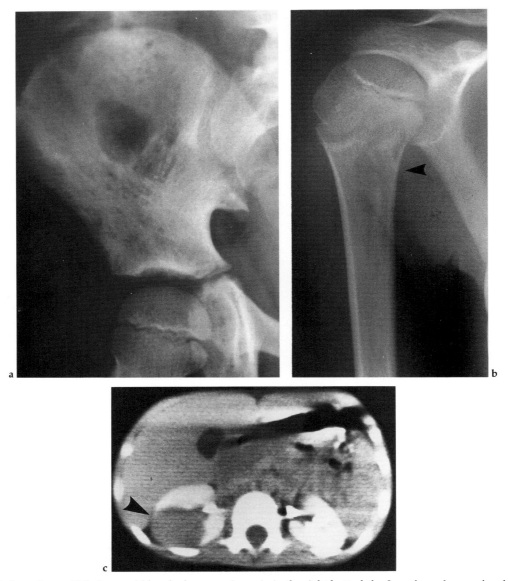

Fig. 4.74. Lymphoma. This 7-year-old boy had progressive pain in the right buttock for 3 weeks and general malaise. **a,b** Osteolytic changes in the lateral lower part of the right iliac bone and in the proximal part of the right humerus (*arrow*). **c** Large infiltration of the enlarged right kidney.

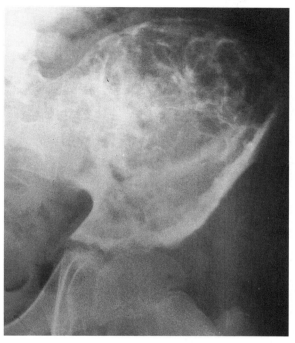

Fig. 4.75. Chondrosarcoma. Irregular, round areas of radiolucency surrounded by sclerotic rims in the upper part of the left ilium, diffuse sclerosis along the sacro-iliac joint, and a band of sclerosis along the outer edge of the iliac bone (11-year-old boy). (Courtesy of Professor A. Pelizza, Instituto G. Gaslini, Genoa, Italy; from Kozlowski et al. 1989, with permission.)

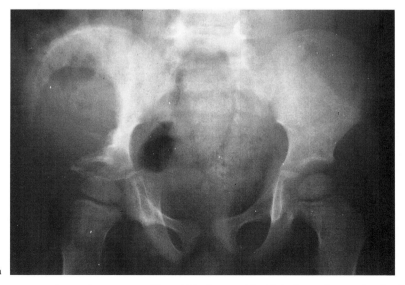

a

Fig. 4.76. Eosinophilic granuloma (histiocytosis X). **a** This 2-year-old girl had an abnormal gait after a fall 2 months previously. There is a large osteolytic defect in the right iliac bone with some sclerotic reaction in the medial aspect. (*continued overleaf*)

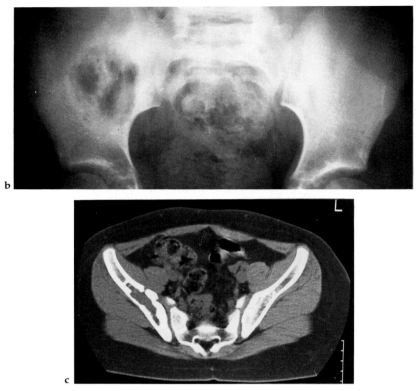

Fig. 4.76 (*continued*) Eosinophilic granuloma (histiocytosis X). **b,c** Eight-year-old girl: **b** radiography shows a large osteolytic lesion with some irregular, sclerotic reaction in the right ilium; **c** CT scan shows more extensive involvement of the ilium with a cortical break but no soft tissue mass. (Courtesy of Professor A. Pelizza, Instituto G. Gaslini, Genoa, Italy; from Kozlowski et al. 1989, with permission.)

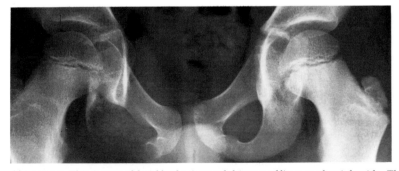

Fig. 4.77. Aneurysmal bone cyst. This 9-year-old girl had a 4-month history of limp on the right side. The radiograph shows a blown out and partly disappearing right ischium and minor, secondary deformity of the right pubis. (From Kozlowski and Middleton 1980, with permission.)

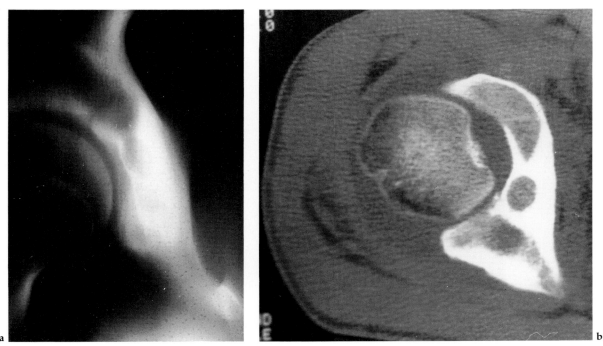

Fig. 4.78. Osteoid osteoma. Extensive sclerosis in the lower part of the right acetabulum (16-year-old boy). (From Kozlowski et al. 1989, with permission.)

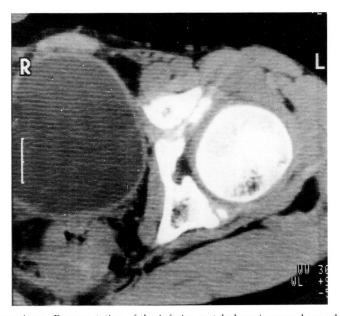

Fig. 4.79. Cavernous hemangioma. Fragmentation of the inferior acetabulum; increased vascularity is present after intravenous contrast (12.5-year-old boy). (From Kozlowski et al. 1989, with permission.)

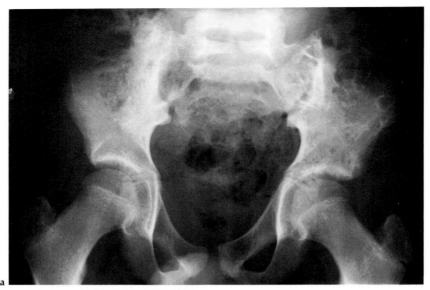

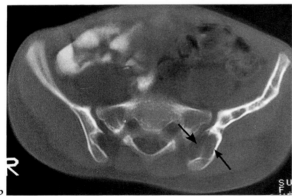

Fig. 4.80. Monostotic fibrous dysplasia (14-year-old boy). a The slightly sclerotic left ilium shows multiple small radiolucencies surrounded by sclerotic rings superiorly. The inferior part shows an irregular trabecular pattern with single, small, irregular radiolucencies. b CT scan shows an expansile lesion in the posterior iliac wing with involvement also of the body of the ilium (*arrows*). (From Kozlowski et al. 1989, with permission.)

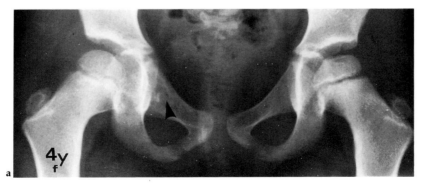

Fig. 4.81. Osteomyelitis. This 4-year-old girl had a history of pain in the right hip for several weeks. Predominantly osteolytic lesions in the acetabular part of the pubic bone (*arrow*) are seen, together with widening of the right hip joint space. (*continued*)

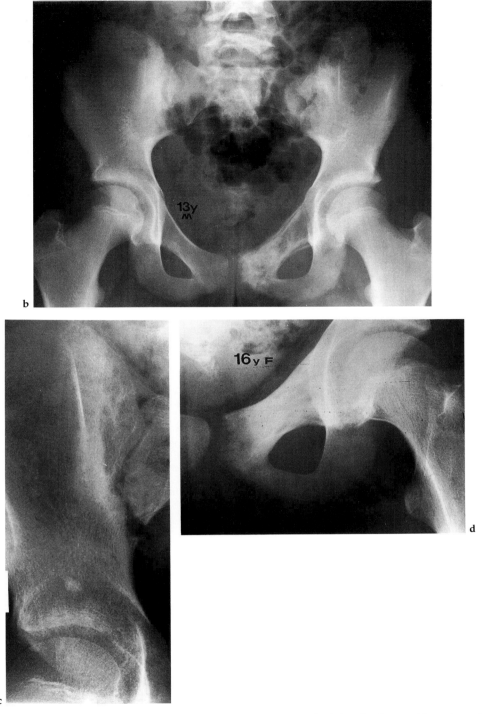

Fig. 4.81 (*continued*) **b** Extensive, predominantly osteosclerotic changes in the left pubic bone with periosteal reaction; without a clinical history typical of inflammatory process Ewing's sarcoma would be seriously considered in this 13-year-old boy. **c** This 13-year-old boy presented with right hip joint pain for 2 weeks, fever, ESR of 82, and positive blood culture. A nuclear scan showed increased uptake along the right sacro-iliac joint. The radiograph shows loss of definition of the bony cortex along the right sacro-iliac joint. **d** Extensive osteosclerotic lesion in the acetabular & pubic regions (16-year-old girl). (From Kozlowski et al. 1985, with permission.)

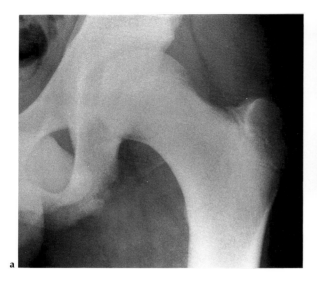

a

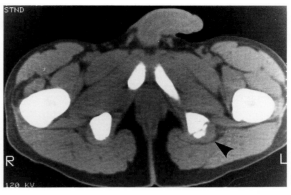

b

Fig. 4.82. Traumatic ischial apophyseolysis (*arrow*). This 14-year-old boy had a 3-month history of left upper posterior thigh pain and was misdiagnosed as having osteosarcoma. (From Kozlowski et al. 1989, with permission.)

LITERATURE
Pelvic Tumors

Appell RG, Willich E. Die Röntgendiagnostik von Strukturveränderungen im Schambeinbereich bei Kindern und Jugendlichen. Eigene Kasuistik. Differentialdiagnose und Literaturübersicht. Radiologe 1983;23:66–71

Beaupre A, Carroll N. The three syndromes of iliac osteomyelitis in children. J Bone Jt Surg 1979;61-A:1087–92

Coombs RJ, Zeiss J, McCann K, Phillips E. Case Report 360. Skeletal Radiol 1986;15:254–7

Crone-Munzebrock W, Brassow F. A comparison of radiographic and bone scan findings in histiocytosis X. Skeletal Radiol 1983;9:170–3

Highland TR, Lamont RL. Osteomyelitis of the pelvis in children. J Bone Jt Surg 1983;65-A:230–4

Jacobs PH. Case Report 7. Skeletal Radiol 1976;1:109–11

Jurik AG, Moller SH, Mosekilde L. Chronic sclerosing osteomyelitis of the iliac bone. Etiologic possibilities. Skeletal Radiol 1988;17:114–18

Kozlowski K, Anderson RJ, Hochberger O, Sacher O. Tumorous osteomyelitis. Pediatr Radiol 1984;14:404–6

Kozlowski K, Beluffi G, Feltham C, James M, Nespoli L, Tamaela L. Multifocal, chronic osteomyelitis of unknown etiology. A further report. Fortschr Röntgenstr 1985;142:440–6

Kozlowski K, Campbell JB, Azouz EM. Traumatised ischial apophysis. Aust Radiol 1989;33:140–3

Kozlowski K, Campbell J, Beluffi G, Hoeffel JC, Morris L, Pelizza A, Sprague P, Taccone A, Arico M, Stevens M. Primary bone tumours of the pelvis in childhood – Ewing's sarcoma of the ilium, pubis and ischium. (Re-

port of 30 cases.) Part I. Austr Radiol 1989;33:354–60

Kozlowski K, Middleton RWD. Aneurysmal bone cyst – review of 10 cases. Aust Radiol 1980;34:170–5

Matsuno T, Hasegawa I, Masuda T. Chondroblastoma arising in the triradiate cartilage. Report of two cases with review of the literature. Skeletal Radiol 1987;16:216–22

MacPherson RI, Halvorsen R. Tumours of the pubis: an analysis by probabilities. J Assoc Can Radiol 1981;32:168–170

Pons A. La dégenerance maligne de la dysplasie fibreuse des os. Revue générale à propos de deux observation. Ann Radiol 1974;17:713–20

Price CHG, Zuber K, Salzer-Kuntschik M, Salzer M, Willert HG, Immenkamp M, Groh P, Matejovsky Z. Osteosarcoma in children. A study of 125 cases. J Bone Jt Surg 57-B:341–5

Reilly JP, Gross RH, Emans JB, Yngve DA. Disorders of the sacro-iliac joint in children. J Bone Jt Surg 1988;70-A:31–40

Schey WL, White H, Conway JJ, Kidd JM. A roentgenographic and clinical evaluation of 60 children. AJR 1973;117:59–72

Schlesinger AE, Glass RBJ, Young S, Fernbach SK. Case Report 342. Skeletal Radiol 1986;15:57–9

Tang TT, Zuege RC, Babbitt DP, Blount WP, McCready SR. Angioglomoid tumor of bone. A case report. J Bone Jt Surg 1976;58-A:873–6

Vanel D, Couanet D, Leclere J, Patte C. Early detection of bone metastases of Ewing's sarcoma by magnetic resonance imaging. Diagn Imag Clin Med 1986;55:381–3

SACRAL TUMORS

All the sacral tumors, with the exception of Ewing's sarcoma, are rare in childhood. The symptomatology of sacral tumors is very uniform. Compression of the spinal nerves presents as a progressive radiculopathy. Sometimes hip, knee or low back pain are the presenting symptoms in early stages.

Plain radiographs may be reported as normal because of overlying gases and fecal masses. The examination of choice is CT and MR, which demonstrate beautifully the anatomic details of the sacrum, sacroiliac joints and surrounding soft tissues. Tumors such as aneurysmal bone cyst, osteoid osteoma and lipoma may present with diagnostic radiographic features.

The radiographic appearance of Ewing's sarcoma is that of a lytic or mixed lesion with soft tissue mass (Figs 4.83 and 4.84). However, an osteosclerotic presentation is not unusual (Fig. 4.85). The primary sites of Ewing's sarcoma are usually the vertebral bodies or lateral masses.

Other malignant sacral tumors – osteosarcoma (Fig. 4.86), lymphoma, malignant vascular tumors (Fig. 4.87) – have been sporadically reported. Their radiographic appearances are usually nonspecific.

Chordoma, a rare tumor of childhood, occurs at either end of the spinal column. The sacral location is extremely rare in children. The position within the sacrum is central and it presents as a lytic lesion with ill-defined, irregular margins. An associated soft tissue mass is present with larger tumors. Metastases into the lungs, liver, lymph nodes and bones occur in about 10% of cases (Fig. 4.88).

Benign sacral tumors are also rare in childhood. They are usually localized in the posterior parts of the vertebrae. Osteoid osteoma is predominantly an osteosclerotic lesion, whereas osteoblastoma has mixed appearances (Fig. 4.89). Aneurysmal bone cyst, giant cell tumor and chondromyxoid fibroma (Fig. 4.90) have also been reported occasionally. All are osteolytic lesions, aneurysmal bone cyst having a tendency to expand and enlarge. A monostotic sacral location is very unusual for eosinophilic granuloma (histiocytosis X). Solitary osteochondromas and enchondromas of the sacrum are extremely rare.

The differential diagnosis of primary sacral bone tumor and osteomyelitis rarely causes difficulties in childhood. The common form of sacral osteomyelitis is sacroiliitis, with the iliac bone being more severely affected (see Fig. 4.81c). The clinical course of sacroiliitis is different from that of primary sacral bone tumors. The nuclear scan is the examination of choice as it enables early detection by increased isotope uptake along the sacroiliac joint. Differential diagnostic difficulties may arise rather with primary iliac bone tumors as the inflammatory process extends more easily into the iliac bone.

Table 4.12. Primary tumors of the sacrum

Common		Rare		Differential diagnosis
Benign	Malignant	Benign	Malignant	
Aneurysmal bone cyst Osteoid osteoma Osteoblastoma Chondroblastoma Eosinophilic granuloma Giant cell tumor	Ewing's sarcoma	All other tumors of the sacrum	Osteosarcoma Lymphoma Malignant vascular tumors Chondrosarcoma	Osteomyelitis Anatomical variants Soft tissue tumors Myelomeningocele

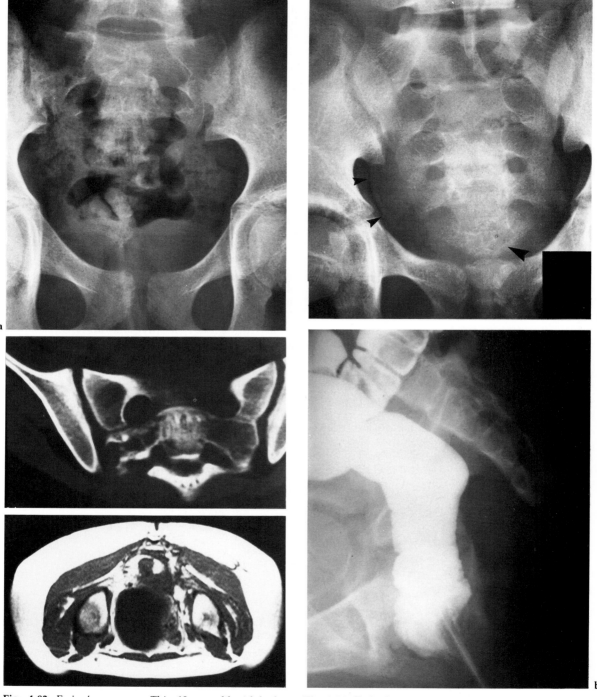

Fig. 4.83. Ewing's sarcoma. This 12-year-old girl had a history of low back pain for 2 months. **a** Fecal masses and gas overly the sacrum; there is some asymmetry of S1/S2 anterior sacral foramina. **b** CT shows extensive destruction of the lateral part of S2. **c** MR shows anterior extansion of the mass with some invasion of the iliac bone and bladder wall.

Fig. 4.84. Ewing's sarcoma. This 8-year-old presented with sacral pain after trauma. **a** Abnormal trabecular pattern of S5 vertebral body (*large arrow*). Note soft tissue mass (*small arrows*). **b** Barium enema shows an impression of the posterior part of the rectum. (*continued*)

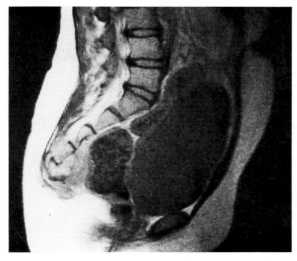

Fig. 4.84 (*continued*) **c** MR shows soft tissue mass confluent with S5 vertebral body (*arrow*). (From Kozlowski et al. 1990, with permission.)

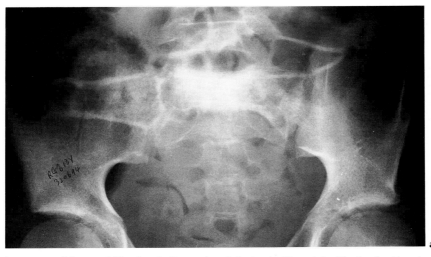

Fig. 4.85. Ewing's sarcoma (13-year-old boy). **a,b** Osteosclerotic lesion in S1 vertebral body. (*continued overleaf*)

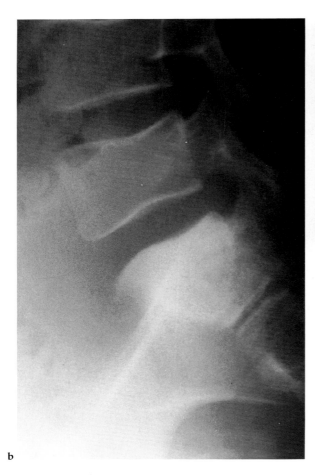

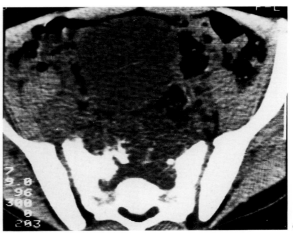

Fig. 4.85 (*continued*) Ewing's sarcoma (13-year-old boy). **c** CT shows a massive destructive process in S1 vertebral body and a large soft tissue mass extending anteriorly. Although the diagnosis of Ewing's sarcoma is evident on plain films, CT demonstrates much better the details of the lesion and presents the soft tissue mass.

b

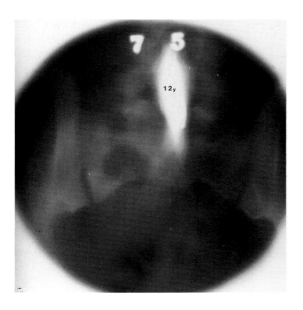

Fig. **4.86.** Osteosarcoma. This 11-year-old girl had pain in the right leg following trauma, and absent right ankle jerk. The radiograph 4 months later shows a large, round radiolucent defect in the sacral bone on the right. (From Kozlowski 1980, with permission.)

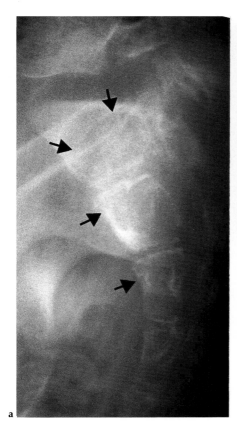

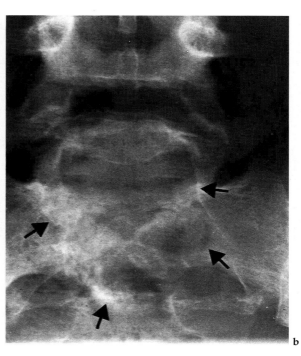

Fig. 4.87. Hemangiopericytoma. This 13-year-old boy had right-sided radiculopathy for 1 year. There is a large osteolytic defect in the sacrum with some osteosclerotic reaction at the right margin (*arrows*). (From Kozlowski et al. 1990, with permission.)

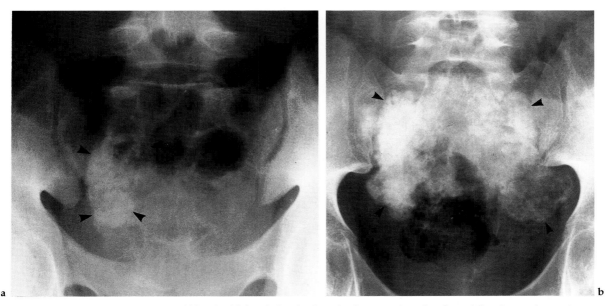

Fig. 4.88. Chordoma. This 12-year-old boy had left-sided radiculopathy for several weeks after a fall. **a** Osteosclerotic lesion on the right lateral aspect of sacrum (*arrows*). **b** Two months after radiotherapy, the mass is situated in the middle and is overlying the sacrum (*arrows*); it is much larger than would be suspected from plain radiography before radiotherapy. (*continued overleaf*)

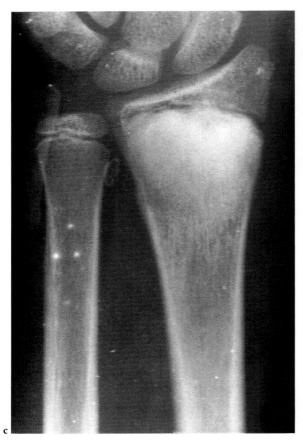

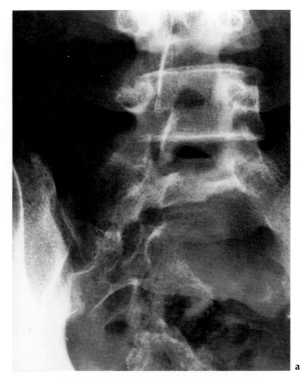

Fig. 4.88 (*continued*) Chordoma. **c** Six months after diagnosis, osteosclerotic metastasis. (From Kozlowski et al. 1990, with permission.)

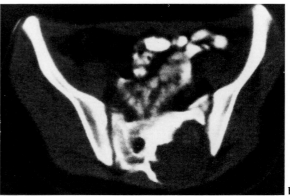

Fig. 4.90. Chondromyxoid fibroma. This girl presented with lower back pain which had lasted 1 year. **a** Extensive lytic lesion on the left side of the sacrum. **b** CT shows destruction of the left side of the sacrum, with extension of the mass into the pelvis and the buttock. (From Shulman 1985, with permission.)

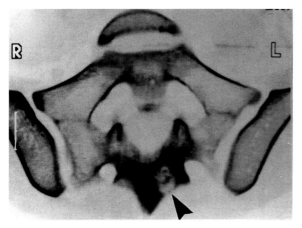

Fig. 4.89. Osteoblastoma. This 16-year-old boy had sacral pain for 18 months. Osteosclerosis of the arch of S3 is seen, with a radiolucent center (*arrow*). (From Kozlowski et al. 1990, with permission.)

LITERATURE
Sacral Tumors

Beltran J, Simon DC, Levy M, Herman L, Weis L, Mueller ChF. Aneurysmal bone cyst: MR imaging at 1.5T[1]. Radiology 1986;158:686–90

Beyer WF, Kraus J, Glückert K, Goldmann AR. Solitaire infantile myofibromatose des os sacrum. Z Orthop 1990; 128:473–6

Braun M, Bracard S, Bernard C, Czorny A, Schmitt M, Hoeffel JC. Les tumeurs primitives du rachis chez l'enfant. A propos de 12 cas. Rev Int Pediatr 1988;179:3–14

Eftekhari F, Wallace S, Chuang VP, Soo CS, Cangir A, Benjamin RS, Murray JA. Interarterial management of giant-cell tumours of the spine in children. Pediatr Radiol 1982;12:289–93

Ehara S, Kattapuram SV. Hemophiliac pseudotumor of the sacrum. Radiation Medicine 1989;7:214–16

Ehara S, Kattapuram SV, Rosenberg AE. Case report 619. Skeletal Radiol 1990;19:375–6

Ehara S, Rosenberg AE, El-Khoury GY. Sacral cyst with exophytic components. A report of two cases. Skeletal Radiol 1990;19:117–19

Firooznia H, Pinto RS, Lin JP, Baruch HH, Zausner J. Chordoma: radiologic evaluation of 20 cases. AJR 1976;

127:797–805

Highland TR, Lamont RL. Osteomyelitis of the pelvis in children. J Bone Jt Surg 1983;65-A:230–4

Kozlowski K. Osteosarcoma with unusual clinical and/or radiographic appearances. Pediatr Radiol 1980;9:167–70

Kozlowski K, Barylak A, Campbell J, Hoeffel JD, Beluffi G, Masel J, Panuel M, Pelizza A, Taccone A, Arico M. Primary sacral bone tumors in children (Report of 16 cases with a short literature review). Austr Radiol 1990;34: 142–9

Pinto RS, Lin JP, Firooznia H, Lefleur RS. The osseous and angiographic features of vertebral chordomas. Neuroradiology 1975;9:231–41

Schaad UB, McCracken GH, Nelson JD. Pyogenic arthritis of the sacroiliac joint in pediatric patients. Pediatrics 1980;66: 375–9

Shulman L, Bale P, M de Silva. Sacral chondromyxoid fibroma. Pediatr Radiol 1985;15:138–40

Vanel D, Rebibo G, Hales H, Lacombe MJ, Masselot J. Contribution of computed tomography in six sacrococcygeal chordomas. Eur J Radiol 1985;5:87–90

LONG-BONE TUMORS

The long bones are the most common location of tumors and tumorous conditions. The radiographic appearances are characteristic in many instances. This has important clinical implications, as most of the patients can be treated on the basis of plain radiographs alone, and the need for biopsy is limited to the malignant neoplasms and patients with unclear radiographic appearances and/or unusual clinical symptoms and signs.

In routine daily work, the benign fibrous tumors and tumorous conditions are the most important benign lesions. They occur most often around the knee, are asymptomatic and are usually discovered on radiographs taken because of trauma, hip or knee pain. Their tendency to regression suggests their developmental or traumatic origin. Some of them are possibly normal anatomic variants.

If the lesion is radiolucent with a more or less sclerotic margin, localized in the metaphyseal region with its long axis parallel to the long axis of the long bone, then it is a cortical defect. A large cortical defect with intramedullary extension is a nonossifying fibroma (Fig. 4.91). These lesions are present in about a third of children in the first decade of life but are uncommon below 2 years of age. They disappear in the second

Table 4.13. Primary benign tumors of the long bones

Common	Rare	Differential diagnosis
Cortical defect	Benign vascular tumors	Anatomic variants
Fibroma	Chondroblastoma	Trauma (periostitis, stress
Exchondroma	Osteoblastoma	fracture, myositis
Eosinophilic granuloma	Chondromyxoid fibroma	ossificans, stress
Osteoid osteoma	Desmoplastic fibroma	apophysis,
Simple bone cyst	Osteoma	apophyseolysis)
Enchondroma	Lipoma	Malignant bone tumors
Fibrous dysplasia		Osteomyelitis
Aneurysmal bone cyst		Metastasis
		Soft tissue tumors

Table 4.14. Primary malignant tumors of the long bones

Common	Rare	Differential diagnosis
Osteosarcoma	Malignant vascular tumors	Osteomyelitis
Ewing's sarcoma	Lymphoma	Eosinophilic granuloma
	Chondrosarcoma	Primary benign bone tumors
		Trauma (periostitis, stress fracture,
		myositis ossificans, stress
		apophysis, apophyseolysis)
		Soft tissue tumors
		Metastases
		Osteolysis (idiopathic, post-
		traumatic)
		Hemophilia

Table 4.15. Single neoplastic cystic bone lesions

Common	Rare	Differential diagnosis
Cortical defect	Chondroblastoma	Benign primary bone tumors
Fibroma	Chondromyxoid fibroma	Malignant primary bone
Simple bone cyst	Desmoplastic fibroma	tumors
Fibrous dysplasia	Giant cell reparative	Osteomyelitis (Brodie's
Eosinophilic granuloma	granuloma	abscess)
Enchondroma	Desmoplastic fibroma	Eosinophilic granuloma
Aneurysmal bone cyst	Teleangiectatic	Metastasis
	osteosarcoma	Soft tissue tumors
	Vascular tumor	Normal anatomical variant
		(pseudocystic lesion)
		Hyperparathyroidism
		Hemophilia
		Trauma

Table 4.16. Multiple cystic bone lesions

Leukemia/lymphoma
Metastasis
Eosinophilic granuloma
Fibrous dysplasia
Enchondromatosis
Osteomyelitis
Angiomatosis (lymphangiomatosis, hemangiomatosis)
Multiple nonossifying fibromas
Hyperparathyroidism

decade of life. The only complication of non-ossifying fibroma is a pathologic fracture (Fig. 4.92), which occurs more commonly in lesions localized in radius and tibia. Nonossifying fibroma of the narrow long tubular bones (radius, ulna, fibula) has a tendency to erode the cortex and expand the bone. On radiographs, it resembles a simple bone cyst or fibrous dysplasia but may show some features of a malignant neoplasm.

The post-traumatic fibrous tumorous lesions are avulsion cortical irregularities (periosteal desmoid) either at the posteromedial border of the distal femur at the attachment of abductor magnus, or in the fossa poplitea at the attachment of gastrocnemius (Fig. 4.93). The latter lesion may simulate osteosarcoma.

Fibrous dysplasia is discussed later in this chapter.

Other than fibrous tumors, osteoid osteoma/osteoblastoma complex is the most common benign tumor or tumorous condition in childhood. Over 50% of osteoid osteoma cases occur in childhood. The upper part of femur, spine and tibia are most often affected. In the femur there is predilection for the upper end. The most characteristic and almost constant clinical feature is pain, often relieved by salicylates. Neurologic (sensory changes, muscular atrophy) and/or musculoskeletal symptoms (athralgia, bone tenderness) may cause a misleading clinical appearance and result in delayed diagnosis. A history of previous trauma may cause additional confusion. It is generally recognized that osteoid osteoma in or near a joint may cause diagnostic problems before it is recognized. Articular or periarticular osteoporosis may be the only or the predominant radiographic sign as it often occurs in osteoid osteoma of the femoral neck.

Although most cases of osteoid osteoma can be recognized on plain films, in doubtful cases the examinations of choice are nuclear scan and CT. A small, round hot spot is pathognomonic if the clinical context is taken into account. When knowledge of the exact location of the nidus is required, CT scan should be performed; CT will show a radiolucent lesion inside a sclerotic area, usually with a dense nidus. These two modalities not only reduce delays in diagnosis but are also extremely helpful in cases with uncharacteristic clinical history and/or unusual tumor location (Fig. 4.94, and see Fig. 4.107).

That there are clinical, radiographic and histologic similarities between osteoid osteoma and osteoblastoma is well recognized. A lesion larger than 1.5–2.0 cm is designated as osteoblastoma. Generally, osteoblastoma is a less painful lesion. It may present as a locally aggressive growth with distant metastases or undergo malignant transformation. Osteoblastoma is much rarer than osteoid osteoma and accounts for about 1% of all bone tumors. It occurs in a slightly older population than osteoid osteoma. It has predilection for the mandibles, spine, femur and tibia. The radiographic appearances of osteoblastoma are less characteristic than those of osteoid osteoma. Cortical expansion, destruction and periosteal reaction often simulate a malignant tumor. In the spine, osteoblastoma may have similar appearances to aneurysmal bone cyst. The radiographic differential diagnosis between these two entities is easy when nuclear scan, CT and MR are performed.

Common benign metaphyseal tumors in childhood are simple bone cyst (Fig. 4.95) and aneurysmal bone cyst (Fig. 4.96). Whereas 75% of simple bone cysts occur in the humerus and femur, only a little over 50% of aneurysmal bone cysts occur in the long bones. A simple bone cyst can usually be recognized as a benign lesion but an aneurysmal bone cyst may mimic a semi-malignant or malignant neoplasm. With new modalities – nuclear scan, CT and MR – it is possible to diagnose aneurysmal bone cyst before the biopsy in most of the cases. Biopsy may be necessary to exclude the presence of a primary lesion, however. Profuse bleeding is a dangerous complication of the aneurysmal bone cyst. Nuclear scan demonstrates localized, increased radionuclide uptake. CT depicts the anatomic details – expansion, cortical erosion and periosteal reaction – as well as increased density after i.v. contrast injection. Fluid levels are characteristic, although not a diagnostic feature of aneurysmal bone cyst. MR is even more specific as it shows not only the internal architecture of the tumor but also depicts the internal content of the cyst.

The rare chondromyxoid fibroma (Fig. 4.97) occurs in the long bones in more than 50% of cases. Typically it is an eccentrically placed, radiolucent lesion with a well-defined margin. Cortical eroding, bone expansion and minor periosteal reaction are frequently seen in larger lesions.

Chondroblastoma (Fig. 4.126), a growth cartilage related lesion, is usually located in the epiphysis but may extend towards the shaft. In rare instances it has a metaphyseal location.

Giant cell tumor occurs very rarely in childhood as typically it develops after the closure of the growth plate.

Solitary enchondroma (Fig. 4.98) of the long bones is easily recognizable when it shows typical mottled or stippled calcification. When calcification is absent, it may simulate any cystic lesion.

Primary bone lipoma (Fig. 4.99) has a characteristic appearance on both plain radiographs and CT. It is a translucent lesion with a sclerotic border and low CT numbers. Lipomas are often located close to the intratrochanteric line.

Osteosarcoma (Figs 4.100 and 4.101) and Ewing's sarcoma are the most common primary malignant long bone tumors in childhood. Usually they present late and already have the radiographic features of malignancy. According to Price et al. (1975), 96% of osteosarcomas occur in the long bones and 68% of these in the knee region. Whereas most types of osteosarcoma (osteoblastic, chondroblastic, fibroblastic) show radiographic appearances of a malignant bone tumor, there are several other forms which radiographically mimic benign entities. Telangiectatic osteosarcoma simulates aneurysmal bone cyst, and central low-grade osteosarcoma mimics fibrous dysplasia or osteoma. Osteosarcoma associated with benign lesions has also been reported.

Ewing's sarcoma (Fig. 4.102), the second most common primary long bone tumor in children, is much rarer in long bones than osteosarcoma. About 50% of Ewing's sarcomas occur in the long bones. Although it usually has malignant features at the first radiographic examination, in the very early stages it may mimic a benign lesion. Protracted pain and a soft tissue mass are important clinical features. Because of the often elevated ESR and osteomyelitis-like radiographic appearances, a misdiagnosis of inflammatory lesion is not uncommon.

Other malignant primary bone tumors of the long bones are very rare in childhood. Chondrosarcoma should be suspected in patients with enchondromatosis. Primary bone lymphoma presents as a solitary, lytic or permeative lesion without characteristic features, or as a poly-

ostotic lytic disorder. The latter often has characteristic appearances – multiple, washed out lytic defects (Fig. 4.103, and see Fig. 4.178c,d). Fracture is a common complication in later stages of lymphoma. The differential diagnosis of the polyostotic form is with other forms of small cell tumors – leukemia, neuroblastoma, Ewing's sarcoma – as well as other polyostotic benign tumors.

Malignant vascular tumors, fibrosarcoma and malignant histiocytoma may occur occasionally.

The most important entity to be considered in the differential of malignant and benign tumors of the long bones, beside osteomyelitis (Fig. 4.104), is histiocytosis X (eosinophilic granuloma). The radiographic appearances of eosinophilic granuloma are very variable. It may present as a benign or a malignant lesion. Any part of the long bone can be affected, though there is a predilection for mid-diaphyseal locations (Fig. 4.105). Two important diagnostic hints are the multifocal tendency of eosinophilic granuloma (apparently more common in preschool age) and elevated eosinophilia (a rare but very characteristic finding, the importance of which is underestimated).

Osteomyelitis can usually be recognized if the clinical history, blood tests, nuclear scan and radiographs are critically evaluated. However, low-grade infections, specifically tuberculosis, mycobacterial and mycotic osteomyelitis, may present very confusing radiographic and clinical appearances. Fortunately, in most cases, the histology is diagnostic.

Trauma, particularly presenting as periostitis, stress fracture and myositis ossificans (Fig. 4.106) may have the appearances of malignant bone tumor. The importance of the clinical history cannot be overemphasized in these situations. Nuclear scan, CT and MR may be decisive in reaching a proper diagnosis in some cases.

There are three anatomic regions in the long bones in which tumors show some features worth a more detailed description: the femoral neck, midfemoral shaft and tibial diaphysis; these are discussed in the following sections.

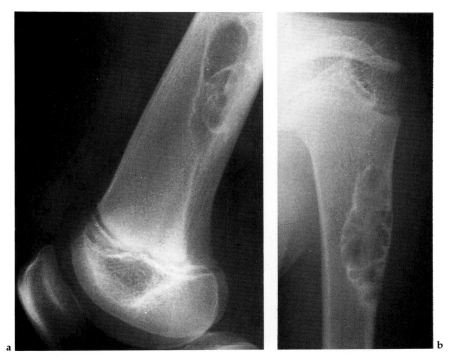

Fig. 4.91. Nonossifying fibroma. **a** Thirteen-year-old boy with knee pain. **b** Eight-year-old girl with shoulder pain.

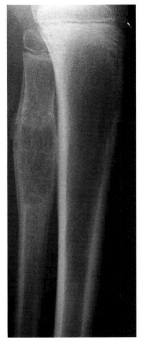

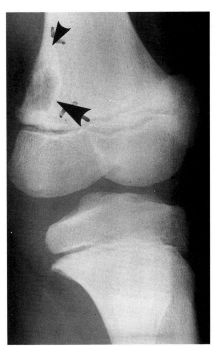

Fig. 4.92. Nonossifying fibroma. This 13-year-old girl injured her leg on a trampoline 3 years previously and had pain on walking. The lesion is radiolucent, slightly expansile, with pathologic fracture and periosteal reaction.

Fig. 4.93. Distal femoral cortical irregularity (*arrows*). This 12-year-old boy active in sport presented with knee pain.

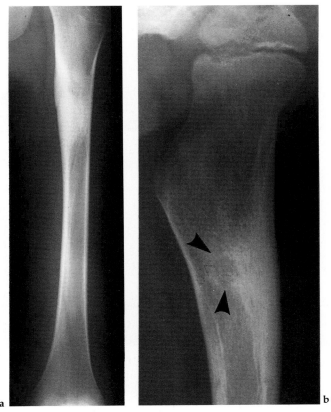

Fig. 4.94. Osteoid osteoma. **a** This 10.5-year-old boy had wasting of the left leg for 1 year; pain in the left knee was worse at night. The myelogram was negative. **b** This 4.5-year-old boy presented with pain in the upper thigh for a period of 18 months; radiography 12 months previously had been reported as normal; the ''aspirin test'' was positive (i.e. pain ceased on taking aspirin). An appointment for operation was cancelled because the pain suddenly stopped. The diagnosis is possible osteoid osteoma (*arrows*).

a   b   c

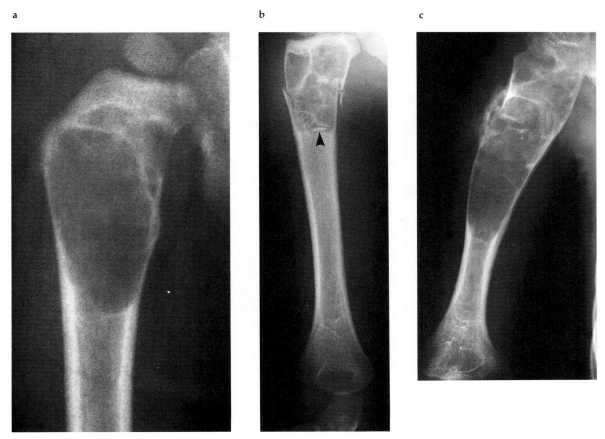

Fig. 4.95. Simple bone cyst. **a** Eighteen-month-old boy with pain in the right shoulder. **b** Three-year-old boy with pain in the right shoulder after a fall; pathological fracture with a loose bony fragment inside the cyst is evident (*arrow*). **c** Eight-year-old boy with pain in the right shoulder after a fall; there is a large cyst with a pathologic fracture and callus formation at the fracture site.

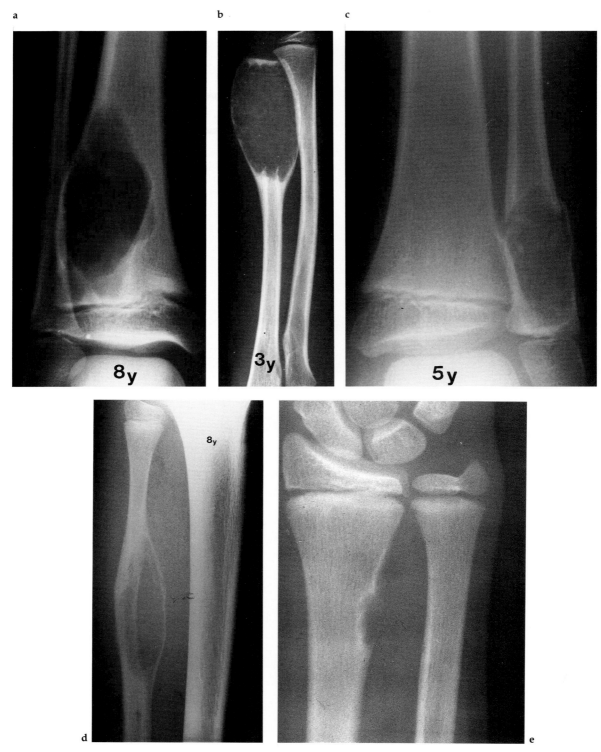

Fig. 4.96. Different appearances of aneurysmal bone syst. **a** Eccentric, lytic expansile lesion with marginal sclerosis and apparent trabeculation (8-year-old boy). Typical appearances are metaphyseal concentric lytic expansion with apparent trabeculation (**b** 3-year-old boy) and pathologic fracture (**c** 5-year-old girl). **d,e** Rare diaphyseal subperiosteal location (8-year-old girl and 11-year-old boy, respectively). (From Kozlowski and Middleton 1980, with permission.)

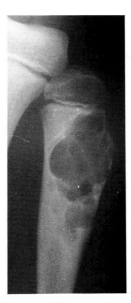

Fig. 4.97. Chondromyxoid fibroma. A lytic, expansile lesion with apparent trabeculation; the cortex is thinned and the margin is scalloped (11-year-old boy).

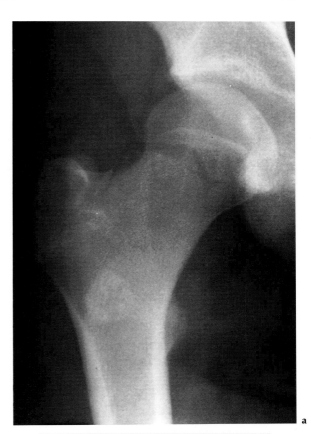

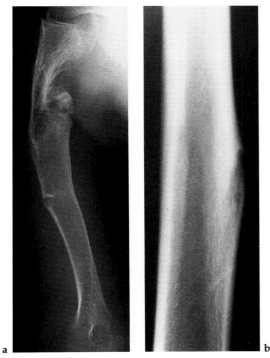

Fig. 4.98. Enchondroma. **a** This 11-year-old boy had deformity of the right shoulder and occasional pain. There is shortening of the right humerus with irregular, radiolucent defects. **b** This 12-year-old boy had a lump over the left femur for 10 days. A small, radiolucent cortical defect is seen at the anterior aspect of the midshaft of the femur.

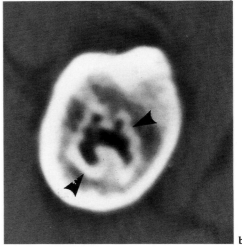

Fig. 4.99. Intraosseous lipoma. This 13-year-old boy presented with pain in the left hip. **a** A round, irregularly sclerotic lesion with single, round, radiolucent spots in the right femur (not expected). **b** CT shows some low-density areas, with CT values compatible with fat inside the round sclerotic lesion (*arrow*). (From Kozlowski and Walshman 1991, with permission.)

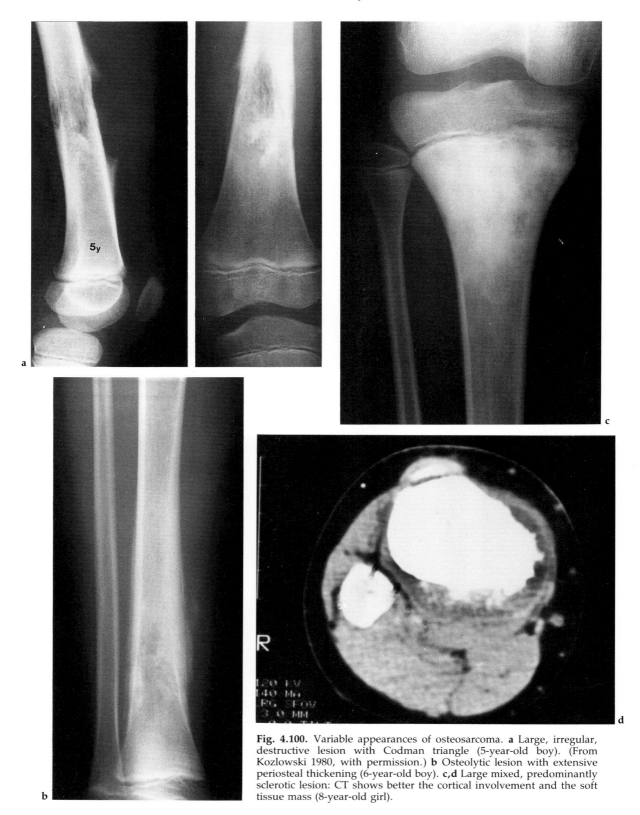

Fig. 4.100. Variable appearances of osteosarcoma. **a** Large, irregular, destructive lesion with Codman triangle (5-year-old boy). (From Kozlowski 1980, with permission.) **b** Osteolytic lesion with extensive periosteal thickening (6-year-old boy). **c,d** Large mixed, predominantly sclerotic lesion: CT shows better the cortical involvement and the soft tissue mass (8-year-old girl).

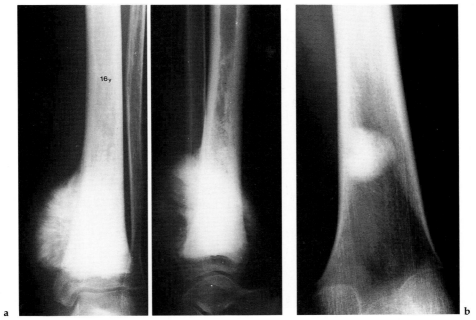

Fig. 4.101. Variable appearances of osteosarcoma. **a** Large osteosclerotic lesion with abundant periosteal reaction (16-year-old girl). **b** Intraosseus lesion resembling osteoma (19-year-old male who presented with increasing pain in the left knee for 3 months). Large osteomas are extremely rare in children and teenagers. (**a** From Kozlowski 1980, **b** from Dr F Diard, Hôpital des Enfant Malades, Bordeaux, France, with permission.)

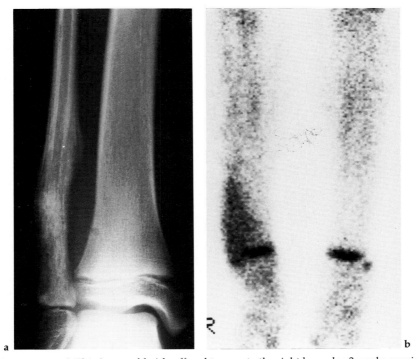

Fig. 4.102. Ewing's sarcoma. **a,b** This 9-year-old girl suffered trauma to the right lower leg 3 weeks previously, followed by increasing swelling and pain. Nuclear scan shows well the extent of the lesion.

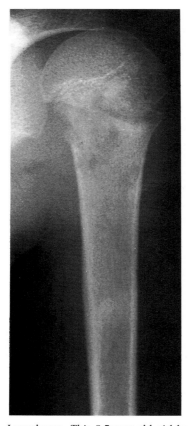

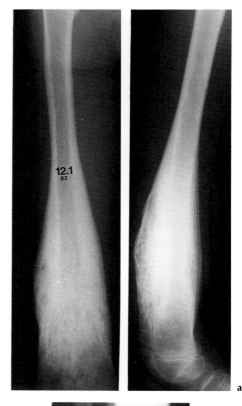

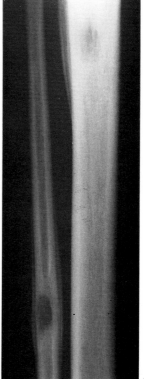

Fig. 4.103. Lymphoma. This 8.5-year-old girl had pain on and off for 1 month and could not move her arm up. No other lesions were present at the time of diagnosis. There is an ill-defined osteolytic lesion at the proximal humeral metaphysis.

Fig. 4.104. Osteomyelitis. **a** Tumorous osteomyelitis in a 10.5-year-old girl who had polyostotic osteomyelitis from the age of 8.5 years; no causative organism was found. (From Kozlowski et al. 1984, with permission.) **b** Atypical *Mycobacterium* osteomyelitis in a 10-year-old boy: there are irregular osteolytic defects in the tibia and fibula, with cortical destruction and periosteal reaction. (From Dr J Andersen, Aarhus, Denmark.)

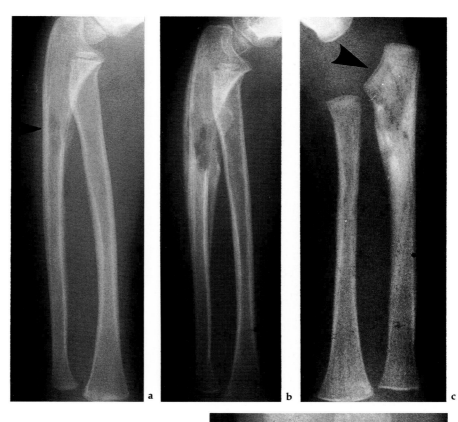

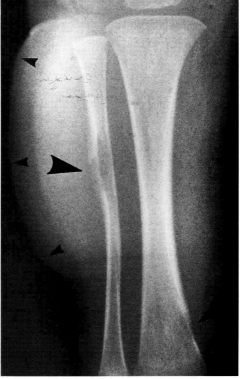

Fig. 4.105. Histiocytosis X. **a,b** Aggressive eosinophilic granuloma in a 6-year-old girl who had pain in the right elbow for 2 weeks. **a** Ill-defined osteolytic lesion with some periosteal reaction (*arrow*). **b** Two weeks later, marked increase of the destructive process, with abundant periosteal reaction. **c,d** Multifocal histiocytosis X (possibly congenital) in a 7-week-old boy. There are soft tissue swellings (*small arrows*) and multiple, destructive bone lesions (*large arrows*); a generalized cutaneous rash was also present. (From Kozlowski and Grigor 1980, with permission.)

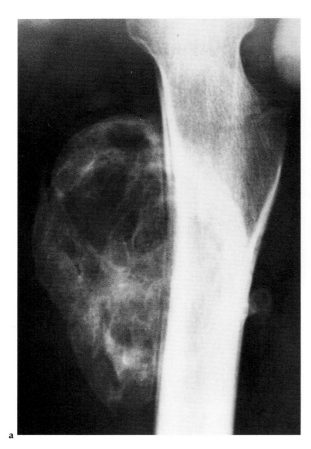

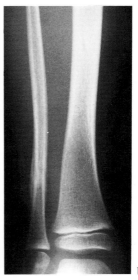

Fig. 4.106. Trauma. **a** Myositis ossificans in a 10-year-old boy with pain and swelling of the right upper thigh and fever (no history of trauma); the radiograph was taken 3 months after the acute episode and shows changes typical of myositis ossificans. **b** Stress fracture of the fibula of a 3.5-year-old girl who had had pain in the lower right leg for 1 week. Medial bowing of the fibula, with minimal localized periosteal reaction at the lateral aspect of distal fibula, is seen. An ill-defined transverse sclerotic band is present at the level of periosteal reaction.

LITERATURE
Long-bone Tumors

Adler CP, Klümper A, Wenz W. Enchondrome aus radiologischer und patologisch-anatomischer Sicht. Radiologe 1979;19:341–9

Alman BA, Goldberg MJ, Naber SP, Galanopoulos T, Antoniades NH, Wolfe HJ. Aggressive fibromatosis. J Pediatr Orthop 1992;12:1–10

Beggs IG, Stoker DJ. Chondromyxoid fibroma of bone. Clinical Radiol 1982;33:671–9

Bonakdarpour A, Levy WM, Aegerter E. Primary and secondary aneurysmal bone cyst: a radiological study of 75 cases. Radiology 1978;126:75–83

Campanacci M, Capanna R, Picci P. Unicameral and aneurysmal bone cysts. Clin Orthop Rel Res 1986;204:25–36

Cohen MD, Harrington TM, Ginsburg WW. Osteoid osteoma: 95 cases and a review of the literature. Semin Arthritis Rheum 1983;12:265–81

Dimentberg RA, Brown KLB. Diagnostic evaluation of patients with histiocytosis X. J Pediatr Orthop 1990;10:733–41

Edeiken J, Raymond AK, Ayala AG, Benjamin RS, Murray JA, Carrasco HC. Small-cell osteosarcoma. Skeletal Radiol 1987;16:621–8

Freyschmidt J, Ostertag H, Saure D. Der fibröse metaphysäre Defekt (fibröser Kortikalisdefekt, nicht-ossifizierendes Knochenfibrom). Fortschr Röntgenstr 1981;134:392–400

Gherlinzoni F, Rock M, Picci P. Chondromyxoid fibroma. J Bone Jt Surg 1983;65-A:198–204

Gutjahr P, Jung H. Fibrosarcom: eine problematische diagnose im Kindesalter. HNO 1974;22:181–5

Unni KK, Dahlin DC. Osteosarcoma: pathology and classification. Seminars in Roentgenology 1989;24:143–52

Kozlowski K. Osteosarcoma with unusual clinical and/or radiographic appearances. Pediatr Radiol 1980;9:167–70

Kozlowski K, Grigor W. Probable congenital histiocytosis X with unusual findings in a 7 week old infant. Pediatr Radiol 1980;9:45–7

Kozlowski K, Anderson RJ, Hochberger O, Sacher O. Tumorous osteomyelitis. Pediatr Radiol 1984;14:404–6

Kozlowski K, Middleton RWD. Aneurysmal bone cyst. Review of 10 cases. Aust Radiol 1980;24:170–5

Kumar R, Swischuk LE, Madewell JE. Benign cortical defect: site for an avulsion fracture. Skeletal Radiol 1986;15:553–5

Mackenzie WG, Morton KS. Eosinophilic granuloma of bone. Can J Surg 1988;31:264–7

Moore TE, King AR, Travis RC, Allen BC. Post-traumatic cysts and cyst-like lesions of bone. Skeletal Radiol 1989;18:93–7

Normal A, Schiffman M. Simple bone cysts: factors of age dependency. Radiology 1977;124:779–82

Nuovo MA, Norman A, Chumas J, Ackerman LV. Myositis ossificans with atypical clinical, radiographic, or pathologic findings: a review of 23 cases. Skeletal Radiol 1992; 21:87–101

Picci P, Gherlinzoni F, Guerra A. Intracortical osteosarcoma. Rare entity or early manifestation of classical osteosarcoma? Skeletal Radiol 1983;9:255–8

Picci P, Manfrini M, Zucchi V, Gherlinzoni F, Rock M, Bertoni F, Neff JR. Giant-cell tumor of bone in skeletally immature patients. J Bone Jt Surg 1983;65-A:486–90

Price CHG, Zhuber K, Salzer-Kuntschik M, Salzer M, Willert HG, Immenkamp M, Groh P, Matejovsky Z, Keyl W. Osteosarcoma in children. A study of 125 cases. J Bone Jt Surg 1975;57-B:341–5

Reider-Grosswasser I, Grunebaum M. Metaphyseal multifocal osteosarcoma. Br J Radiol 1978;61:627–81

Rigault P, Mouterde P, Padovani JP, Jaubert F, Guyonvarch

G. Ostéome ostéoide chez enfant. A propos de 29 cas. Rev Chir Orthop 1975;61:627–46

Ritts GD, Pritchard DJ, Unni KK, Beabout JW, Eckardt JJ. Periosteal osteosarcoma. Clinical Orthop 1987;219: 299–307

Rousselin B, Vanel D, Terrier-Lacombe MJ, Istria BJM, Spielman M, Masselot J. Clinical and radiologic analysis of 13 cases of primary neuroectodermal tumours of bone. Skeletal Radiol 1989;18:115–20

Schajowicz F. Chondromyxoid fibroma: report of three cases with predominant cortical involvement. Radiology 1987; 164:783–6

Schajowicz F, Mcguire MH, Araujo ES, Muscolo DL, Gitelis S. Osteosarcomas arising on the surface of long bones. J Bone Jt Surg 1988;70-A:555–64

Siddiqui AS, Tashjian JH, Lazarus K, Wellman HN, Baehner RL. Nuclear medicine studies in evaluation of skeletal lesions in children with Histiocytosis X. Radiology 1981; 140:787–9

Sklar DH, Phillips JJ, Lachman RS. Case report 683. Skeletal Radiol 1991;20:394–6

Taconis WK, Mudler JD. Fibrosarcoma and malignant fibrous histiocytoma of long bones: radiographic features and grading. Skeletal Radiol 1984;11:237–45

Thijn CJP, Martijn A, Postma A, Molenaar WM. Case report 615. Skeletal Radiol 1990;19:309–11

Vanel D, Tcheng S, Contesso G, Zafrani B, Kalifa C, Dubousset J, Kron P. The radiological appearances of telangiectatic osteosarcoma. A study of 14 cases. Skeletal Radiol 1987; 16:196–200

Wilkins RM, Pritchard DJ, Burgert EO, Unni KK. Ewing's sarcoma of bone. Experience with 140 patients. Cancer 1986;58:2551–5

Wilson AJ, Kyriakos M, Ackerman LV. Chondromyxoid fibroma: radiographic appearance in 38 cases and in a review of the literature. Radiology 1991;179:513–8

Young CL, Sim FH, Unni KK, McLeod RA. Case report 559. Skeletal Radiol 1989;18:403–5

FEMORAL NECK TUMORS

Whereas malignant bone lesions of the femoral neck are very rare in childhood, benign ones are common. However, because of their location, even a benign lesion is potentially serious. Complications such as pathologic fracture, coxa vara and leg shortening are to be expected. Diagnosis in many cases is by radiography, as the femoral neck is not easily accessible to surgery and biopsy increases the possibility of com-

plications. The "wait and see" approach is common in cases diagnosed radiographically as benign lesions.

The most common femoral neck tumors are osteoid osteoma, simple bone cyst, aneurysmal bone cyst and fibrous dysplasia. Osteoid osteoma of the femoral neck was often difficult to diagnose before the advent of nuclear scan and CT. The plain radiographs may be normal

Table 4.17. Femoral neck tumors

Common	Differential diagnosis
Fibrous dysplasia	Osteomyelitis
Simple bone cyst	Trauma
Osteoid osteoma	
Chondroblastoma	
Aneurysmal bone cyst	

or nearly normal. Osteopenia, ill-defined cortical thickening and/or hip-joint widening may be the only radiographic signs in a child with long-standing femoral neck osteoid osteoma. Both nuclear scan and CT show characteristic appearances – a hot spot at the lesion and a low-density nidus, often with central calcification (Fig. 4.107). Simple bone cyst, aneurysmal bone cyst and fibrous dysplasia usually image as a radiolucent lesion. If the lytic lesion does not contain trabecular pattern and a sclerotic rim, the diagnosis is simple bone cyst

(Fig. 4.108). If both those features are present, a diagnosis of fibrous dysplasia is more appropriate (Fig. 4.109). We have seen aneurysmal bone cysts which at first examination presented as a simple bone cyst: follow-up studies several months later showed typical features of aneurysmal bone cyst – extension of the lesion, expansion of the femoral neck, trabecular pattern inside the defect and, often, pathologic fracture (Fig. 4.110).

If a radiolucent lesion abuts the growth cartilage chondroblastoma should be considered.

Other benign and malignant bone tumors are occasionally found in the femoral neck. However their rarity and uncharacteristic radiographic appearances rarely allow radiographic diagnosis (Fig. 4.111).

The most common disorder to be differentiated from the benign and malignant primary tumors of the femoral neck is osteomyelitis (Fig. 4.112). Single femoral neck metastases are extremely rare in children.

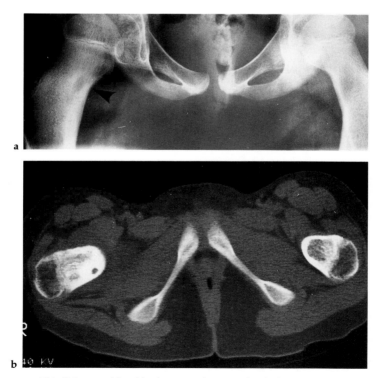

Fig. 4.107. Osteoid osteoma. This 7.5-year-old girl had a 1-year history of right knee pain and had been limping for several months. **a** Radiolucent defect surrounded by sclerotic bone (*arrow*). **b** CT scan demonstrates well the radiolucent nidus surrounded by sclerotic bone.

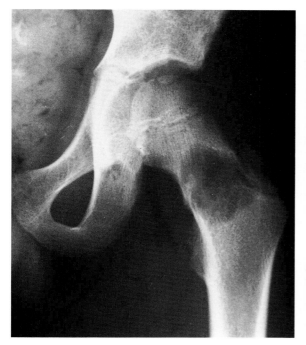

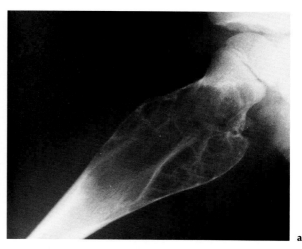

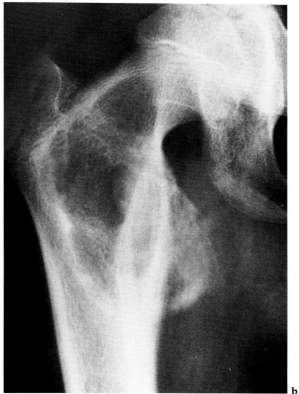

Fig. 4.108. Possible simple bone cyst. This 7-year-old boy had a 4-week history of left knee and hip pain. There is a radiolucent defect in the femoral neck, with a pathologic fracture.

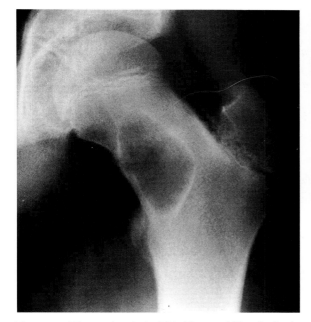

Fig. 4.109. Fibrous dysplasia. This 13-year-old boy had pain in the left hip and limp for 4 months. There is a radiolucent defect with sclerotic border in the femoral neck, with pathologic fracture.

Fig. 4.110. Aneurysmal bone cyst. **a** This 4.5-year-old girl presented with pain in the right hip after a fall 6 months previously. The diagnosis was cystic lesion. The lesion increased in size and expanded during the 9-month observation period. **b** This 9.5-year-old girl presented with right hip pain and limp over a 4-month period. There is a large radiolucent lesion with medial expansion.

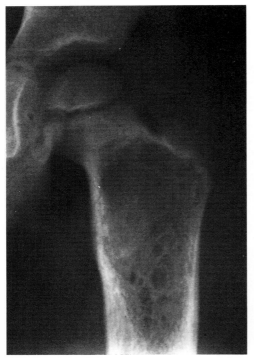

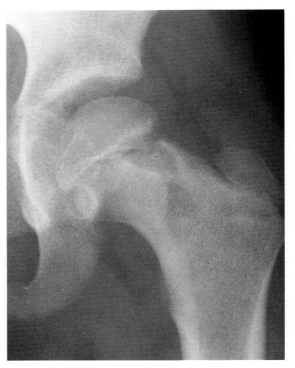

Fig. 4.111. Small cell malignant tumor, possibly hemangiopericytoma. This 5-year-old boy had pain in the left lower limb, experienced loss of weight over 2 weeks, and had a temperature of 38.5°C and a white cell count of 17 000. There is a large radiolucent defect in the proximal part of the left femur extending into the femoral neck. The borders of the lesion are indistinct and there is some septation in the distal part.

Fig. 4.112. Osteomyelitis. This 6-year-old boy experienced pain in the left hip for several weeks after a fall. Two oval defects in the neck of the left femur extend into the growth cartilage.

LITERATURE
Femoral Neck Tumors

Enneking WF, Gearen PF. Fibrous dysplasia of the femoral neck. J Bone Jr Surg 1986;68-A:1415–22

Goldman AB, Vigorita VJ. Case Report 245. Skeletal Radiol 1983;10:179–200

Howie JL. CT of osteoid osteoma of the femoral neck: the value of oblique reformating. J Assoc Can Radiol 1985;36: 254–6

Lichtman EA, Klein MJ. Case Report 302. Skeletal Radiol 1985;13:160–3

Pignatti G, Nigrisoli M. Case report 537. Skeletal Radiol 1989;18:225–7

Savage PE, Stoker DJ. Fibrous dysplasia of the femoral neck. Skeletal Radiol 1984;11:119–23

Sotelo-Avila C, Sundaram M, Kyriakos M, Graviss ER, Tayob AA. Case report 373. Skeletal Radiol 1986;15: 387–90

Theros EG, Mirra JM, Smasson J, Cove K, Paladugu R. Case Report 95. Skeletal Radiol 1979:4:157–62

MIDFEMORAL PERIOSTEAL THICKENING

Protracted thigh pain in a child with mid-femoral, periosteal new bone formation is an important finding which requires a prompt clinical explanation. It is of little diagnostic significance if clinical symptoms and signs of another disease are present or the diagnosis is already known, but it may be the most significant sign in a patient with a life-threatening disease.

The two most common disorders causing midfemoral periosteal thickening are Ewing's sarcoma and eosinophilic granuloma. They often have common symptoms and signs – protracted thigh pain, midthigh swelling and local tenderness. The ESR may be increased in both. The child with Ewing's sarcoma is usually, but not always, more severely ill.

Characteristic features of Ewing's sarcoma are permeative bone destruction, subperiosteal erosions, spicules, periosteal onion skin layering, Codman's triangle, soft tissue mass and pulmonary metastases (Fig. 4.113). However, it is not unusual for it to present as a localized intramedullary lesion simulating eosinophilic granuloma. Soft tissue mass, an important sign of Ewing's sarcoma, is absent in the early stages of midfemoral Ewing's sarcoma.

Eosinophilic granuloma usually has a more uniform pattern of changes: a circumscribed, intramedullary lucent lesion, endosteal cortical scalloping and periosteal reaction. In atypical forms, radiographic features resembling Ewing's sarcoma, such as poorly delineated intramedullary lesion, permeative bone destruction and periosteal reaction, resembling onion skin layering, may be present (Fig. 4.114). In the very early stages, both Ewing's sarcoma and eosinophilic granuloma cannot be differentiated not only from each other but also from the anatomical variants of normal bone.

Neither nuclear scan nor CT is helpful in differentiating early stages of Ewing's sarcoma from eosinophilic granuloma.

Another common cause of midfemoral periosteal thickening is osteoid osteoma. Often it has a characteristic history and the diagnosis is evident on plain radiographs. The nuclear scan and CT have diagnostic radiographic features (Fig. 4.115).

Other bone tumours (e.g. osteosarcoma and chondrosarcoma) may in some instances present as midfemoral periosteal thickening. Chondrosarcoma is often accompanied by chondromatous lesions elsewhere.

Contrary to general opinion, osteomyelitis is very rare as a cause of midfemoral periosteal thickening. We have encountered midfemoral periosteal thickening in other disorders – leukemia, neuroblastoma, rhabdomyosarcoma and as a post-traumatic lesion. Stress fracture, in particular, may mimic malignant bone lesion. Here, the diagnosis may initially be very difficult if a history of athletic activity is not disclosed. In other disorders, the primary disease is usually already known.

We would like to stress the value of skeletal survey and/or nuclear scan in children with midfemoral periosteal thickening. In cases of leukemia, neuroblastoma and rhabdomyosarcoma, even if the basic disorder is not recognized, a multifocal process will be at once diagnosed. Eosinophilic granuloma is often a multifocal process.

Table 4.18. Midfemoral tumors

Common	Rare	Differential diagnosis
Ewing's sarcoma	Osteosarcoma	Osteomyelitis (Brodie's abscess)
Eosinophilic granuloma	Chondrosarcoma	Myositis ossificans
Osteoid osteoma		Trauma – stress fracture – fibroblastic periosteal reaction
		Leukemia
		Soft tissue tumors

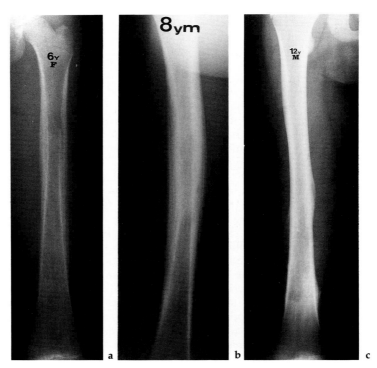

Fig. 4.113

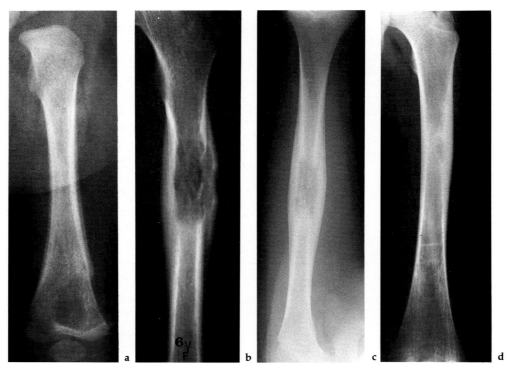

Fig. 4.114

Fig. 4.113. Ewing's sarcoma. **a** 6-year-old girl had left thigh pain for 2 months with intermittent fever and general malaise. On examination, the thigh was hot, swollen and tender. There are extensive destructive changes in the femoral shaft, with onion-like periosteal layering and Codman's triangle. Lung metastases were found. **b** This 8-year-old boy had a painful right thigh for 7 months; on examination, no abnormality was detected, her ESR was 16/42. There is onion-like periosteal layering with permeative cortical destruction. **c** This 12-year-old boy had episodic right thigh pain for 5 months; his right thigh was painfull and swollen and he had an ESR of 79/122. There is a slightly wavy contour with spiculations and Codman's triangle. (From Kozlowski et al. 1986, with permission.)

Fig. 4.114. Eosinophilic granuloma. **a** This 11-month-old boy had fever and pain in his left thigh for 3 weeks. He refused to move his left leg. There was swelling in the midthigh and enlargement of the left groin lymph nodes. There is a large osteolytic defect at the distal end of the femur, periosteal reaction along the femoral shaft. The trabecular pattern was abnormal. Bone biopsy indicated osteomyelitis or histiocytosis X, lymph node biopsy eosinophilic granuloma. **b** This 6-year-old girl had a painful left thigh for 3 months; her left thigh was swollen. A large osteolytic defect is present in the midshaft of the femur, with periosteal reaction and cortical destruction at the lateral aspect. **c** This 7.5-year-old boy presented with pain in the left thigh over a period of 2 weeks and weight loss despite a normal appetite. The thigh was swollen and warm, and the groin nodes enlarged; the ESR was 37. An irregular, lucent defect in the midpart of the left femur with some cortical erosions and periosteal thickening. **d** This 3.5-year-old girl had pain in the left thigh for several months. A small ill-defined radiolucent defect with sclerosis is seen in the midshaft of the femur. The presence of other bone lesions made the diagnosis of eosinophilic granuloma easy. (From Kozlowski et al. 1986, with permission.)

◄

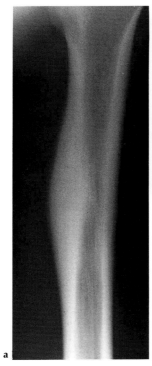
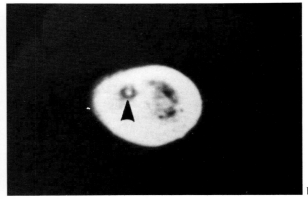

Fig. 4.115. Osteoid osteoma. This 13-year-old girl had pain in the left midthigh for 2 months; it was worse at night and was relieved by aspirin. **a** Unilateral periosteal thickening in the midshaft of the femur. **b** CT scan shows very well the low-density nidus with central calcification (*arrow*). (From Kozlowski et al. 1986, with permission.)

LITERATURE
Midfemoral Periosteal Thickening

Davies AM, Carter SR, Grimer RJ, Sneath RS. Fatigue frac-
    tures of the femoral diaphysis in the skeletally immature
    simulating malignancy. Br J Radiol 1989;62:893–6
Kozlowski K, Diard F, Padovani J, Sprague P, Pietron K.
    Unilateral mid-femoral periosteal newbone of varying

aetiology in children. Radiographic analysis of 25 cases.
    Pediatr Radiol 1986;16:475–82
Weisberg AL, Haller JO. Radiological case of the month. Am
    J Dis Child 1989;143:379–80

MIDSHAFT TIBIAL TUMORS

The tibial diaphysis is the location of some unique lesions. Bowing of the tibia in infancy and childhood, once congenital bowing is excluded, is most likely the result of one of two conditions, neurofibromatosis or fibro-osseous dysplasia.

Congenital bowing of the tibia and/or fibula with or without pseudoarthrosis is a well-known finding in neurofibromatosis and it may be the first sign of this disorder. There is sclerosis of the tibia with varying narrowing of the meduallary canal at the site of the lesion (Fig. 4.116).

Osteofibrous dysplasia (Fig. 4.117) is most often a midtibial lesion, with ipsilateral fibular involvement in about 20%. The radiographic appearances in early infancy are a unilocular, expansile, lytic lesion with some ill-defined sclerotic, patchy areas. A lesion presenting later in infancy or early childhood is lytic but eccentric and intracortical with multisatellites. The outer cortex is thinned and expanded.

Often there is reactive sclerosis, with narrowing of the medullary canal at the site of the lesion. Associated pathologic fractures have been reported. Osteofibrous dysplasia localized in the lower tibia may have similar appearances to nonossifying fibroma. The natural history is that of regression, and the treatment of choice is conservative therapy. The most important entity in differential diagnosis is adamantinoma.

Adamantinoma (Fig. 4.118) is a mid-diaphyseal, eccentric, solitary or multicystic tibial tumor similar in appearances to a late-presenting osteofibrous dysplasia. Both the tibia and fibula can be affected. Adamantinoma usually presents after the second decade of life.

In rare instances, other lesions such as fibrous dysplasia, eosinophilic granuloma and malignant bone tumors (Fig. 4.119) have a mid-diaphyseal location and can mimic osteofibrous dysplasia or adamantinoma. Midshaft tibial periosteal thickening with localized sclerosis is one of the common presentations of osteoid

Table 4.19. Midshaft tibial bone tumors

Benign	Malignant	Differential diagnosis
Osteoid osteoma	Osteosarcoma	Trauma – stress fracture
Eosinophilic granuloma	Ewing's sarcoma	Myositis ossificans
Neurofibromatosis		Osteomyelitis
Osteofibrous dysplasia		Soft tissue tumors
Fibrous dysplasia		Nonopaque foreign body with
Adamantinoma		osseous reaction

osteoma (Fig. 4.120). The tibia is also the most common site of the rare neuroectodermal tumor of bone.

Tibia vara subsequent to localized fibrocartilaginous dysplasia has diagnostic radiographic features, being characterized by local, proximal medial fibrocartilaginous dysplasia. The recognition of this is important, as biopsy and surgical treatment are contraindicated.

Other characteristic and not uncommon midshaft entities are osteomyelitis and post-traumatic lesions. Osteomyelitis has variable appearances (Fig. 4.121). If the marrow cavity is involved, osteolytic changes will predominate, with early periosteal reaction. A type of osteomyelitis with isolated sclerotic periosteal reaction and Brodie's abscess can also occur.

Post-traumatic lesions – periosteal thickening, stress fracture and myositis ossificans – have characteristic clinical histories. The most common sites of tibial stress fracture in children are the proximal part of the tibial shaft, the distal part and, more rarely, the midshaft (Fig. 4.122). The latter occurs often in adult weight-lifters and ballet dancers. It is usually bilateral. Midshaft osteosarcoma may in the early stages simulate stress fracture (Fig. 4.123). Diagnostic difficulties in the early stages of myositis ossificans are well known. Follow-up examination usually demonstrates typical appearances (Fig. 4.124). Tumoral calcinosis (Fig. 4.125) a disorder of uncertain etiology, may occasionally have a peridiaphyseal location.

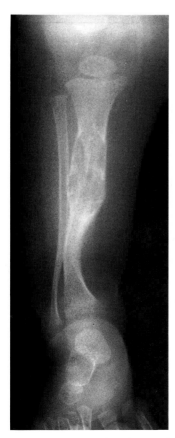

Fig. 4.116. Neurofibromatosis. This aboriginal 5-month-old girl with extensive skin and bony changes and deformity of the right leg from birth.

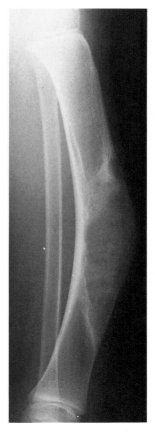

Fig. 4.117. Osteofibrous dysplasia. Deformity of the left leg noted in the first year of this 4-year-old boy's life. The deformity increased after he started to walk.

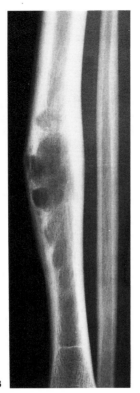

Fig. 4.118

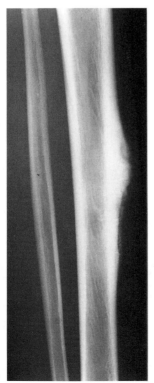

Fig. 4.119

Fig. 4.118. Adamantinoma. This 9-year-old boy had pain in the left leg for 1 year, gradually increasing in severity.

Fig. 4.119. Osteosarcoma. This 9-year-old girl had had a lump on the left leg for 10 weeks following trauma 2.5–3.0 months previously and 2 weeks after the initial trauma. There is superficial erosion of the cortex, with coarse periosteal bone formation and irregular spicula. (From Kozlowski 1980a, with permission.)

←————————————————————————

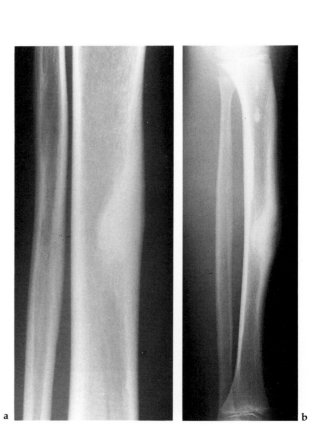

a   b

Fig. 4.120. Osteoid osteoma. **a** There was a 1 year history of lump on the left tibia of this 9-year-old boy. The increase in size was minimal. Initially he was asymptomatic, but later experienced occasional pain with increased exercise or trauma. **b** This 13-year-old boy had a history of pain in the left leg, relieved by aspirin, for several months.

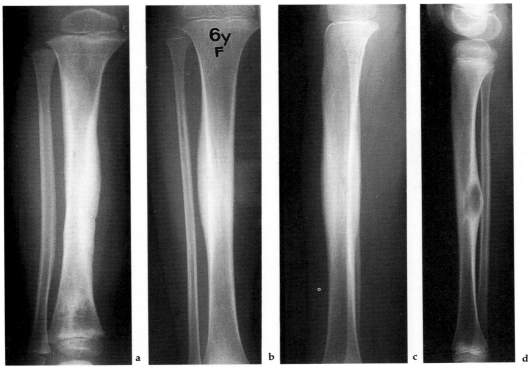

Fig. 4.121. Osteomyelitis. **a** Sclerosis and periosteal thickening in the midshaft of the right tibia (3-year-old boy). **b,c** 6-year-old girl, 4 weeks after cardiac catheterization. **d** This 9-year-old girl had pain in the right hip and lower back for 6 months. There is a large defect (3 × 1 cm) in the posterior part of the right tibial shaft (Brodie's abscess). (**b,c** From Kozlowski 1980, with permission.)

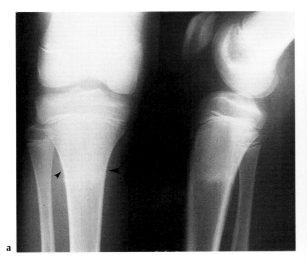

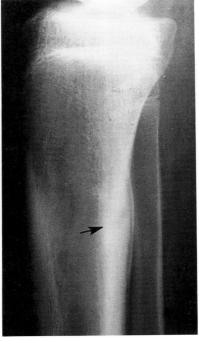

Fig. 4.122. Stress fracture. **a** This 10-year-old girl presented with pain in the right knee for 3 weeks. There is minimal periosteal reaction with sclerotic transverse band (*arrows*). **b** This 13-year-old boy had pain in the right leg for several weeks. There is a fracture line with periosteal bone formation (*arrow*).

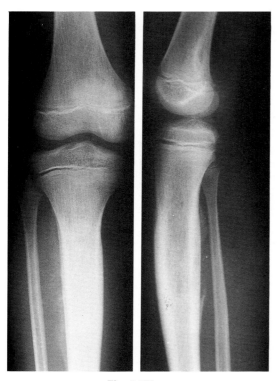

Fig. 4.123. Osteosarcoma. This 11-year-old boy presented with pain in the right leg for several months. There is extensive periosteal new bone formation, with multiple spiculae and Codman's triangle.

Fig. 4.124. Myositis ossificans. There had been a greenstick fracture of the left tibia of this 7-year-old boy 6 months before the radiograph was taken. (From Kozlowski et al. 1976, with permission.)

Fig. 4.123

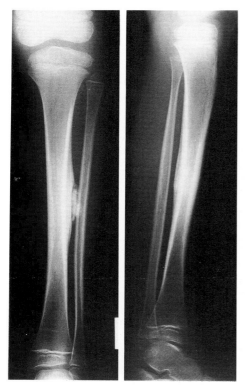

Fig. 4.124

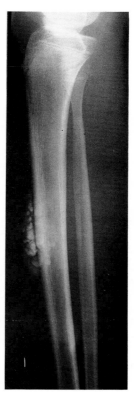

Fig. 4.125. Tumoral calcinosis in the midshaft, a rare location. This 14-year-old boy had tumors in several other periarticular locations. (From Kozlowski et al. 1988, with permission.)

LITERATURE
Midshaft Tibial Tumors

Adler CP. Case report 587. Skeletal Radiol 1990;19:55–8

Anderson RB, McAlister JA, Wrenn RN. Case report 585. Skeletal Radiol 1989;18:627–30

Bloem JL, van der Heul RO, Schuttevaer HM, Kuipers D. Fibrous dysplasia vs adamantinoma of the tibia: differentiation based on discriminant analysis of clinical and plain film findings. AJR 1991;156:1017–23

Bradish CF, Davies SJM, Malone M. Tibia vara due to focal fibrocartilaginous dysplasia. J Bone Jt Surg 1988;70B:106–8

Capusten BM, Rochon L, Rosman MA, Marton D. Osteofibrous dysplasia. J Assoc Can Radiol 1980;31:50–3

Davies AM, Evans N, Grimer RJ. Fatigue fractures of the proximal tibia simulating malignancy. Br J Radiol 1988; 61:903–8

Faure C, Boccon-Gibod L, Bercovy M. Case Report 257. Skeletal Radiol 1984;11:73–6

Gwinn JL, Barnes GR, Castro de FJ. Radiological case of the month. Am J Dis Child 1967;114:401–2

Haberman ET, Stern RE. Osteiod-osteoma of the tibia in an eight month old boy. J Bone Jt Surg 1974;56-A:633–6

Herman TE, Siegel MJ, McAlister WH. Focal fibrocartilaginous dysplasia associated with tibia vara. Radiology 1990;177:767–8

Keeney GL, Krishnan U, Beabout JW, Douglas JP. Adamantinoma of long bones. A clinicopathologic study of 85 cases. Cancer 1989;64:730–7

Kozlowski K. Osteosarcoma with unusual clinical and/or radiographic appearances. Pediatr Radiol 1980a;9:167–170

Kozlowski K. Brodie's abscess in the first decade of life. Report of eleven cases. Pediatr Radiol 1980;b10:33–7

Kozlowski K, Bale P, Reye DK. Difficultés du diagnostic radiographique des tumeurs primitives et secondaires de l'os chez l'enfant. Ann Radiol 1976;19:781–90

Kozlowski K, BarylakA, Campbell J, Diard F, Masel J, Massen R, Kan AE. Tumoral calcinosis in children. Report of 13 cases. Aust Radiol 1988;32:448

Kozlowski K, Azouz M, Barrett IR, Hoff D, Scougall JS. Midshaft tibial stress fractures in children (report of four cases). Australas Radiol 1992;36:131–4

Labrune M, Guinard J, Rengeval JP, Carlioz N, Dubousset JF, Queneau P. L'ostéofibrodysplasie des os longs à évolution regressive. Arch Fr Pediatr 1979;36:134–43

Malghem J, Maldague B. Transient fatty cortical defects following fractures in children. Skeletal Radiol 1986; 15:368–71

Malghem J, Maldague B. Post-traumatic cyst-like lesions. Skeletal Radiol 1987;16:403–6

Olney BW, Cole WG, Menelaus MB. Three additional cases of focal fibrocartilaginous dysplasia causing tibia vara. J Pediatr Orthop 1990;10:405–7

Rousselin B, Vanel D, Terrier-Lacombe MJ, Istria BJM, Spielman M, Masselot J. Clinical and radiologic analysis of 13 cases of primary neuroectodermal tumors of bone. Skeletal Radiol 1989;18:115–20

Smith NM, Byard RW, Foster B, Morris L, Clark B, Bourne AJ. Congenital ossifying fibroma (osteofibrous dysplasia) of the tibia – a case report. Pediatr Radiol 1991;21:449–51

EPIPHYSEAL TUMORS

There are only few reports on the primary tumors of the epiphyses in children. They usually present as a radiolucent or oval defect. The exact histological diagnosis is essential for appropriate treatment of these important regions of the skeletal system.

The clinical symptoms of the epiphyseal tumors are pain, rarely swelling and joint effusion. Radiologically they show little specificity. They present usually as well-demarcated, radiolucent, round defects. The most common lesion is chondroblastoma (Fig. 4.126). Enchondroma, osteoblastoma, chondromyxoid fibroma and eosinophilic granuloma have been reported occasionally. Nuclear scan and CT rarely add additional diagnostic data. The common osteoid osteoma is rarely localized in the epiphyses, and when it is it has less characteristic features than it does in the shaft. The lesion is round, lytic and surrounded by a sclerotic rim, but sometimes it has a dense, central calcification. The reactive sclerosis is much less marked. Soft tissue swelling, synovial effusion and local osteoporosis may be present. CT shows the anatomic details better than radiography. We observed a case of epiphyseal osteoid osteoma which presented as a round, lytic defect with local osteoporosis but without any sclerotic reaction (Fig. 4.127). Exchondroma can be recognized easily (Fig. 4.128); however, Trevor's disease and metachondromatosis should be excluded before its diagnosis is accepted.

Most important in the differential diagnosis of primary epiphyseal tumours is osteomyelitis (Brodie's abscess). This is the most frequent cause of a radiolucent, cyst-like defect in the epiphysis (Fig. 4.129). Brodie's abscess may present with general and local signs and symptoms and positive blood findings; nevertheless there is often only some swelling and pain in the region of the affected epiphysis. In cases of a chronic inflammatory process, both radiologic and histologic distinction from eosinophilic granuloma may be difficult. Transepiphyseal extension into the metaphysis has been reported in both disorders.

Normal anatomic variants should be borne in mind in differential diagnosis of epiphyseal tumors. They may sometimes cause confusion (Fig. 4.130).

Table 4.20. Epiphyseal tumors

"Common"	Rare	Differential diagnosis of cystic lesions	Radiographic clues to the diagnosis of Brodie's abscess
Enchondroma Chondroblastoma Osteoid osteoma Eosinophilic granuloma Fibrous dysplasia (usually as part of multifocal disease)	Other tumors: non-ossifying fibroma, chondromyxoid fibroma and unicameral and aneurysmal bone cyst have been sporadically reported	Brodie's abscess (chronic or subacute osteomyelitis)	Radiolucent, cystic lesion Soft tissue swelling Little periosteal reaction Sequestrum (demonstrated only on CT) Multiple epi- and metaphyseal cavities with connecting channels

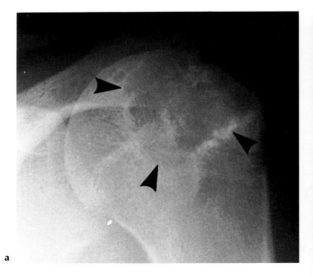

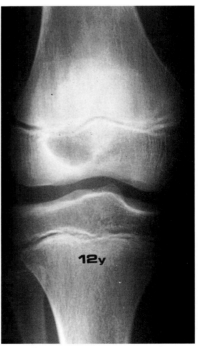

Fig. 4.126. Chondroblastoma. **a** This 12-year-old girl had pain in the left shoulder radiating into the left wrist for the previous 18 months. The great tuberosity was tender. There is a large radiolucent defect with an irregular sclerotic rim and some ill-defined calcification inside the lesion (*arrows*). **b** This 12-year-old boy had increasing pain in the right knee for several months. A radiolucent defect can be seen in the distal femoral epiphysis, with surrounding sclerosis.

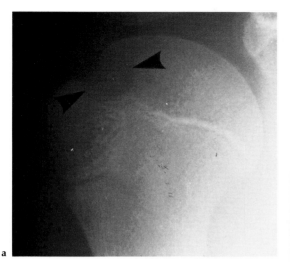

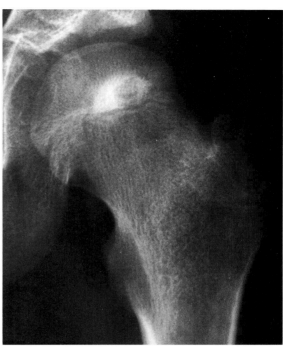

Fig. 4.127. Osteoid osteoma. **a** This 11-year-old girl had pain in the right shoulder for 1 month. There is an osteolytic defect in the right humeral epiphysis (*arrows*). **b** This 8-year-old girl had pain in the left hip for 2 years. Here a radiolucent defect with a sclerotic border is seen (diagnosis uncertain – case not proved by biopsy). A radiograph taken 20 months later was normal.

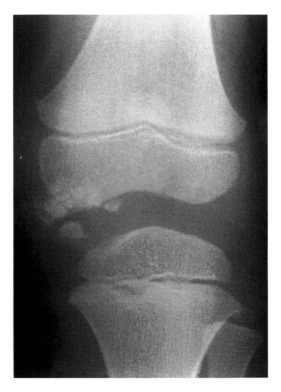

Fig. 4.128. Osteochondroma. This 5.5-year-old boy had a stiff knee. There is a large lesion with multiple ossification centers.

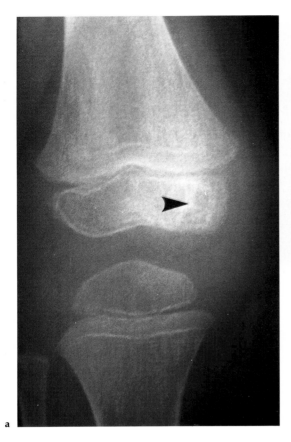

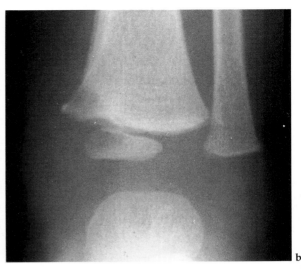

Fig. 4.129. Osteomyelitis (Brodie's abscess). **a** There had been trauma to the right knee of this 4-year-old boy 6 weeks ago. Increasing swelling, with little pain, had occurred for 5 weeks. There is an ill-defined defect in the medial part of the distal femoral epiphysis (*arrow*), and soft tissue swelling and regional osteopenia. **b** This 20-month-old boy had ankle pain for several weeks. Radiolucent defects are seen in the distal tibial epiphysis and metaphysis, with minimal periosteal reaction and soft tissue swelling.

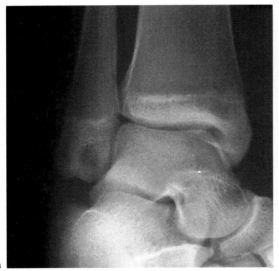

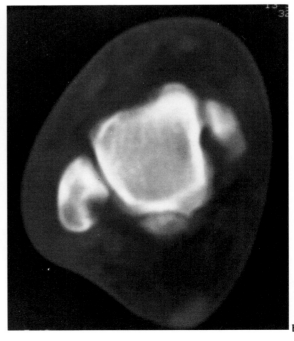

Fig. 4.130. Anatomic variant. This 13.5-year-old girl was in pain after twisting her ankle. **a** There is a radiolucency in the distal fibular epiphysis which could be mistaken for a Brodie's abscess or osteoid osteoma. **b** CT scan shows a deep cortical defect. The "lesion" was present bilaterally.

LITERATURE
Epiphyseal Tumors

Bogoch E, Thompson G, Salter RB. Foci of chronic circum-scribed osteomyelitis (Brodies's abscess) that traverse the epiphyseal plate. J Pediatr Orthop 1984;4:162–9

Destian S, Hernanax-Schulman M, Raskin K, Genieser N, Becker M, Crider R, Alba Greco M. Case Report 468. Skeletal Radiol 1988;17:141–143

Dunlap H, Martin DJ. Osteoid osteoma of the femoral head. Pediatr Radiol 1985;15:262–3

Fassier F, Duhaime M, Marton D, Brochu P. Un cas d'ostéome ostéoide de l'ésiphyse de la tête fémorale chez un enfant de 9 ans. Rev Chir Orthop 1986;72:215–17

Fobben ES, Dalinka MK, Schiebler ML, Burk DL, Fallon MD, Schmidt RG, Kressel HY. The magnetic resonance imaging appearance at 1.5 Tesla of cartilaginous tumors involving the epiphysis. Skeletal Radiol 1987;16:647–51

Gardner DJ, Azouz MA. Solitary epiphyseal lesions in children. Skeletal Radiol 1988;17:497–504

Giudici MAL, Eggli KD, Moser RP, Roloff JS, Frauenhoffer EE, Kransdorf MJ. Case report 730. Skeletal Radiol 1992;

21:260–5

Kozlowski K. Brodie's abscess in the first decade of life. Pediatr Radiol 1980;10:33–7

Kozlowski K. Osteoid osteoma (some diagnostic problems). Radiol Diagn 1982;23:317–25

Laurent F, Diard F, Calabet A, Chabane M. Les ostéomyelites circonscrites non tuberculeuses de l'enfant. A propos de 31 cas. J Radiol 1984;65:545–553

Lebarbier P, Cahuzac JP, Eymeri JC, Verge JH, Pasquie M. Les lacunes épiphysaires de l'enfant. Chir Pediatr 1979; 20:95–7

Leeson MC, Smith A, Carter JR, Makley JT. Eosinophilic granuloma of bone in the growing epiphysis. J Pediatr Orthop 1985;5:147–50

Miller WB, Murphy WA, Gilula LA. Brodie's abscess: re-appraisal. Radiology 1979;132:15–23

Rosenbaum DM, Blumhagen JD. Acute epiphyseal osteomyelitis in children. Radiology 1985;156:89–92

PATELLAR TUMORS

Primary tumors of the patella are extremely rare in childhood and almost all reports describe adult patients. In 42 cases reviewed by Kransdorf et al. (1989) there were only three children; the tumors were chondroblastoma, angioma and lipoma and the youngest patient was 13 years old.

In a case of patellar lesion, congenital anomaly and stress reaction should be excluded. The congenital anomaly is usually a part of a generalized bone dysplasia, bone dysostosis, malformation syndrome or chromosomal abnormality. The most common stress ractions are the dorsal defect and osteochondritis dissecans. The dorsal defect presents as a round, radiolucent lesion with a sclerotic border, located in the superolateral quadrant of the patella. It is a stress-induced anomaly of ossification. Osteochondritis dissecans is the result of minor injuries to the articular surface of the patella.

Larsen–Johansson syndrome is an aseptic necrosis of the patellar tip. Usually a clinical diagnosis is made and the radiographs are normal.

When congenital and stress-related disorders have been excluded, an inflammatory lesion is a most likely diagnosis, especially if clinical signs

Table 4.21. Patellar tumors: all are very rare in childhood

Differential diagnosis
Osteomyelitis
Trauma
Congenital malformation

and symptoms – constant pain, pyrexia, hot red tender swelling over the patella – are present. Depending on the stage of the inflammatory process and the causative organism, the radiographic examination may reveal any appearance between that of a small, localized, destructive lesion and that of an osteosclerotic overgrowth of the patella (Figs 4.131 and 4.132).

A malignant patellar tumor or metastases as a first manifestation of a malignant tumor are unlikely diagnoses in childhood.

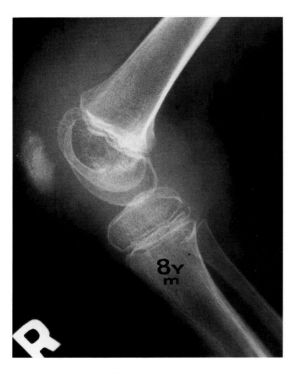

Fig. 4.131. Osteomyelitis. This 8-year-old boy had pain and swelling of the right knee for 3 weeks. The patella is osteosclerotic and irregular in outline, with an ill-defined osteolytic area in the upper part. There is marked soft tissue swelling and osteoporosis.

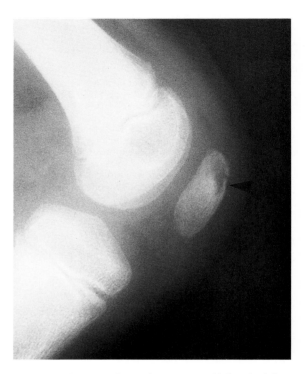

Fig. 4.132. Osteomyelitis. This 10-year-old boy had knee pain for 2 weeks. An osteolytic defect is seen in the anterior, upper part of the patella.

LITERATURE

Patellar Tumors

Denham RH. Dorsal defect of the patella. J Bone Jt Surg 1984;66-A:116–20

Desai SS, Michelli LJ, Patel MR, Silver JW, Lidge RT. Osteochondritis dissecans of the patella. J Bone Jt Surg 1987;69-B:320–5

Holsbeeck van M, Vandamme B, Marchal G, Martens M, Victor J, Baert AL. Doral defect of the patella: concept of its origin and relationship with bipartite and multipartite patella. Skeletal Radiol 1987;16:304–11

Kransdorf MJ, Moser RP, Vinh TN, Aoki J, Callaghan JJ. Primary tumors of the patella. A review of 42 cases. Skeletal Radiol 1989;18:365–71

Linscheid RL, Dahlin DC. Unusual lesions of the patella. J Bone Jt Surg 1966;48-A:1359–66

Meyer St, Dick W, Fliegel CP. Zystische Aufhellungen der Patella im Wachstumsalter. Z Kinderchir 1978;24:46–55

Remagen W, Schäfer R, Roggatz J. Chondroblastoma of the patella. Arch Orthop Trauma Surg 1980;96:157–8

HAND TUMORS

Primary bone tumors of the hands, with the exception of enchondromatosis and exchondromatosis, are rare in childhood. In these instances they are part of a generalized disease. Single enchondromas (Fig. 4.133) and single exchondromas (Fig. 4.134) are much rarer, and the former may cause diagnostic difficulties.

Although almost all tumors can be encountered in the hand, some of them are so rare (Fig. 4.135) that they will never be seen even in a large pediatric hospital. There is however a group of relatively common tumors with fairly characteristic radiographic findings. This includes osteoid osteoma, aneurysmal bone cyst and Ewing's sarcoma. Radiographic recognition of the other tumors is rather the result of good luck than a thorough clinical and radiographic analysis.

Osteoid osteoma of the hand, which comprises about 5% of the adult and pediatric patients with tumors of the hand, usually presents with characteristic clinical features: recurrent pain, swelling, tenderness, bone enlargement and nail hypertrophy when the distal phalanx is involved (Fig. 4.136a). The radiographic appearances in the distal phalanx are those of sclerotic nidus with radiolucent halo (ring sequestrum). In the remaining short tubular bones, an intense sclerotic reaction is usually present. Carpal osteoma presents with intense local sclerosis (Fig. 4.136b–d).

Aneurysmal bone cyst of the hands comprises about 2% of the adult and pediatric patients with tumors of the hand. In the terminal phalanges, it often causes extensive bone destruc-

tion simulating malignant bone tumor. In the remaining short tubular bones, aneurysmal bone cyst presents as a more or less destructive and expansile lesion sometimes involving the whole bone (Fig. 4.137).

The radiographic appearances of fibrous lesions of the hand are uncharacteristic (Fig. 4.138) and the histology is often confusing.

Epidermoid cyst is a rare finding in children. It shows characteristic cystic radiolucency in the distal phalanx (Fig. 4.139).

Recently, giant reparative granuloma in the hands and feet has been reported with increased frequency. It is predominantly a lesion of young adults and teenagers. Radiologically it typically presents as a lytic expansile lesion with cortical thinning but without cortical destruction or periosteal reaction. It resembles aneurysmal bone cyst. Recurrences are common after surgery but no metastases have been reported.

Ewing's sarcoma represents 1–2% of combined adult and pediatric cases involving the hands. It shows the typical permeative destruction and osteosclerotic changes with periosteal bone formation. A honeycomb destructive pattern may be seen occasionally. A large soft tissue mass is a constant finding in later stages (Fig. 4.140).

Other malignant (osteosarcoma, malignant vascular tumors – Fig. 4.141) and benign (simple bone cyst, osteoma, chondroblastoma, glomus tumor) tumors have been reported occasionally. Osteosarcoma and glomus tumor of the hand are common in adults but are rarely encountered in children.

Table 4.22. Hand tumors

Common		Rare		Differential diagnosis
Benign	Malignant	Benign	Malignant	
Enchondroma	Ewing's sarcoma	Epidermoid cyst	Osteosarcoma	Osteomyelitis (including
Exchondroma		Fibro-osseous tumors	Malignant vascular	tuberculosis)
Aneurysmal bone cyst		Osteoblastoma	tumors	Soft tissue tumors
Osteoid osteoma		Chondromyxoid fibroma		Sarcoidosis
		Giant cell reparative granuloma		

In the differential diagnosis of primary bone tumors of the hand nontumorous but tumor-simulating bone lesions and osteomyelitis should be considered. Primary hematogenous osteomyelitis of the hand without any underlying disorder (including sepsis) is extremely rare in childhood (Fig. 4.142). Usually it is secondary to a soft tissue inflammation and/or penetrating traumatic lesion. Spina ventosa (Fig. 4.143) and chronic granulomatous disease are usually multifocal. The systemic manifestations of the latter are evident and most often the diagnosis is known when the bone complications occur. The osseous appearances of hemophilia may be very similar to those of aneurysmal bone cyst (Fig. 4.144). Idiopathic osteolysis presents under many different forms. Its main radiographic feature is multifocal, progressive osteolysis.

Systemic diseases of unknown etiology, such as sarcoidosis or tuberous sclerosis, may present very rarely as a single bony lesion. Usually bone involvement is multifocal and the disorder has been already diagnosed (Fig. 4.145).

Metastases to the hand bones are not unusual in leukemia, neuroblastoma and reticuloendotheliosis (Fig. 4.146). Usually the involvement is multifocal and the disorder has been already diagnosed. Surprisingly, the hands and the feet are not affected in eosinophilic granuloma.

The diagnosis of the primary bone tumors may be extremely difficult when two different tumors or osteomyelitis and a tumor are present. Such circumstances, with the exception of secondary aneurysmal bone cyst, are however extremely rare.

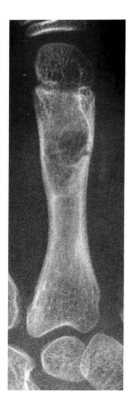

Fig. 4.133. Enchondroma. This 10-year-old boy had a painful second metacarpal for several weeks. A large, radiolucent, slightly expansile lesion crosses the growth cartilage and extends into the epiphysis. (From Kozlowski et al. 1988, with permission.)

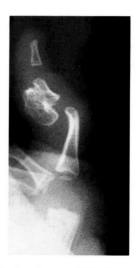

Fig. 4.134. Exchondroma. This 8-month-old girl had a painless, enlarging hard swelling of the midpart of the 4th finger. No other bony lesions were present. (From Dr D. Marton, Montreal, Canada, with permission.)

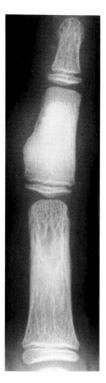

Fig. 4.135. Osteocondensant osteoma. Osteosclerotic, slightly expansile lesion in the middle phalanx of the right 3rd finger of a 12-year-old boy. (From Kozlowski et al. 1988 with permission.)

Fig. 4.136. Osteoid osteoma. **a,b** Overgrowth of the left thumb including nail, and osteolytic defect in the distal phalanx with sclerotic nidus (12-year-old boy). **c** This 17-year-old girl had a painful wrist for several months. Sclerotic and enlarged trapezium can be seen. **d** Massive sclerotic reaction at the proximal phalanx of the left index finger (16-year-old boy). (From Kozlowski et al. 1988, with permission.)
▼

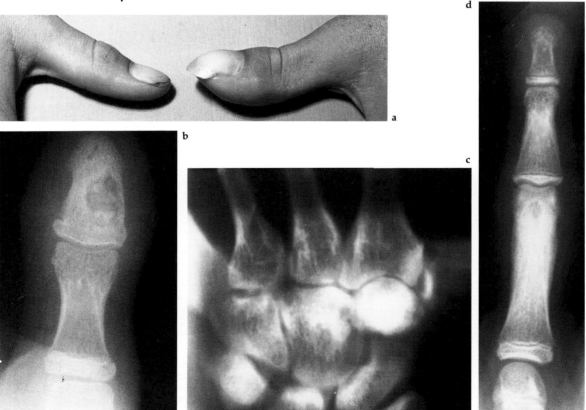

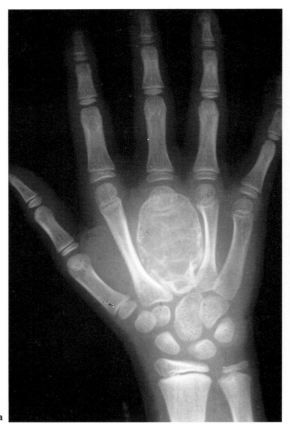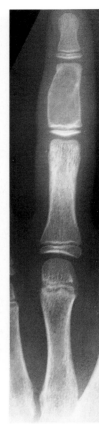

Fig. 4.137. Aneurysmal bone cyst. **a** Ballooned-out distention of the 3rd metacarpals with "soap bubble" pattern of the affected bone, and paper thin cortex; no periosteal reaction is present (8-year-old boy). **b** A slightly expansile lesion involving the second phalanx of the left middle finger, with some "soap bubble" trabecular pattern (10-year-old boy). (From Kozlowski et al. 1988, with permission.)

a   b

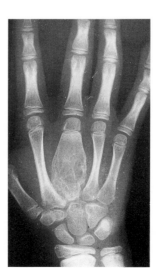

Fig. 4.138. Possible osteoblastoma or benign ossifying fibroma. This 10-year-old girl had pain in the right hand for several months. There is an expansile lesion in the 3rd metacarpal, with cortical thinning and irregular medullary destruction and deformity of the adjacent metacarpals. (From Kozlowski et al. 1988, with permission.)

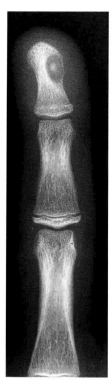

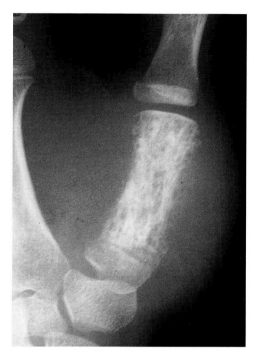

Fig. 4.139. Epidermoid cyst. Asymptomatic, round, cystic lesion in the distal phalanx of the second finger (15.5-year-old boy). (From Kozlowski et al. 1988, with permission.)

Fig. 4.140. Ewing's sarcoma. In this 12-year-old boy's 1st metacarpal there is a widespread osteolytic and osteosclerotic lesion extending through the whole of the metacarpal, cortical destruction with spiculae, and a large soft tissue mass. (From Kozlowski et al. 1988, with permission.)

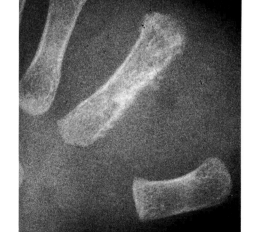

Fig. 4.141. Malignant hemangiopericytoma. In this 6-year-old girl's 2nd metacarpal there is a widespread osteolytic and osteosclerotic lesion and cortical destruction with spiculae. The appearances are similar to Fig. 4.140. (From Kozlowski et al. 1988, with permission.)

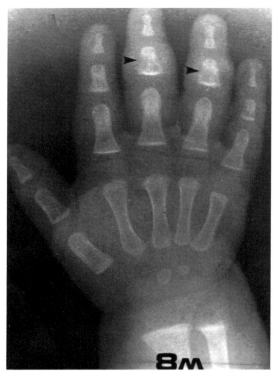

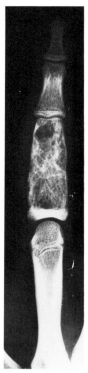

Fig. 4.142. Osteomyelitis. This 8-month-old girl had swelling of the 3rd and 4th fingers for 2 months without preceding illness.

Fig. 4.143. Spina ventosa. This 15-year-old boy displayed the signs and symptoms of low-grade osteomyelitis. There is an irregular osteolytic lesion in the basal phalanx of the index finger; no other bony lesion was found and there was no detectable pulmonary lesion. (From Kozlowski et al. 1988, with permission.)

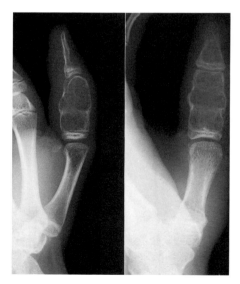

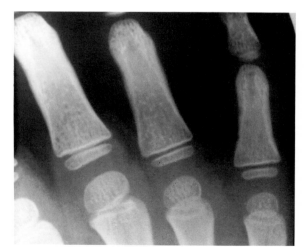

Fig. 4.144. Hemophilia. This 17-year-old boy presented with swelling of the left thumb over a period of 2 years after a minor trauma. There is an expansile radiolucent lesion with cortical thinning in the basal phalanx of the thumb. A destructive lesion is seen in the distal phalanx. (From Kozlowski et al. 1988, with permission.)

Fig. 4.145. Sarcoidosis. Multiple, small osteolytic lesions in the proximal phalanx of the little finger (5-year-old boy).

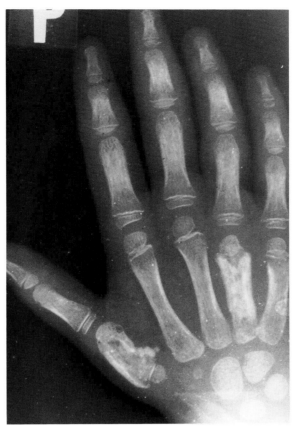

Fig. 4.146. Reticuloendotheliosis. Multifocal, mixed osteolytic and osteosclerotic lesions (6-year-old boy). (From Kozlowski et al. 1988, with permission.)

LITERATURE
Hand Tumors

Bücheler E, Klammer HHL. Ossäre hämophilie Pseudotumoren. Forschr Röntgenstr 1974;120:468–73

Byers P, Mantle J, Salm R. Epidermal cysts of phalanges. J Bone Jt Surg 1966;48-B:577–81

Carrol RE, Berman AT. Glomus tumors of the hand. J Bone Jt Surg 1972;54-A:691–703

Diard F, Kozlowski K, Masel J, Marc J. Multifocal, chronic, non-staphylococcal osteomyelitis in children (Report of four cases – Aspergillosis, Klebsiella, Tuberculosis). Aust Radiol 1983;27:39–44

Dick HM, Francis KC, Johnston AD. Ewing's sarcoma of the hand. J Bone Jt Surg 1971;53-A:345–8

Drompp BW. Bilateral osteosarcoma in the phalanges of the hand. J Bone Jt Surg 1961;43-A:199–204

Dunitz NL, Lipscomb PR, Ivins JC. Osteoid osteoma of the hands and wrist. Am Jt Surg 1957;94:65–9

Ewald FC. Bone cyst in a phalanx of a two- and a-half-year-old child. Case report and discussion. J Bone Jt Surg 1972;54-A:399–402

Ghiam GF, Bora FW. Osteoid osteoma of the carpal bones. J Hand Surg 1978;3:280–3

Hoeffel JC, Germain E, Bretagne MC, Bernard C, Galloy

MA. Tumeurs osseuses primitives de la main chez l'enfant aspects radiologiques. Med Infant 1989;96:49–57

Kozlowski K. Dactylitis secondary to chronic granulomatous disease Report of a case. Radiol Diagn 1976;3:347–50

Kozlowski K, Azouz EM, Campbell J, Marton D, Morris L, Padovani J, Spraque P, Beluffi G, Berzero GF, Cherubino P. Primary bone tumours of the hand. Report of 21 cases. Pediatr Radiol 1988;18:140–8

Kozlowski K, Hanicka M, Garapich M. Neurogene ulcerierende akropathie. (Akroosteolyse-Syndrome). Monatschr Kinderheilk 1971;119:169–75

Lacey SH, Danish EH, Thompson GH, Joyce MJ. Ewing's sarcoma of the proximal phalanx of a finger. A case report. J Bone Jt Surg 1987;69-A:931–4.

Mangini U. Tumors of the skeleton of the hand. Bull Hosp Jt Dis 1967;28:61–102

Monsees B, Murphy WA. Distal phalangeal erosive lesions. Arthritis Rheum 1984;27:449–55

Nidecker A, Remangen W, Elke M. Korrelation radio-logischer and pathologischer Befunde bei Tumoren und tumorähnlichen Läsionen der Hand. Radiologe 1982; 22:222–9

Picci P, Baldini N, Sudanese A, Boriani S, Campanacci M. Giant cell reparative granuloma and other giant cell lesions of the bones of the hands and feet. Skeletal Radiol 1986;15:415–21

Reinus WR, Gilula LA, Shirley SK, Askin FB, Siegal GP. Radiographic appearance of Ewing's sarcoma of the hands and feet: report from the intergroup Ewing's sarcoma study. AJR 1985;144:331–6

Schajowicz F, Atello CL, Slullitel I. Cystic and pseudocystic lesions of the terminal phalanx with special reference to epidermoid cyst. Clin Orthop 1970;68:84–92

Scutellari PN, Orzincolo C, Trotta F. Case report 375. Skeletal Radiol 1986;15:394–7

Tillman BP, Dahlin DC, Lipscomb PR, Stewart JR. Aneurysmal bone cyst. An analysis of ninety five cases. Mayo Clin Proc 1968;43:478–95

FOOT TUMORS

Primary bone tumors of the foot are more common than those of the hands. Some differences between them are due to anatomic particularities. In the first decade to life, tumors of the foot are very rare.

Two recent papers have analysed the bone tumors of the feet. Ochsner reviewed 512 cases (among them 132 children up to 16 years old) and Richter et al. (1986) 554 cases. The text that here follows is principally on these two publications.

In our experience, osteochondroma and enchondroma are the most common tumors of the foot, and according to Richter et al. they represent 90% of all adult and child cases; however, they account for only 3% of the pediatric cases reviewed by Ochsner. This discrepancy can be explained by the fact that Ochsner's paper was based to a great extent on the literature and his specialized clinic did not attract many simple cases. He also included in his material 28 children with calcaneal cyst and four children with metastases.

The rare benign tumors of the feet are osteoid osteoma (Fig. 4.147), aneurysmal bone cyst (Fig. 4.148), osteoblastoma, chondroblastoma and

Table 4.23. Foot tumors

Common		Rare		Differential diagnosis
Benign	Malignant	Benign	Malignant	
Enchondroma	Ewing's sarcoma	Chondroblastoma	Osteosarcoma	Osteomyelitis
Exchondroma		Chondromyxoid fibroma	Malignant vascular tumors	Trauma – stress fracture
Simple bone cyst (calcanear cyst)		Fibro-osseous tumors		Soft tissue tumors
Osteoid osteoma		Giant cell tumor		Nonopaque foreign bodies with osseous reaction
Aneurysmal bone cyst		Giant cell reparative granuloma		
Osteoblastoma				

chondromyxoid fibroma. In a review of 40 pediatric and adult patients with osteoid osteoma and osteoblastoma of the talus, a predilection for a subperiosteal, pare-articular location, in the area of the capsular attachment at the junction between the articular surface and the neck, was found in 25 of 32 cases of osteoid osteoma. The radiographic appearances, usually characteristic, were those of a target lesion (central calcification), peripheral calcification or small, irregular osteolytic excavation of the cortex. Osteoblastoma is more common in the talar neck, whereas chondroblastoma and chondromyxoid fibroma tend to be localized in the posterior part. Giant cell tumor may occur sporadically.

In the calcaneus the most common lesion is a bone cyst, which may be difficult to differentiate on plain radiographs from normal anatomic variant or calcanear lipoma. Chondroblastoma, chondromyxoid fibroma and aneurysmal bone cyst are the other benign bone tumors encountered in the foot. CT and MR can be extremely useful in the differential diagnosis of tarsal bone tumors.

The small tarsal bones are a site of bone tumor in very rare instances. Aneurysmal bone cyst and chondromyxoid fibroma are the most common of primary metatarsal tumors. Giant cell reparative granuloma has recently been reported as an entity which has to be differentiated from aneurysmal bone cyst. This tumor-like condition has predilection for the small tubular bones of the hands and feet.

The only common malignant tumor of the feet is Ewing's sarcoma (Fig. 4.149). Like its counterpart in the hand it has a poor prognosis. Other malignant primary bone tumors of the foot are very rare in children.

Leukemia and neuroblastoma are the most common metastatic neoplasms.

Calcaneal spur and ungual spur are most likely post-traumatic lesions. The latter is extremely rare in children.

In the differential diagnosis of primary bone tumors, inflammatory lesions and trauma should be considered. The former may easily cause confusion, particularly in cases of primary bone tumors of the talus and calcaneus (Fig. 4.150); the latter should particularly be considered in morbid diseases of the metatarsals and phalanges (Fig. 4.151). Normal anatomic variants should cause no confusion (Fig. 4.152). In rare instances a malignant soft tissue tumor such as aggressive fibromatosis/fibrosarcoma complex can be diagnosed as primary bone tumor. CT and MR studies should be performed for both diagnostic and therapeutic purposes in patients with primary malignant soft tissue tumors.

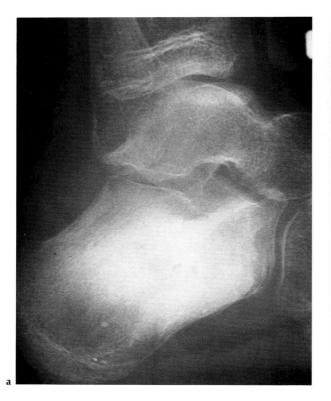

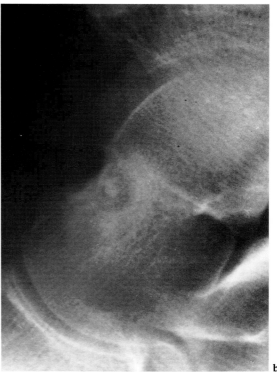

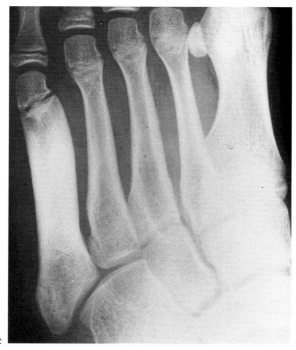

Fig. 4.147. Osteoid osteoma. **a** This 14-year-old boy had pain in the heel for 3 years. There is diffuse sclerosis of the calcaneus. **b** This 13-year-old girl had ankle pain for 2 years, with increasing ankle swelling. The ossified nidus is separated from the surrounding, slightly sclerotic bone by a ring of radiolucency representing the unossified nidus. **c** This 13-year-old boy had a painful foot for 1 year. There is massive overgrowth and sclerosis of the 5th metatarsal.

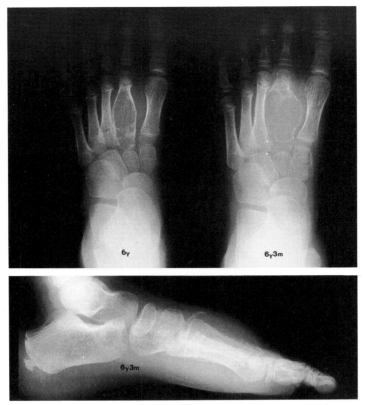

Fig. 4.148. Aneurysmal bone cyst. This 6-year-old boy had a 3-month history of a painful left foot since stubbing his toes. There is a radiolucent, expansile lesion in the left second metatarsal with "soap buble" pattern. Note the increase in size of the lesion in 3 months. (From Kozlowski and Middleton 1980, with permission.)

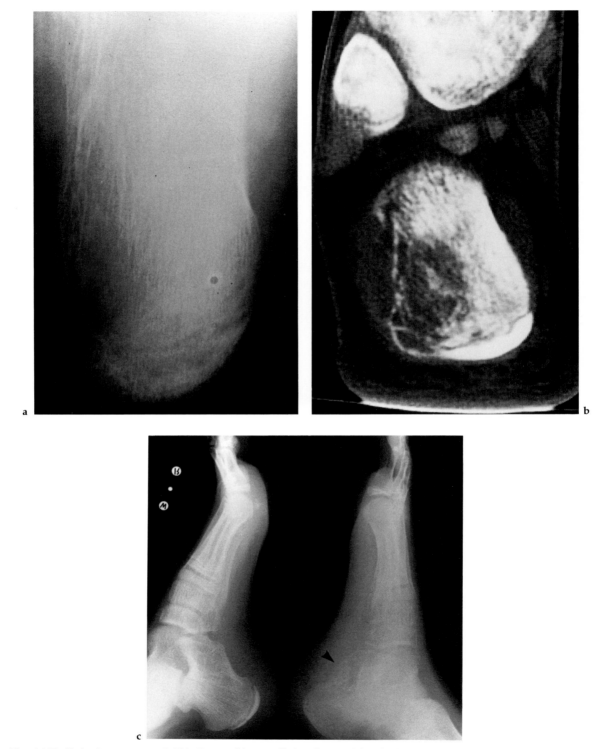

Fig. 4.149. Ewing's sarcoma. **a,b** This 7-year-old mentally handicapped boy had dysmorphic features and an unbalanced translocation of the long arm of chromosome 11. CT shows much better than the radiograph the extent of the lytic lesion as well as the adjacent soft tissue mass. **c** This 11-year-old boy injured his left ankle 3 months previously and was treated for lateral ligament injury. There is a lytic lesion in the left calcaneus (*arrow*) and osteoporosis of the left foot.

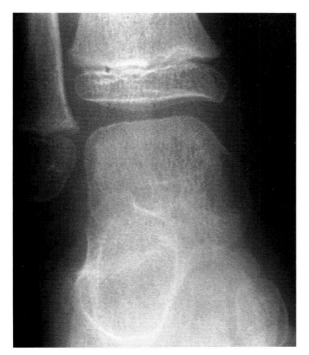

Fig. 4.150. Osteomyelitis (Brodie's abscess). This 4-year-old girl had a painful, swollen right ankle for several weeks. A radiolucent defect is seen at the medial aspect of talus. (From Kozlowski 1980, with permission.)

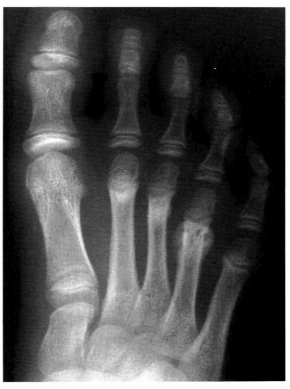

Fig. 4.151. Stress fractures. Metatarsal fractures were discovered accidentally during skeletal survey of this mentally handicapped 12-year-old boy.

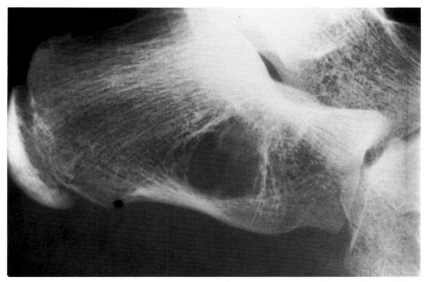

Fig. 4.152. Normal variant. Normal pseudocystic radiolucency due to a deficiency of spongy bone (11-year-old boy). (From Kozlowski 1980, with permission.)

LITERATURE
Foot Tumors

Capanna R, Van Horn JR, Ayala A et al. Osteoid osteoma and osteoblastoma of the talus. A report of 40 cases. Skeletal Radiol 1986;15:360–4

Glass TA, Mills SE, Fechner RE et al. Giant-cell reparative granuloma of the hands and feet. Radiology 1983;149: 65–8

Jongeward RH, Martel W, Louis DS et al. Case report 304. Skeletal Radiol 1985;13:169–73

Kozlowski K. Brodie's abscess in the first decade of life. Pediatr Radiol 1980;10:33–7

Kozlowski K, Middleton RWD. Aneurysmal bone cyst. Review of 10 cases. Aust Radiol 1980;24:170–5

Landon GC, Johnson KA, Dahlin DC. Subungual exostosis. J Bone Jt Surg 1979;61A:256–9

Mechlin MB, Kricun ME, Stead J, Schwamm HA. Giant cell tumor of tarsal bones. Report of three cases and review of

the literature. Skeletal Radiol 1984:11:266–70

Ochsner PE. Tumoren des kindlichen Fusses. Orthopäde 1986;15:227–32

Ohno T, Kadoya H, Park P et al. Case report 382. Skeletal Radiol 1986:15:478–3

Richter GM, Ernst HU, Dinkel E, Adler CP. Morphologie und Diagnostik von Knochentumoren des Fusses. Radiologe 1986;26:341–52

Sartoris DJ, Haghighi P, Resnick D. Painful swelling of the toe in a young boy. Invest Radiol 1987;22:170–4

Tang J, Gold RH, Mirra JM. Case report 454. Skeletal Radiol 1987;16:675–8

Van Horn JR, Lemmens JAM. Chondromyxoid fibroma of the foot. A report of a missed diagnosis. Acta Orthop Scand 1986;57:375–7

PRIMARY TUMORS IN INFANTS

Primary bone tumors in infants are very rare. Ewing's sarcoma is probably the most common malignant primary tumor in the first year of life. Radiologically it presents as a widespread, expansile, osteolytic lesion. The usual "onion peel" periosteal reaction was absent in two cases in the long bones seen by us (Fig. 4.153). In a case of Ewing's sarcoma of the the rib, the appearances were that of "vanishing bone". Osteosarcoma (Fig. 4.154) and chondrosarcoma have also been reported sporadically. They do not show any characteristic radiographic features.

Infantile fibrosarcoma/fibromatosis complex (Fig. 4.155) is diagnosed at birth or soon after. In newborns it is characterized by swelling of the limb. It is often difficult to decide if the lesion is a primary bone tumor or if bone involvement is secondary to a soft tissue tumor.

Of benign lesions are several which show characteristic clinical and/or radiographic appearances. These include diffuse hemangiomatosis (Fig. 4.156), congenital multiple fibromatosis (Fig. 4.157), hamartoma (mesen-

chymoma) of the chest wall (Fig. 4.158), osteochondroma (Fig. 4.159), enchondroma, simple bone cyst (Fig. 4.160) and progonoma (see Fig. 4.9). Other primary benign tumors have been reported; accurate radiographic diagnosis of these seems unlikely.

Large hemangiomas and their variants [diffuse hemangiomas (angiomatosis)] show often bone changes. The diagnosis of angiomatosis is a clinical one, the radiographic examination only confirming the diagnosis and showing the extent of bone involvement. The radiographic changes of bone angiomatosis in infancy and early childhood present as sunburst pattern, radiating pattern, periosteal thickening, cyst-like defects, and expansion and deformity of the affected bones (Fig. 4.156). Angiomatosis is one of the few congenital bone tumors for which biopsy is not only unnecessary but may be dangerous.

There are three angiodysplastic syndromes of clinical significance – the Kasabach–Merritt, Maffucci's and Klippel–Trenaunay syndromes. The Kasabach–Merritt syndrome is a complication of a pre-existing pathology. Intra-vascular thrombosis in any angiodysplasia with entrapment of clotting factor presents clinically as sudden growth of hemangiomata and systemic hemorrhagic symptoms. The Kasabach–Merritt syndrome is rare after the first year of life. The Klippel–Trenaunay syndrome is characterized by the classic triad of cutaneous hemangiomas, bone and soft tissue hypertrophy, and varicose veins. The latter may develop later in life. The diagnosis of Klippel–Trenaunay syndrome can be established only after venography is performed. Maffucci's syndrome is characterized by coexisting hemangiomas and enchondromas. Whereas the former are usually detected at or shortly after the birth, the latter appear later.

Congenital multiple fibromatosis is characterized by benign fibrous tumors which present clinically in two forms. In the multiple, diffuse form, predominantly the muscles and frequently the bones are affected. The lesions grow in the first few months of life but complete regression is then observed. In the generalized form, in which the visceral organs are affected, the prognosis is unfavorable, with most of the patients dying in infancy. The radiographic findings are the same in both forms: cystic lesions with smooth, well-demarcated margins located in the metaphyses of the long bones. The ribs, pelvis and spine are frequently involved (Fig. 4.157). The differential diagnosis includes histiocytosis X, the neonatal form of enchondromatosis and syphilis. If the clinical context is considered, there should be no diagnostic difficulties in recognition of congenital multiple fibromatosis with bone involvement.

Mesenchymal hamartoma of the chest wall is a destructive lesion presenting at birth or soon after as a chest mass which may cause cardiorespiratory symptoms. Radiographically the mass, which may contain calcification, is accompanied by spectacular rib deformities, erosions and periosteal reaction (Fig. 4.158). Radiographic recognition of the tumor is important as a hamartomatous malformation often spontaneuosly regresses. It is, however, often misdiagnosed histologically as osteochondroma, aneurysmal bone cyst or even malignant bone tumor. In one of our patients, the histologic diagnosis was chondroblastoma. Malignant, undifferentiated mesenchymal tumors have also been reported (Fig. 4.161).

The differential diagnosis of primary neonatal and infantile bone tumors comprises histiocytosis X, Caffey's disease, osteomyelitis and metastases.

In infancy histiocytosis X usually presents as Letterer–Siwe disease, with generalized symptoms including fever, cutaneous lesions, hepatosplenomegaly, lymphadenopathy, otitis media, pulmonary involvement, anemia, leukopenia, trombocytopenia and often multiple osteolytic lesions. We have never seen a monostotic histiocytosis X in infancy.

Caffey's disease is a polyostotic disease, the mandible and clavicles being most often affected. Monostotic involvement has been reported.

Osteomyelitis (Fig. 4.162) in the first year of life usually presents as a septic, multifocal process in a metaphyseal location and with articular involvement. The ESR and WBC are usually elevated. Chronic, subacute osteomyelitis in the form of Brodie's abscess may cause some confusion. A history of febrile illness, local swelling and elevated WBC are characteristic features of Brodie's abscess.

Metastatic disease – usually leukemia and neuroblastoma – is easily recognizable because the underlying disorder has already been diagnosed. Metastases are usually multifocal, symmetrical, osteolytic and often with periosteal reaction. Metastases from soft tissue tumors also rarely cause diagnostic difficulties (Fig. 4.163). Only in rare instances does the primary site remain unknown.

Osteofibrous dysplasia and fibrocartilaginous dysplasia are discussed earlier in this chapter (Midshaft Tibial Tumors) as is progonoma (Skull Tumors).

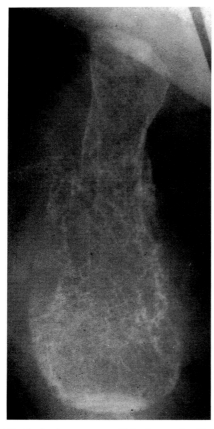

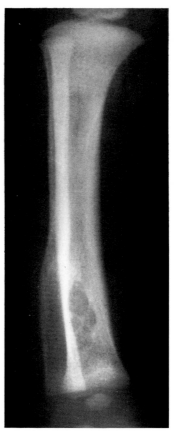

Fig. 4.153. Ewing's sarcoma. This 6-month-old girl had swelling of the right thigh for 2 weeks. There is expansion of the distal three-quarters of the right femur with peculiar honeycomb pattern. (From Kozlowski et al. 1985, with permission.)

Fig. 4.155. Fibrosarcoma or aggressive fibromatosis. This 4-month-old presented with swelling of the right leg. There is a lytic lesion in the distal tibia and deformity of the distal fibula. (From Kozlowski et al. 1976, with permission.)

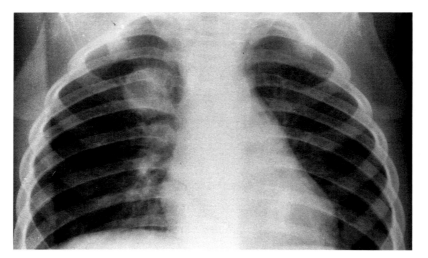

Fig. 4.154. Osteosarcoma. Routine chest radiography showed around opacity attached to the 4th rib of this 14-month-old boy. (From Kozlowski et al. 1985, with permission.)

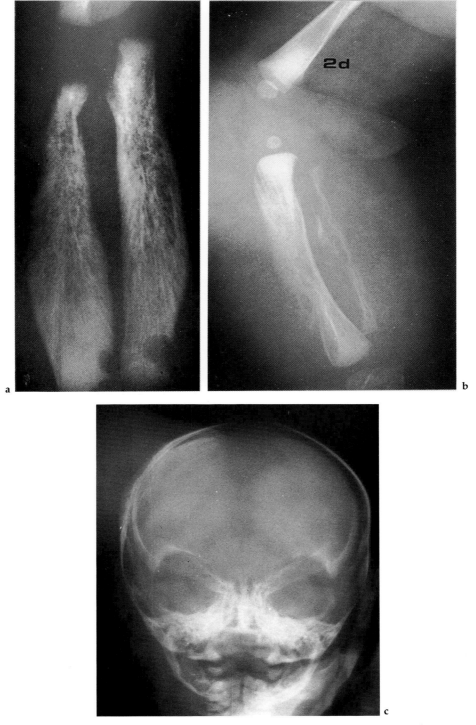

Fig. 4.156. Hemangiomatosis. **a** This newborn girl had a swollen right forearm. The typical "sunburst" radial pattern of intraosseous hemangioma is seen; there are cystic defects in the distal end of the forearm. **b** Cystic and radial pattern of intraosseous hemangioma are seen in this newborn girl who had a swollen leg. (From Kozlowski 1985, with permission.) **c** In this newborn boy there are destructive changes in the right parietal bone with some "sunburst" radial pattern; there is overlying soft tissue swelling. (From Kozlowski et al. 1970, with permission.)

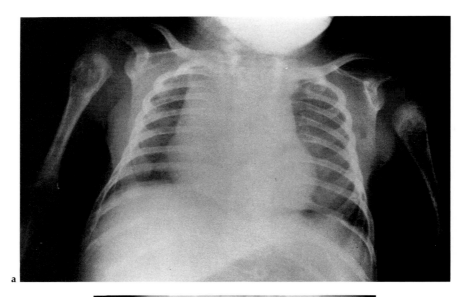

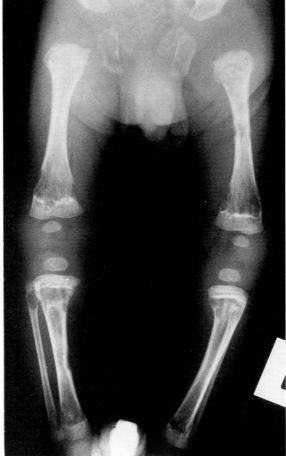

Fig. 4.157. Congenital multiple fibromatosis. Symmetrical ovoid defects in diametaphyses of the long bones of a neonate. Small lesions are present in the left scapula, midshaft of the right tibia and left femur.

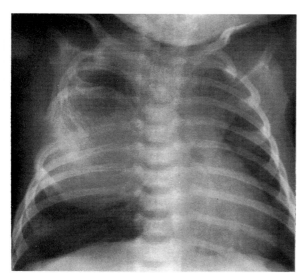

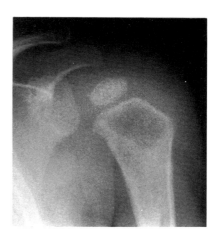

Fig. 4.160. Possible simple bone cyst in a 10-month-old boy with a painful shoulder.

Fig. 4.158. Benign mesenchymoma. This 3-year-old girl displayed restlessness, pallor, sweating and screaming for several hours' duration. There is a large, soft tissue mass in the right hemithorax, with destruction of the 2nd to 5th ribs. (From Kozlowski et al. 1985, with permission.)

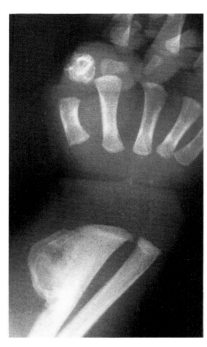

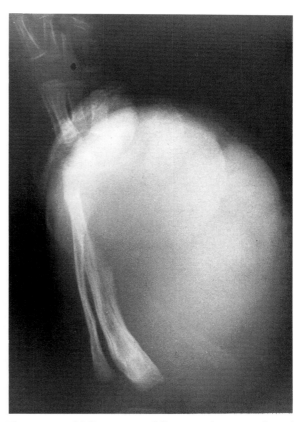

Fig. 4.159. Osteochondroma. Deformity of the arm of a 2-year-old boy, noted at birth. (From Dr M Braune, Kinderkrankenhaus, Kassel, Germany.)

Fig. 4.161. Malignant undifferentiated mesenchymal tumor. This 6-month-old boy had swelling of the left forearm since birth, which increased with age. (From Kozlowski et al. 1970, with permission.)

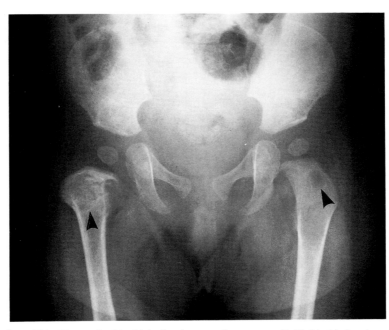

Fig. 4.162. Osteomyelitis. This 10-month-old girl had a fever and was unwell. Right-sided osteoarthritis and left-sided osteomyelitis (*arrows*).

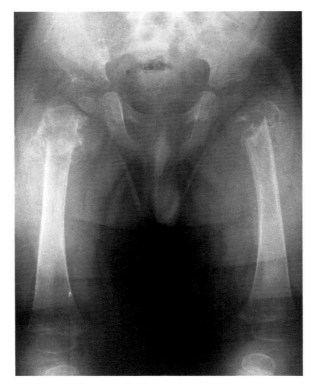

Fig. 4.163. Metastases from embryonal carcinoma. Operated on at the age of 7 months for a malignant tumor of the left testicle, this 12-month-old boy has a lytic lesion in the proximal femoral metaphyses. (From Kozlowski et al. 1970, with permission.)

LITERATURE
Primary Tumors in Infants

Baer JW, Radknowski MA. Congenital multiple fibromatosis. A case report with review of the world literature. AJR 1973;118:200–5

Bernard C, Ishihara K, Sirinelli D, Faure C. Les lésions fibreuses du squelette chez le nourrison et l'enfant. Ann Radiol 1987;30:307–22

Branue M. Personal communication.

Dahlin DC. Case report 189. Skeletal Radiol 1982;7:282–5

Ewerbeck V, Bolkenius M, Braun A, Brandeis WE. Knochentumoren und tumorähnliche Veränderungen im Neugeborenen- und Säuglingsalter. Z. Orthop 123:895–90

Faure C, Gruner M, Boccon-Gibod L. Case report 149. Skeletal Radiol 6:208–11

Ginsburg LD. Congenital aneurysmal bone cyst. Radiology 1974;110:175–6

Hall DP, Ellison RG. Osteosarcoma of the chest wall in a newborn infant: a case report six years after surgery. Am Surg 1964;30:745–7

Habermann ET. Stern RE. Osteoid-osteoma of the tibia in an eigth-month-old boy. A case report. J Bone Jt Surg 1974; 56-A:633–6

Hofmann P, Galanski M. Kongenitale Unterschenkelverbiegung bei Neurofibromatose von Recklinghausen. Fortschr Röntgenstr 1976;125:417–21

Holdsworth CM, Favara BE, Holton CP, Rainer WG. Malignant mesenchymoma in infants. Am J Dis Child 1974;128:847–50

Hopkins SM, Freitas EL. Bilateral osteochondroma of the ribs in an infant: an unusual cause of cyanosis. J Thorac Cardiovasc Surg 1965;49:247–9

Hütting G. Rittmeyer K. Multiple aneurismatische Knochenzysten bei 3 Monate altem Säugling. Fortschr Röntgenstr 1978;129:796–7

Kadell BM, Coulson WF, Desilets DT, Fonkalsrud EW. Congenital atypical benign chondroblastoma of a rib. J Pediatr Surg 1970;5:46–52

Kozlowski K, Bale P, Reye RDK. Difficultés du diagnostic radiographique des tumeurs primitives et secondaires de l'os chez l'enfant. Ann Radiol 1976;19:781–90

Kozlowski K, Beluffi G, Cohen DH et al. Primary bone tumours in infants. Short literature review and report of 10 cases. Pediatr Radiol 1985;15:359–67

Kozlowski K, Gorska M, Depowski M, Sikorska B. Tumeurs osséuses rares primitives ou secondaires de l'enfant. A propos de neuf observation. Ann Radiol 1970;13:219–28

Kubicz S. Olbrzymi naczyniak z maloplytkowoscia u dzieci. Pol Przegl Radiol Med Nukl 1978;42:23–7

Lauras B, Freycon F, Nivelon JL et al. Fibromatose congenital generalisee. A propos de trois observation. Pediatrie 1976;31:327–35

Leiber B, Riemann A. Klippel–Trenaunay syndrome. Pediatr Prax 1976;17:771–5

McLeod RA, Dahlin DC. Hamartoma (mesenchymoma) of the chest wall in infancy. Radiology 1979;131:657–61

Morettin LB, Mueller E, Schreiber M. Generalised hamartomatosis (congenital generalised fibromatosis). AJR 1972;114:722–34

Rolain G, Olive D, Marchal C et al. Etude radiologique d'angiomes multiples hépatiques et osséuse chez un nourrisson. J Radiol Electrol 1978;59:109–11

Safar J. Chondrosarcom steny hrudni u trimesiciniho kojence s dlouhodobym prezitim. Ceskoslov Pediatr 1964;19:422–4

Vinik M, Altman D. Congenital malignant tumors. Cancer 1966;19:967–79

Wickenhauser J. Das Maffucci–Kast Syndrome. Pediatr Prax 1974;14:677–83

Willich E, Daum R. Die aneurysmatische Knochenzyste der Rippen. Übersicht und Fallbericht. Z Kinderchir 1979; 28:22–8

Visscher DW, Alexander RW, Dempsey TR. Case report 472. Skeletal Radiol 1988;17:285–8

FIBROUS DYSPLASIA

Fibrous dysplasia is a fibro-osseous developmental abnormality of the skeletal system. Its frequency is about 2–3% of benign osseous tumors in combined child and adult series. It presents radiologically in monofocal, multifocal or more rarely in generalized forms.

The monofocal (monostotic) form is difficult to diagnose. It presents as an incidental finding or with symptoms such as pain, fracture or rarely localized deformity. In children the femur, tibia, fibula and facial bones are most often affected (Fig. 4.164, and see Fig. 4.109). On radiographs a lesion in the long bones presents as a well-defined radiolucent area with smooth borders due to thinning of the cortex. The appearances are that of a cystic lesion. Sometimes the appearance is multilocular as a result of endosteal erosion or scalloping. More characteristic is the ground glass appearance, the result of diffuse trabecular calcification. The differential diagnosis includes other monostotic, radiolucent lesions of bone.

The diagnosis of monofocal fibrous dysplasia can be accepted only after a positive biopsy.

In the multifocal (polyostotic) forms involvement tends to be unilateral (Fig. 4.165), whereas in the generalized form of fibrous dysplasia most of the skeletal system is affected (Fig. 4.166). The clinical course of multifocal (polyostotic) and generalized forms is more severe than that of the monostotic form. Café-au-lait spots are always present, local deformities are much more common (leg discrepancy) and extraskeletal symptoms are not unusual. These include endocrine abnormalities (McCune–Albright syndrome (Fig. 4.165b,c), hyperthyroidism, diabetes mellitus, hyperparathyroidism), soft tissue myxomas and coarctation of the aorta. Radiologically the changes are much more severe. Expansion and bowing of the shafts of the long bones, coxa vara, shephard's crook deformity of the femur, acetabular protrusions, facial bone deformities, sclerosis of the base of the skull are diagnostic radiographic features. Advanced bone age is often present in the generalized forms. Increased serum alkaline phosphatase levels are not uncommon in the more severe forms.

In general, patients with more extensive involvement may expect a more severe course, with ensuing serious complications. Facial bone and proximal femoral involvement presents especially difficult therapeutic problems. At puberty the course of the disease is usually slowed down, but regression of the existing lesions can rarely be expected. Malignant degeneration very rarely occurs in children; in most instances, it is subsequent to radiation therapy.

The differential diagnosis of the polyostotic fibrous dysplasia includes other benign polyostotic lesions, particularly multiple nonossifying fibroma (Fig. 4.167), enchondromatosis and neurofibromatosis, as well as other radiolucent, polyostotic lesions.

There are several lesions like or related to fibrous dysplasia. Some of them present characteristic radiographic appearances, others diagnostic microscopic appearances and some can be diagnosed by both radiology and histology.

Fibrocartilaginous dysplasia (fibrochondroplasia; Fig. 4.168) presents as cartilaginous overgrowth with secondary calcification in areas of authenticated fibrous dysplasia. It is a benign complication, occurring espec-

Table 4.24. Differential diagnosis of fibrous dysplasia

Monostotic		Polyostotic	
Common	Rare	Common	Rare
Simple bone cyst	Desmoid fibroma	McCune–Albright syndrome	Multifocal osteomyelitis
Nonossifying fibroma	Hyperparathyroidism	Neurofibromatosis	Polyostotic angiomatosis
Aneurysmal bone cyst		Eosinophilic granuloma	Enchondromatosis
Eosinophilic granuloma		Multiple nonossifying fibroma	Metastases
Osteomyelitis		Multiple cortical defects	Hyperparathyroidism
Post-traumatic repair			
Malignant bone tumor			

ially in the femoral neck. The chondroid features of the lesion may cause misdiagnosis of enchondromatosis (Ollier's disease) or chondrosarcoma.

Fibrocartilaginous mesenchymoma with low-grade malignancy, reported by Dahlin et al. (1984) resembles fibrocartilaginous dysplasia, but the fibrous elements resemble dermoid tumor or low-grade fibrosarcoma rather than fibrous dysplasia. Radiologically the lesion is expansile, with a thinned cortex on the endosteal surface with areas of cortical destruction, but with little or no periosteal formation. Mineralization has been present in the three of the five reported cases; recurrence occurred in three patients; there were no metastases.

Aggressive fibromatosis (desmoid fibroma of the soft tissues) is usually situated in the abdominal region. The most frequent juxtaosseous location is in the upper extremities. The appearances are those of soft tissue tumor which invades and destroys the bones. The intraosseous form corresponds to desmoid fibroma of bone. The tumor is well demonstrated on CT after contrast injection (Fig. 4.169) but the examination of choice is MR.

Juvenile hyaline fibromatosis is a rare disease characterized by skin lesions, gum hypertrophy, muscle weakness and flexion contracture of the large joints. Symmetrical medial defects at the proximal ends of the long bones (Fig. 4.170), particularly the tibia and humerus, and acro-osteolytic changes have been described.

Ill-defined and/or strange fibrous dysplasia-like lesions have been described in the cranial vault. Most patients are asymptomatic and present with an incidental finding of lumps on the head. The lesions may be radiolucent and cystic, with or without a dense border, or may resemble the "doughnut lesions" reported by Keats and Holt (1969). A case of "doughnut lesions" with osteoporosis and multiple fractures was reported by Colavita et al. (1984). Blood biochemistry may show increased alkaline phosphatase levels.

The histology of the lesions is often not easy to categorize, and they are reported as fibrous dysplasia, desmoid fibroma, fibromatosis or osteofibrous dysplasia.

Cherubism, a familial form of fibrous dysplasia, is limited to the jaws and has a good prognosis (see Fig. 4.21).

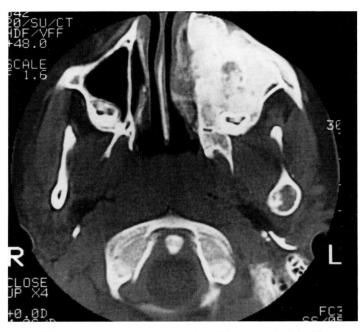

Fig. 4.164. Fibrous dysplasia. This girl presented with asymmetry of the face, which had been present for 1.5 years, and of the upper gum and left palate, present for 2 months. A large lesion in the left maxillary sinus concentrically expands the sinus, partly destroying the walls and invading the neighboring spaces.

a   b   c

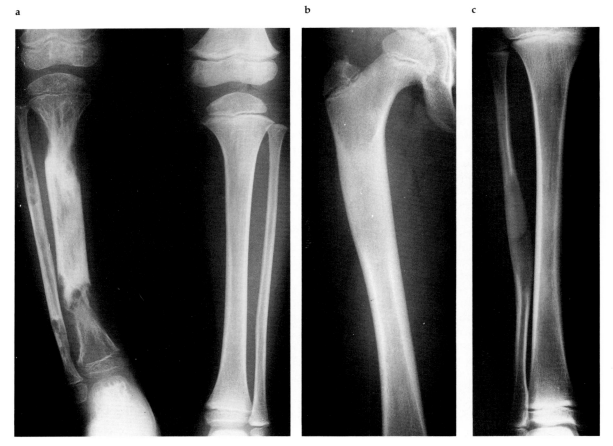

Fig. 4.165. Polyostotic fibrous dysplasia. **a** Extensive involvement of the right leg (4-year-old boy). **b,c** Large, localized slightly expanded areas of ground-glass appearance in the right femur and right fibula, and disappearing cortex (McCune–Albright syndrome) (7-year-old girl).

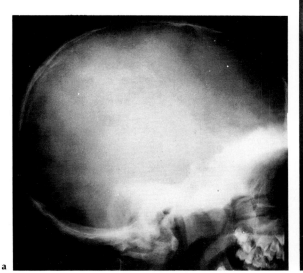

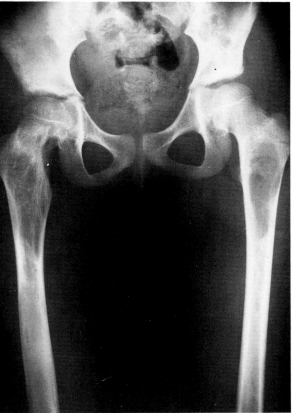

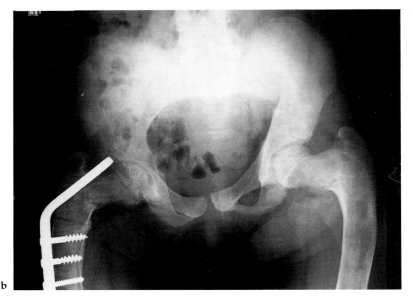

Fig. 4.166. Generalized fibrous dysplasia. **a** Prominent sclerosis at the base of the skull and in the temporoparietal region, and multiple cystic areas of rarefaction in the bones of the cranial vault (9-year-old girl). **b** Abnormal trabecular pattern in the pelvis and femora of the same patient, with irregular areas or rarefaction and bilateral shepherd's crook deformity with fractures. **c** Extensive involvement of the femora and pelvis of an 8-year-old girl, with radiolucent defects in the proximal femora, ground-glass appearance of the midshaft of the right femur, sclerosis of the midshaft of the left femur and sclerotic areas in the iliac bones.

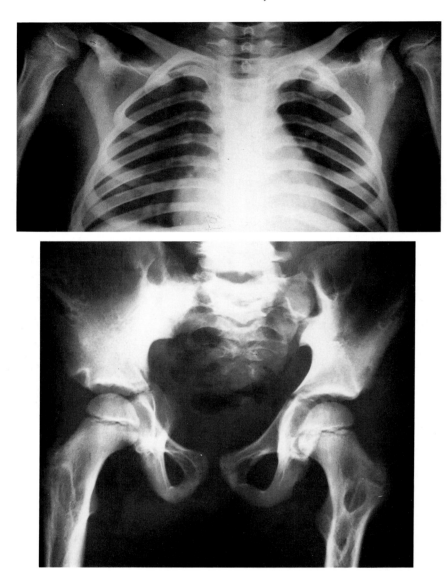

Fig. 4.167. Multiple nonosifying fibroma. This 10-year-old boy had leg pain after a fall. There are multiple radiolucent lesions, predominantly in the long bones. (*continued*)

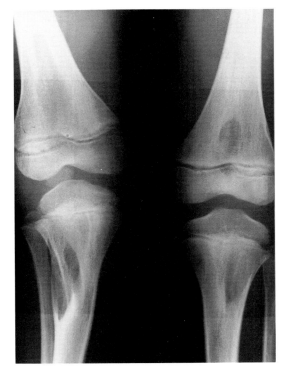

Fig. 4.167 (*continued*)

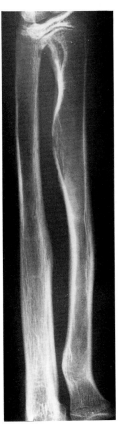

a

Fig. 4.169. Aggressive fibromatosis. This 14-year-old boy had pain in the right wrist for 6 months, with decreasing pronation and supination. Over the 4 weeks prior to radiography he had developed a soft tissue mass over the volar aspect of the right wrist. **a** Deformity of the distal radius by an extrinsic mass, and abnormal trabecular pattern in both the distal parts of the left forearm bones, particularly the radius. (*continued overleaf*)

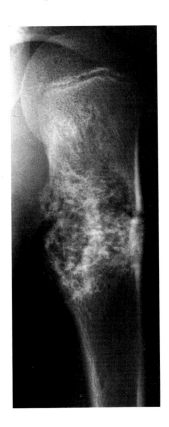

Fig. 4.168. Fibrocartilaginous dysplasia. This 11-year-old girl experienced pain in the left humerus after trauma. Multiple chondroid calcifications are present in a large lytic area with fracture.

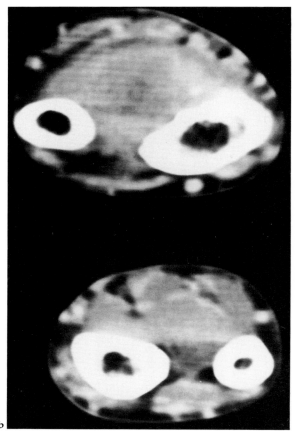

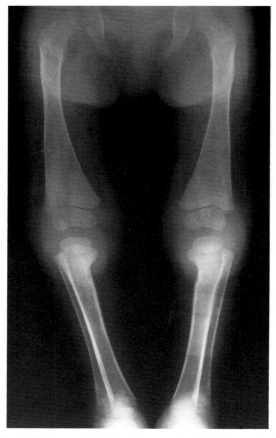

Fig. 4.169 (*continued*) Aggressive fibromatosis. **b** CT shows the volar soft tissue mass with radial extrinsic cortical erosions. Ulnar cortical erosions were also present in other CT sections.

Fig. 4.170. Juvenile hyaline fibromatosis. This 15-month-old girl had chronic arthropathy with contractures from birth, coarse facial features, large liver, anal condyloma, failure to thrive and developmental delay. Osteopenia, a thin cortex and symmetrical defects are seen at the proximal and medial tibial metaphyses, together with hypotubulation of the femora.

LITERATURE
Fibrous Dysplasia

Bernard C, Ishihara K, Sirinelli D, Faure C. Les lésions fibreuses du squelette chez le nourrisson et l'enfant. Ann Radiol 1987;30:307–22

Colavita N, Kozlowski K, La Vecchia G, Fileni A, Ricci R. Calvarial doughnut lesions with osteoporosis, multiple fractures, dentinogenesis imperfecta and tumorous changes in the jaws (report of a case). Aust Radiol 1984; 28:226–31

Daffner RH, Kirks DR, Gehweiler JA, Heaston DK. Computed tomography of fibrous dysplasia. AJR 1982;

139:943–8

Dahlin DC, Bertoni F, Beabout JW, Campanacci M. Fibro-cartilaginous mesenchymoma with low-grade malignancy. Skeletal Radiol 1984;12:263–9

Friedel B, Weickert H. Verlauf und Differentialdiagnostik des McCune-Albright-Syndroms. Fortschr Röntgenstr 1986;144:552–7

Giovannelli G, Bernasconi S, Banchini G. McCune–Albright syndrome in a male child: a clinical and endocrinologic enigma. J Pediatr 1978;92:220–6

Harris WH, Dudley HR, Barry RJ. The natural history of fibrous dysplasia. An orthopaedic, pathological and roentgenographic study. J Bone Jt Surg 1962;44-A:207–33

Keats TE, Holt JF. The calvarial "doughnut lesion". A previously undescribed entity. AJR 1969;105:314–18

Machida K, Makita K, Nishikawa J, Ohtake T, Iio M.

Scintigraphic manifestation of fibrous dysplasia. Clin Nuclear Med 1986;11:426–9

Malin JP, Wende S. Beitrag zur fibrösen Knochendysplasie. Fortschr Röntgenstr 1974;121:12–20

Mouterde P, Rigault P, Padovani JP, et al. Les problemes orthopediques de la dysplasie fibreuse des os chez l'enfant a propos de 23 observations. Chir Pediatr 1973; 19:169–78

Nixon GW, Condon VR. Epiphyseal involvement in polyostotic fibrous dysplasia. A report of two cases. Radiology 1972;106:167–70

Vanel D, Couanet D, Doppfer E, et al. Dysplasie fibreuse des os. In: Encyclopedie Medico-Chirurgicale. Paris, 1980

Warrick CK. Some aspects of polyostotic fibrous dysplasia. Possible hypothesis to account for the associated endocrinological changes. Clin Radiol 1973;24:125–38

NEUROFIBROMATOSIS

Neurofibromatosis is the most common phacomatosis and the one by which bones are most commonly affected. Mesodermal and endodermal derivatives are affected to a lesser degree.

Neurofibromatosis is the most common autosomal, dominant genetic disorder of bone, with a frequency about 1/3000 live births and a variable penetrance. Any part of the body can be affected, and great variability of clinical and radiographic manifestations is characteristic of the disease. Although some authors claim that there is a high percentage of new mutations (up to 50%), other believe, following detailed study of patients and their families, that new mutations are rarely accountable.

The proportion of neurofibromatosis patients who have bone changes increases with age, probably to 100% of adult patients if changes are carefully sought. A variable incidence of bone changes is cited in the literature: 28–88%. From the radiologist's point of view, this inexorably progressive disease should be suspected in any "strange looking" bone abnormality in any patient, regardless of the reason for presentation. Neurofibromatosis is a great imitator of other diseases. The explanation of the sometimes bizzare radiographic appearances is easy if the diagnosis of neuro-

fibromatosis is known or if there is a positive family history. Lesions of other systems, specifically of neuroectodermal origin are always present.

There are two established forms of neurofibromatosis and some variant forms. Neurofibromatosis 1 (von Recklinghausen's disease) is determined by a gene on chromosome 17 and neurofibromatosis 2 (central neurofibromatosis) by a gene on chromosome 22. The exact frequency of the latter is not known, but it is much the rarer of the two. It is characterized by acoustic neurofibroma and other tumors of the nervous system, nerve sheath and enveloping membranes (glioma, ependymoma, schwannoma, meningioma). Presenile lens opacities and subcapsular cataracts are common findings in neurofibromatosis 2, whereas café-au-lait spots and skin neurofibromas are less common.

Some individuals with neurofibromatosis also show manifestations of Noonan's syndrome (short stature, mid-facial hypoplasia, ptosis, short webbed neck, learning disabilities and weakness). The cause of this association is uncertain. The neurofibromatosis/Noonan's syndrome phenotype may be a single disorder or a chance occurrence of two causally separate syndromes. It has been also suggested

Table 4.25. Radiographic changes in neurofibromatosis

Mesodermal dysplastic changes	Erosions	Uncharacteristic lesions
1. Kyphoscoliosis (a) mild (b) severe (short, angular scoliosis, secondary to vertebral hypoplasia/dysplasia) 2. Other hypoplastic/dysplastic spinal changes: pedicular hypoplasia or agenesis, widening of the vertebral foramina, narrowing and elongation of the transverse processes, posterior vertebral scalloping, vertebral body dislocation 3. Cervical kyphosis (rare) 4. Lateral thoracic meningocoele (rare) 5. "Twisted ribbon" rib deformity, rib narrowing and elongation 6. Pseudoarthrosis (usually tibial, rarely in other long bones) 7. Subperiosteal defects (fibromas) 8. Subperiosteal hemorrhage (rare) 9. Intraosseous cysts (rare) 10. "Blank orbit" (defect in the posterosuperior wall of the orbit, deepening of the middle cranial fossa) (rare) 11. Cranial suture defects (left lambdoid suture most often affected) 12. Dysplasia of os temporale and facial bones 13. J-shaped pituitary fossa 14. Abnormalities of growth (hyperplasia or hypoplasia) – macrocrania 15. Modelling errors (over tubulation, undertubulation)	1. Optic canal – orbital bones 2. Spine – widening of the vertebral foramina, pedicle erosions, central and peripheral vertebral body erosions, widening of the spinal canal 3. Ribs 4. Other bones	1. Rickets, osteomalacia, osteopenia 2. Congenital abnormalities

that Noonan's syndrome predisposes to a variety of neurocristopathies, including neurofibromatosis, and that Noonan's syndrome-like phenotype is nonspecific and occurs as an occasional feature in many disorders including neurofibromatosis.

The skeletal changes in neurofibromatosis can be categorized as mesodermal dysplastic changes, secondary erosive changes, and uncharacteristic changes, often coincidental (Figs 4.171–4.173). Mesodermal dysplasia presents as hypoplastic/dysplastic changes in the skeleton. Any bone can be affected. The bone changes in neurofibromatosis 2 are erosive changes secondary to soft tissue tumors growth.

The most common and best known radiographic abnormalities in neurofibromatosis are presented in Table 4.25, along with secondary erosive changes and uncharacteristic changes.

Fig. 4.171. Neurofibromatosis. **a** Congenital pre-pseudoarthrotic kyphoscoliotic tibia and fibula (2-year-old boy). **b** Congenital pseudoarthrosis of the left tibia diagnosed after fracture occurred (7-year-old boy).

Fig. 4.172. Neurofibromatosis. This 10-year-old boy had a greenstick fracture of the right ulna at the age of 6 years; pseudoarthrosis was possibly present but was not diagnosed. **a** There has been "disappearance" of the distal ulna. **b** Widening of the thoracolumbar spinal canal and narrow pedicles in the same patient.

Fig. 4.171

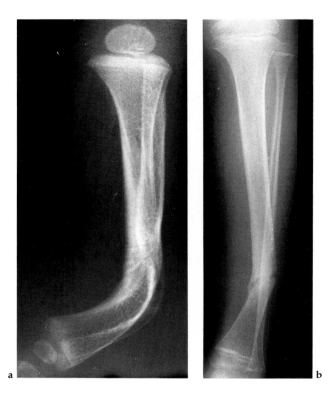

a   b

Fig. 4.172

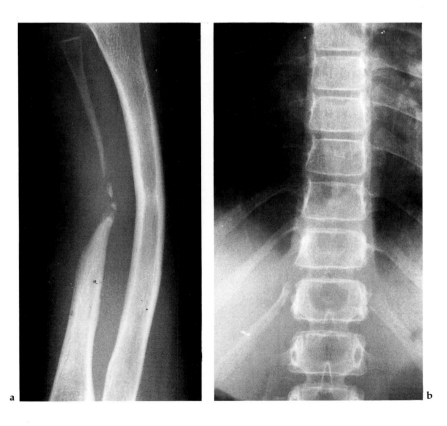

a   b

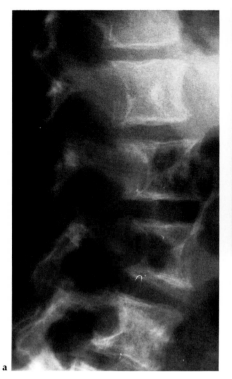

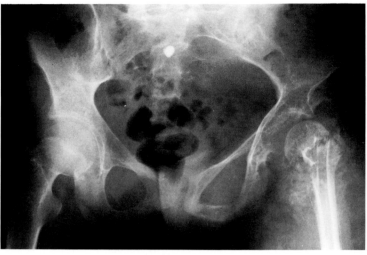

Fig. 4.173. Neurofibromatosis. This 14-year-old boy was correctly diagnosed at the age of 4 years. **a** Marked scalloping of the posterior portion of the bodies of the lumbar vertebrae. **b** Hypoplastic/dysplastic changes in the pelvis, and fracture of the left femoral neck with abundant callus formation.

LITERATURE
Neurofibromatosis

Bader JL. Neurofibromatosis and cancer: an overview. Dysmorphol Clin Genet 1987;1:43–8

Baltzell JW, Davis DO, Condon VR. Unusual manifestations of neurofibromatosis. Med Radiogr Photogr 1974;50:2–15

Casselman ES, Miller WT, Lin SR, Mandell GA. Von Recklinghausen's disease: incidence of roentgenographic findings with a clinical review of the literature. CRC Crit Rev Diagn Imaging 1977;4:387–419

Chaglassian JH, Rieseborough EJ, Hall JE. Neurofibromatosis scoliosis. Natural history and results of treatment in thirty seven cases. J Bone Jt Surg 1976; 58-A:695–702

Crawford AH. Neurofibromatosis in children. Acta Orthop Scand 1986;57 (suppl 218)

Diard F, Guibert F, Cadier L, Garel L. Manifestations radiologiques de la neurofibromatose chez l'enfant. Med Infant 1980;87:825–41

Ender A, Weickert H, Braun HSt, Franz U, Ender I. Sippenunter-suchungen bei der Neurofibromatose von Recklinghausen – Eine klinische Studie. Beitr Orthop Traumatol 1984;31:290–8

Ferris NJ, Siu KH. Neurofibromatosis 2: report of an affected kindred with a discussion of imaging strategy. Austr Radiol 1990;34:229–33

Galanski M, Cramer BM, Thun F, Peters PE, Vogelsang H. Radiologische Befunde bei der Neurofibromatose von Recklinghausen. Radiologe 1983;23:437–50

Holt JF. Neurofibromatosis in children. AJR 1977;130:615–39

Kameyama O, Ogawa R. Pseudoarthrosis of the radius associated with neurofibromatosis: report of a case and review of the literature. J Pediatr Orthop 1990;10:128–31

Klatte CE, Franken EA, Smith JA. The radiographic spectrum of Neurofibromatosis. Semin Roentgenol 1976;11:17–33

Mendez HMM. The neurofibromatosis–Noonan syndrome. Am J Med Genet 1985;21:471–6

Riccardi VM. Von Recklinghausen Neurofibromatosis. N Engl J Med 1981;305:1617–27

Zanella U, Mödder U, Benz-Bohm G, Thun F. Die Neurofibromatose im Kindesalter. CT Befunde im Schädel- und Halsbereich. Fortschr Röntgenstr 1984;141:498–504

METASTATIC BONE DISEASE

Metastases as the first manifestation of a primary bone tumor are much rarer in children than in adults and the primary site of the tumor is usually already known. If the primary site has not yet been recognized, this is the result of unsufficient clinical history, superficial clinical examination or failure to perform appropriate radiographic or biochemical examinations.

Bone involvement may follow the direct encroachment of the tumor on the bone, as often happens in patients with ganglioneuroma and allied tumors. More often it is the result of hematogenous or lymphatic spread. Bone marrow, the bone itself or both can be affected. The changes may be microscopic or macroscopic. The latter will be usually detected on nuclear scan, MR or radiography. Wide variations in incidence of metastatic disease in different reports are probably due partly to different criteria of detection and analysis.

As the most common metastases in children are those of small cell round tumors, specifically leukemia (Fig. 4.174) and neuroblastoma (Fig. 4.175), the radiographic appearances are predominantly those of osteolytic lesions – "moth-eaten" or permeative appearances with periosteal reaction. The bone changes in leukemia are reported to occur between 20% and 100% of cases and are characterized by osteoporosis, radiolucent bands, osteolytic lesions, periostitis and, rarely, osteosclerosis. Unusual features are severe periosteal thickening involving all the long bones as the only major sign and localized vertical radiolucent lines (Fig. 4.174).

Early neuroblastoma metastases may be similar to those of leukemia, with a tendency for greater cortical destruction in the former. Later, an "onion-skin" periosteal reaction, spiculae and osteosclerotic metastases make the diagnosis of neuroblastoma more likely.

Single bone lesions may occur in leukemia and occasionally in neuroblastoma. We have seen children in whom it was the first positive finding. A local bone or articular pain, lasting sometimes for weeks was the only complaint (Fig. 4.176). However, when skeletal survey was performed the changes, although discrete, were usually polyostotic.

Metastatic lesions as the first manifestation of neoplastic disease are very rare in other tumors, such as Wilms' tumor, rhabdomyosarcoma (Fig. 4.177) and retinoblastoma. Bone metastasis from primary renal tumor in children is probably different from classic Wilms' tumor. In some cases of lymphoma, it can be very difficult to decide whether the bone lesion is primary or metastatic (Fig. 4.178, and see Fig. 4.74). Usually, metastases are osteolytic with a sclerotic border, but they may be mixed and even, though rarely, osteosclerotic. Osteosclerotic lesions are characteristic in medulloblastoma.

Single cases of metastases have been reported for glioblastoma, fibrosarcoma, synovial sarcoma and lung carcinoma in children.

The methods of choice for detecting bone metastases are bone biopsy, MR, nuclear scan and skeletal survey. Although MR is the most sensitive method for detecting bone marrow changes it is also the most expensive and time-

Table 4.26. Metastases

Common (Usually multiple)	Rare (Single or multiple)	Differential diagnosis	
		Single	Multiple
Leukemia	Soft tissue tumors	Primary benign bone tumor	Histiocytosis X
Neuroblastoma	All other primary bone tumors	Primary malignant bone tumor	Multifocal osteomyelitis
Lymphoma		Histiocytosis X	Polyostotic fibrous dysplasia
Ewing's sarcoma		Normal anatomic variant	Multiple osteosarcoma
Osteosarcoma		Trauma	Multiple nonossifying fibroma
		Osteomyelitis	Polyostotic angiomatosis
			Enchondromatosis
			Hyperparathyroidism

consuming method, and is more limited in its availability. The nuclear scan is much easier to perform and much more accessible. Therefore, in children with small cell tumor metastases, nuclear scan or MR should be performed, followed, if clinically indicated, by marrow biopsy. Plain radiography is useful for complete evaluation of the involved bone. This unified approach – nuclear scan and skeletal survey – is often most desirable as it reflects physiologic and morphologic alterations and decreases false-positive and false-negative nuclear scan and radiographic readings.

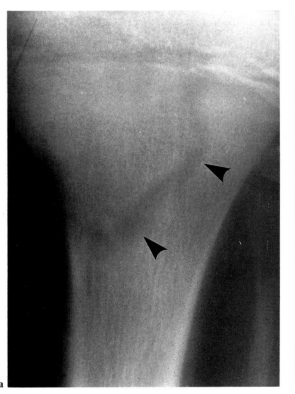

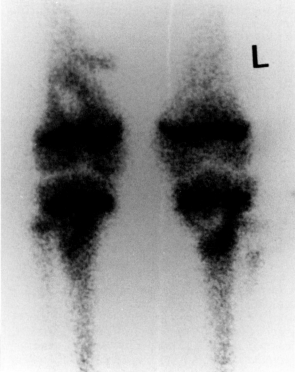

a

b

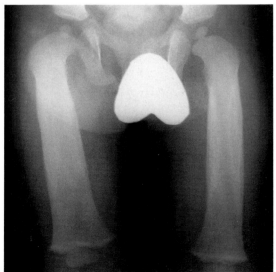

c

Fig. 4.174. Leukemia. **a** Oblique radiolucent line and subperiosteal destruction at the medial aspect of the proximal shaft of the left tibia (9-year-old girl). **b** Nuclear scan in the same patient demonstrates the oblique and vertical lines of increased uptake. **c** Abundant, symmetrical new bone formation, and ill-defined changes at the end of the shafts (18-month-old boy). (From Kozlowski et al. 1987, with permission.)

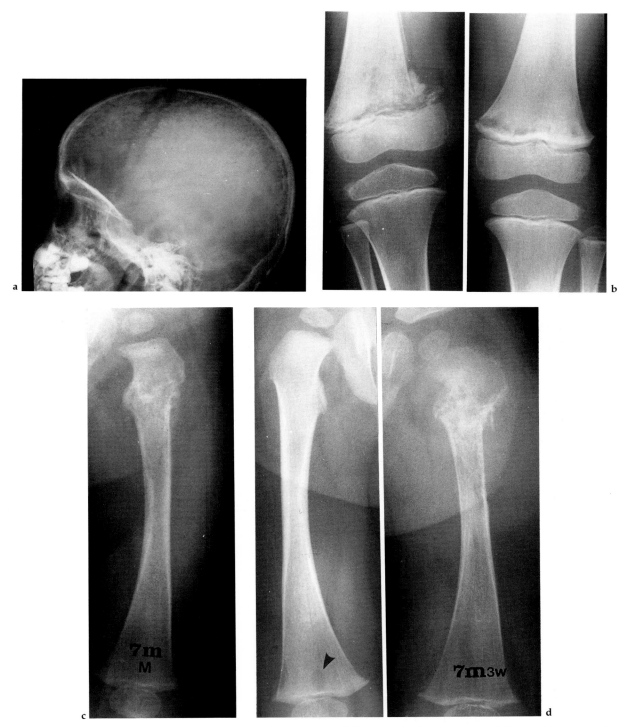

Fig. 4.175. Disseminated neuroblastoma. **a** Multiple, irregular radiolucencies in the outer part of the cranial vault, and widened coronal suture (4.5-year-old girl). **b** Irregular metaphyseal defects in the distal femoral metaphyses, with trans-metaphyseal fracture and epiphyseal dislocation on the right, and osteopenia of the right tibia and fibula (4.5-year-old boy). **c** Destructive changes in the proximal part of the left femur diagnosed as osteomyelitis (7-month-old boy). **d** In the same patient there is marked progress of the destructive process 3 weeks later, and metastases are seen in the distal right femoral metaphysis (*arrow*).

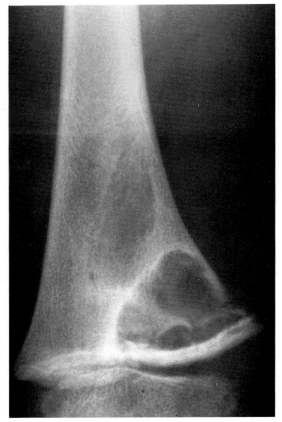

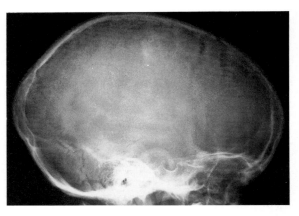

Fig. 4.177. Disseminated rhabdomyosarcoma. Multiple, irregular radiolucencies in the outer part of the cranial vault, and an area of irregular sclerosis in the anterior part of the parietal region (5-year-old boy).

Fig. 4.176. Neuroblastoma. Metastasis in a 4.5-year-old boy who had limp and mid-lumbar pain for 3 weeks. A large osteolytic defect is seen in the distal part of the right femur.

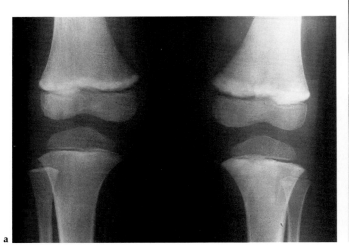

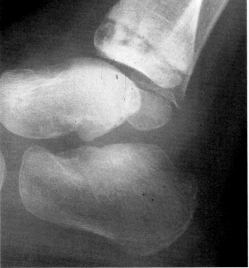

Fig. 4.178. Disseminated lymphoma. The variable radiographic appearances of lymphoma are well demonstrated in these two patients, **a,b** Predominantly osteosclerotic form in a 6-year-old boy. Some lytic lesions are also present. (*continued*)

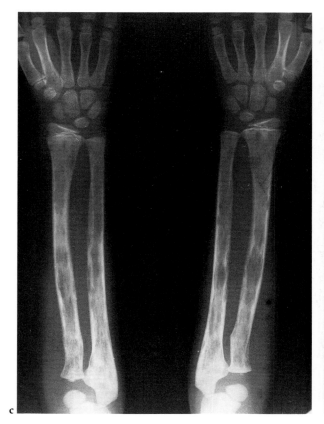
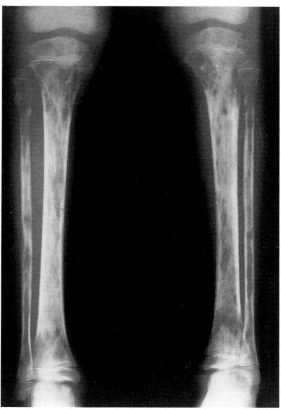

c

d

Fig. 4.178 (*continued*) **c,d** Predominantly lytic form in a 7-year-old boy. (From Kozlowski et al. 1976, with permission.)

LITERATURE
Metastatic Bone Disease

Beluffi G, Kozlowski K, Arico M. Simultaneous (synchronous) occurrence of Ewing sarcoma. Pediatr Radiol 1991;21:452–4

Greinacher I, Neidhardt M. Generalised osteosclerotic metastases secondary to operated medulloblastoma of the cerebellum. Ann Radiol 1968;11:470–4

Herman G, Feldman F, Abdelwahab IF, Klein MJ. Skeletal manifestations of granulocytic sarcoma (chloroma). Skeletal Radiol 1991;20:509–12

Hope JW, Borns PF Borns. Radiologic diagnosis of primary and metastatic cancer in infants and children. Radiol Clin N Am 1965;3:353–74

Kozlowski K, Bale P, Reye Dk. Difficultés du diagnostic radiographique des tumeurs primitives et secondaires de l'os chez l'enfant. Ann Radiol 1976;19:781

Kozlowski K, Campbell JB, Leonidas JC, Stevens M. Unusual radiographic bone abnormalities in leukaemia. Report of three cases. J Belge Radiol 1987;70:229–33

Kremens B, Roessner A, Decking D. Solitäre Knochenläsion als radiologische Erstmanifestation einer akuten lymphatischen Leukämie. Pediatr Prax 1982;26:67–72

Lamego CMB, Zerbini MCN. Bone-metastasizing primary renal tumours in children. Radiology 1983;147:449–54

Leeson MC, Makley JT, Carter JR. Metastatic skeletal disease in the pediatric population. J Pediatr Orthop 1985;5:261–7

Ogden J, Ogden D. Skeletal metastasis: the effect on the immature skeleton. Skeletal Radiol 1982;9:73–82

Olson PN, Prewitt L, Griffiths HJ, Cherkna B. Case report 703. Skeletal Radiol 1991;20:624–7

McLean RG, Murray PC. Case report 292. Skeletal Radiol 1984;12:288–93

Simmons M, Tucker AK. The radiology of bone changes in rhabdomyosarcoma. Clin Radiol 1978;29:47–52

Slavc I, Urban Ch, Kaulfersch W, Mutz I. Wirbelkörperveränderungen als Initialsymptom einer Leukämie. Pediatr Pädolog 1987;22:59–65

Willich E, Appell RG, Brandeis WE. Skelettmanifestationen von malignen, nichtossären Tumoren im Kindesalter. Radiologe 1985;25:166–76

SECONDARY MALIGNANT NEOPLASMS

The definition of secondary tumor is that it has a different histologic diagnosis from the first one. It has been known for a long time that both benign and malignant secondary neoplasms can occur in patients who have been treated successfully for a primary tumor. As the number of survivors of primary neoplasms increases, so does the incidence of malignancy later in life. A child cured of a malignant tumour has about a 10% chance of developing a second malignant neoplasm in the next 20 years. The development of secondary tumor is favoured by radiotherapy, genetic susceptibility and chemotherapy.

An international study by Meadows et al. (1977) of 102 children with secondary malignant tumors revealed that sarcoma of bone (osteosarcoma, chondrosarcoma, fibrosarcoma) was the most common secondary malignant neoplasm in irradiated tissues in children with no known disposition for cancer (13/54 cases). The interval between radiation therapy and development of the secondary neoplasm ranged between 5 months and 24 years. In a similar study by Gutjahr of 100 children with secondary malignant neoplasms, most of whom had had radiotherapy, osteosarcoma (18/100 cases) and leukemia (18/100 cases) were the most common malignant secondaries. The interval between the primary and secondary tumor, in cases of osteosarcoma, was between 1.0 and 14.5 years.

The genetic disorders retinoblastoma, neurofibromatosis, nevoid basal cell carcinoma syndrome and xeroderma pigmentosum are known to be associated with multiple neoplasia. In the study by Meadows et al. (1977, 1980) of

27 children with one of these diseases, bone sarcoma was the most frequent tumor in the 17 children with retinoblastoma; the most common location was the long bones, distant from the sites of radiotherapy. The other 10 children with genetic disorders did not show this high association with bone sarcoma. The only members of "families at risk" – siblings of patients with cancer – who showed increased incidence of bone sarcoma were those from families with a history of retinoblastoma. It is presumed that members of predisposed families are already carriers of a mutant gene in some somatic cells. The possibility of a second tumor occurring increases if radiotherapy is applied.

The carcinogenic effect of chemotherapy in the development of secondary, localized solid tumors is more difficult to determine. Carcinogenic effects of some antitumorous drugs have been shown in animals. An elevated incidence of malignant tumors is proved in immunodeficient patients (ataxia-telangiectasia, Wiskott–Aldrich syndrome, Rothmund–Thomson syndrome). Chromosomal abnormalities have been demonstrated in patients treated for Hodgkin's disease and leukemia.

The risk of malignant degeneration in pure bone dysplasias is negligible. There is a high probability of malignancy in disorders which are both bone dysplasias and benign multifocal tumors – exchondromatosis, enchondromatosis, including Maffucci's syndrome, and fibrous dysplasia. However, it occurs only very rarely in childhood.

The possibility of inducing osteosarcoma or other malignant bone tumors by radiation can never be excluded, but the oncogenic effect of modern radiotherapy is so low that this is not a contraindication for its use in patients with life-threatening malignant neoplastic conditions.

The risk is even smaller with chemotherapy. Leukemia, non-Hodgkin's lymphoma and soft tissue tumors are the most common secondary neoplasms.

LITERATURE
Secondary Malignant Neoplasms

Constine LS. Late effects of radiation therapy. Pediatrician 1991;18:37–48

Forte V, Shimotakahara S, Crysdale WS, Thorner P. Recurring giant-cell granuloma at the site of previous radiation therapy. J Otolaryngol 1990;19:285–7

Freeman C, Gledhill R, Chevalier LM, Whitehead VM, Esseltine DL. Osteogenic sarcoma following treatment with megavoltage radiation and chemotherapy for bone tumours in children. Med Pediatr Oncol 1980;8:375–82

Gutjahr P. EEG Befunde bei ALL Patienten 10 Jahre nach Bestrahlungund Cytostatikatherapie. Klin Ped 1990;202:153–6

Li FP. Second malignant tumours after cancer in childhood. Cancer 1977;40:1899–902

Meadows AT, D'Angio GJ, Mike V, et al. Patterns of second malignant neoplasms in children. Cancer 1977;40:1903–11

Meadows AT, Strong LC, Li FP, et al. Bone sarcoma as a second malignant neoplasm in children: influence of radiation and genetic predisposition. Cancer 1980;46:2603–6

Mike V, Meadows AT, D'Angio GJ. Incidence of second malignant neoplasms in children: results of an international study. Lancet 1982;2:1326–31

Mulvihill JJ, McKeen EA. Discussion: genetics of multiple primary tumors. A clinical etiologic approach illustrated by three patients. Cancer 1977;40:1867–71

Oberlin O, Bernard A, Flamant O, et al. Les secondes tumeurs malignes de l'enfant. Etude de 38 cas. Arch Fr Pediatr 1984;41:241–8

Penn I. Second malignant neoplasms associated with immunosupressive medications. Cancer 1976;37:1024–32

Pons A, Arlet J, Alibellis MJ. La dégénerescence maligne de la dysplasie fibreuse des os. Revue générale à propos de deux observations. Ann Radiol 1974;17:713–20

Smith J. Postradiation sarcoma of bone in Hodgkin's disease. Skeletal Radiol 1987;16:524–32

Toorkey BC, Unni KK, Dahlin DC. Case report 714. Skeletal Radiol 1992;21:121–3

Tountas AA, Fornasier VL, Hardwood AR, Leung PMK. Postirradiation sarcoma of bone. A perspective. Cancer 1979;43:182–7

Tsuruta T, Ogihara Y. Malignant tumours arising in patients with congenital bone disease. Investigation by a questionnaire. Jap J Hum Genet 1984;29:31–7

Vanel D, Coffre C, Zemoura L, Oberlin O. Chondrosarcoma in children subsequent to other malignant tumours in different localtions. Skeletal Radiol 1984;11:96–101

Vanel D, Hagay C, Rebibo G, Oberlin O, Masselot J. Study of three radio-induced malignant fibrohistiocytomas of bone. Skeletal Radiol 1983;9:174–8

RICKETS SECONDARY TO NEOPLASIA

Hypophosphatemic rickets secondary to neoplasia is a rare but well-recognized entity. The disease is characterized clinically by fatigue, muscular weakness and bone pain. Biochemical investigations show hypophosphatemia, hyperphosphaturia, normocalcemia and often aminoaciduria, most frequently glycinuria and glycosuria. Serum levels of 25-hydroxycholecalciferol are normal, those of 1,25-dihydroxycholecalciferol are low.

The radiographic examination shows in younger patients signs of active rickets; after the closure of the epiphseal plates there is evidence of osteomalacia (osteopenia, stress fractures).

Most patients are young and middle-aged adults. About a dozen cases have been reported in children. The tumors are usually localized in the bones, but soft tissue location is not unusual. Different tumor types are responsible for rickets/osteomalacia. Their common feature is mesenchymal derivation.

The most common tumor responsible for rickets in children is nonossifying fibroma.

After tumor removal there is dramatic regression of the clinical symptoms and biochemical changes. It takes several weeks for radiographic abnormalities to return to normal.

LITERATURE
Rickets Secondary to Neoplasia

Aschinberg LC, Solomon LM, Zeis PM, Justice P, Rosenthal IM. Vitamin D-resistant rickets associated with epidermal nevus syndrome: demonstration of a phosphaturic substance in the dermal lesions. J Pediatr 1977;91:56–60

Asnes RS, Berdon WE, Bassett CA. Hypophosphatemic rickets in an adolescent cured by excision of a nonossifying fibroma. Clinical Pediatr 1981;20:646–8

Carey DE, Drezner MK, Hamdan JA, et al. Hypophosphatemic rickets/osteomalacia in linear sebaceous nevus syndrome: a variant of tumour-induced osteomalacia. J Pediatr 1986;109:994–1000

Cotton GE, Van Puffelen P. Hypophosphatemic osteomalacia secondary to neoplasia. J Bone Jt Surg 1986;68-A:129–33

Parker MS, Klein I, Haussler MR, Mintz DH. Tumor-induced osteomalacia. Evidence of a surgically correctable alteration in vitamin D metabolism. JAMA 1981;245:492–4

Pollack JA, Schiller AL, Crawford JD. Rickets and myopathy cured by removal of a nonossifying fibroma of bone. Pediatrics 1973;52:364–71

Prader A, Illig R, Uehlinger E, Stalder G. Rachitis infolge Knochentumors. Helv Paediatr Acta 1960;5/6:554–79

Renton P, Shaw DG. Hypophosphatemic osteomalacia secondary to vascular tumors of bone and soft tissue. Skeletal Radiol 1976;1:21–4

Willhoite DR. Acquired rickets and solitary bone tumor: the question of a causal relationship. Clin Orthop 1975;109:210–11

Yoshikawa S, Nakamura T, Takagi M, et al. Benign osteoblastoma as a cause of osteomalacia. Report of two cases. J Bone Jt Surg 1977;59B:279–86

PERIOSTITIS

The periosteum is a dense membrane of connective tissue that covers all but the articular surfaces of bones. It is composed of two layers. The thicker, more active inner layer contains osteoblasts in developing bones and also in adults with pathologic conditions. Collagenous fibres extend from the deeper layer into the bone (Sharpey's fibers). In children the periosteum is bound more loosely to the underlying cortex than it is in adults and is more prone to separation and subperiosteal hemorrhage. As the result of these anatomic differences, periosteal reactions are more common and play a more important role in the bone pathology of children than in that of adults.

Periosteal thickening is one of the most important radiographic signs of inflammatory bone disease in children. It is also present, often as the most significant sign, in scores of other conditions. The differential diagnosis of periosteal reactions in children has been thoroughly reviewed by Kaufmann (1962).

Before diagnosing a periosteal reaction, pseudoperiostitis should be excluded (Table 4.27). Pseudoperiostitis encompasses the following:

1. Physiological thickening of periosteum secondary to increased osteoblastic activity without underlying disease as an expression of exuberant growth; this is a common finding in the long bones of normal newborns between 2 and 3 months of age and in prematures.

2. Increased osteoclastic activity of the inner layer of the periosteum, presenting as a radiolucent line parallel to the diaphysis and simulateing periostitis; this is observed after rapid bone demineralization secondary to immobilization, severe debilitating disease and use of corticosteroids.

3. Faulty projection, specifically of the legs and forearms, in which adjacent bones are covering each other (ulna and radius, tibia and fibula).

4. Misinterpretion of normal anatomical features, e.g. linea poplitea tibiae.

5. Wiberg's sign: periosteal thickening at the medial aspect of the femoral neck as a resut of mechanical malfunction of the hip joint (subluxation, epiphyseolysis).

The character and distribution of the periosteal thickening may have some features that give clues to the etiology and diagnosis. Three types of periosteal reaction are generally recognized: solid, onion-skin and sunburst. Soft tissue abnormalities, the character of subperiosteal calcifications and, especially, associated bone abnormalities give further important diagnostic information. However, a firm conclusion cannot be made until the clinical findings and history are correlated with the radiographic abnormalities. This three-step approach, radiographic findings + history + clinical

findings, is of primary importance in analyzing periosteal thickening in children. Further imaging – nuclear scan, ultrasound, CT and

Table 4.27. Features of pseudoperiostitis

Increased osteoblastic activity (prematures, newborns)
Rapid bone demineralization (immobilization, debilitating disease, corticosteroids)
Faulty projection
Misinterpretation of normal anatomical features
Wiberg's sign

Table 4.28. Differential diagnosis of periosteal thickening in childhood

Inflammatory periostitis
Pyogenic infections
Syphilis
Tuberculosis
BCG
Mycobacteriae
Sarcoidosis
Mycoses
Juvenile rheumatoid arthritis and other rheumatoid diseases

Tumors and tumorous conditions
Ewing's sarcoma, osteosarcoma, lymphoma, neuroblastoma and other malignant primary or secondary tumors
Leukemia
Histiocytosis X
Hemangioma of soft tissue and bone, osteoid osteoma and other benign primary tumors

Traumatic periostitis
Prolonged, complicated delivery
Ordinary handling of premature and newborn babies
Abused child
Direct trauma
Stress fracture

Bone disease
Caffey's disease
Osteogenesis imperfecta
Neurofibromatosis
Engelmann's disease
Familial idiopathic osteoarthropathy
Osteopoikilosis with hyperostosis
Melorheostosis

Hypo- and hypervitaminosis
Hypovitaminosis D
Hypervitaminosis D
Vitamin C deficiency
Hypervitaminosis A

Endocrine and metabolic disorders
Hypoparathyroidism
Pseudohypoparathyroidism
Hyperparathyroidism
Thyroid acropathy
Pancreatitis
Menkes' syndrome
I-cell disease
Prostaglandin therapy

Neurogenic disorders
Meningocele
Congenital insensitivity to pain (congenital analgesia)

Others
Skin disease (ichthyosis, urticaria, pyodermia, progressive scleroderma, pachydermoperiostosis)
Soft tissue tumors
Vascular insufficiency
Foreign bodies
Cardiopulmonary hypertrophic osteoarthropathy
Thermal injuries

MR – may be useful in some instances. The list of differential diagnosis of the most common periosteal thickenings in children is presented in Table 4.28.

Periosteal thickening can appear in many different diseases, such as Paget's disease, acromegaly, tuberous sclerosis, Gardner's syndrome, fluorosis, mother-of-pearl disease, and leprosy. However, most of these entities are adult disorders, usually with a clear-cut clinical picture. If present in childhood, some of these diseases rarely cause periosteal thickening. (e.g. tuberous sclerosis). Some, such as fluorosis, are limited to certain geographical areas. Most are rarely seen by medical practitioners caring for children.

LITERATURE
Periostitis

Ameri MR, Alebouyeh M, Donner WM. Hypertrophic osteoarthropathy in childhood malignancy. AJR 1978; 130:992–3

Appel W, Schulz RD, Barth V, Wissmann C. Radiologische Befunde des Periostes bei enzündlichen Knochenerkrankungen. Radiologe 1979;19:317–20

Baert AL, Casteels-Van Daele M, Broeckx J, et al. Generalised juvenile polyposis with pulmonary arteriovenous malformations and hypertrophic osteoarthropathy. AJR 1983;141;661–2

Beluffi G, Marseglia GL, Monafo V, et al. Pulmonary hypertrophic osteoarthropathy in a child with late-onset agammaglobulinemia. Eur J Pediatr 1982;139:199–201

Bloom RA, Libson E, Husband JE, Stocker DJ. The periosteal sunburst reaction to bone metastases. A literature review and report of 20 additional cases. Skeletal Radiol 1987; 16:629–34

Bretagne MC, Mouton JN, Pierson M, et al. A propos de periostite ou plutot d'appositions periostées en pediatrie. J Radiol Electrol 1977;58:119–23

Brower AC, Moser RP, Kransdorf MJ. The frequency and diagnostic significance of periostitis in chondroblastoma. AJR 1990;154:309–14

Cavanaugh JJA, Holman GH. Hypertrophic osteoarthropathy in childhood. J Pediatr 1965;66:27–40

Forrester DM, Kirkpatrick J. Periostitis and pseudoperiostitis. Radiology 1976;118:597–601

Glaser K. Double contous, cupping and spurring in roentgenograms of long bones in infants. AJR 1949; 61:482–92

Heuck F. Zum Thema "Periostreactionen". Radiologe 1979;19:289–90

Heuck F. Periostale Reaktionen bei Knochentumoren. Radiologe 1979;19:329–40

Hooper G, McMaster MJ. Neurofibromatosis with tibial cyst caused by recurrent hemorrhage. J Bone Jt Surg 1979; 61-B:247–75

Kaufmann HJ. Differentialdiagnose periostaler Reactionen im Säuglings- und Kleinkindesalter. Radiol Clin 1962; 31:337–56

Kay CJ, Rosenberg MA, Burd R. Hypertrophic osteoarthropathy and childhood Hodgkin's disease. Radiology 1974;112:177–8

Kleinman MB, Elfenbein DS, Wolf EL, Hemphill M, Kurlinski JP. Periosteal reaction due to foreign body – induced inflammation of soft tissue. Pediatrics 1977; 60:638–41

Kozlowski K, Posen S. Idiopathic hypertrophic osteoarthropathy (Report of a further case with brief literature review). Austr Radiol 1983;27:291–4

Lemaitre L, Remy J, Farriaux JP, Dhondt JL, Walbaum R. Radiological signs of mucolipidosis II or I-cell disease. A study of nine cases. Pediatr Radiol 1978;7:97–105

Lipnick RN, Glass RBJ. Bone changes associated with cystic fibrosis. Skeletal Radiol 1992;21:115–6

Nathanson I, Riddlesberger MM. Pulmonary hypertrophic osteoarthropathy in cystic fibrosis. Radiology 1980; 135:649–51

Rowley RF, Lawson JP. Case report 701. Skeletal Radiol 1991;617–9

Poznanski AK, Fernbach SK, Berry TE. Bone changes from prostaglandin therapy. Skeletal Radiol 1985;14:20–5

Schiliro G, Russo A. Radiological case of the month. Am J Dis Child 1979;133:323–4

Spjut HJ, Dorfman HD. Florid reactive periostitis of the tubular bones of the hands and feet. Am J Surg Pathol 1981;5:423–8

Subject Index